CORONARY CARE UNITS

DEVELOPMENTS IN CARDIOVASCULAR MEDICINE

VOLUME 10

CORONARY CARE UNITS

Proceedings of a European Seminar
held in Pisa, Italy

Sponsored by European Economic Communities
CMSI
(ad hoc Committee for monitoring the seriously ill)

edited by

ATTILIO MASERI, MD
Director of the Cardiovascular Research Unit,
Royal Postgraduate Medical School,
Hammersmith Hospital,
London, England

and

CARLO MARCHESI, D.Engr.
SERGIO CHIERCHIA, MD
MARIA GIOVANNA TRIVELLA, MD
Clinical Physiology Institute and
Patologia Medica I, University of Pisa,
Pisa, Italy

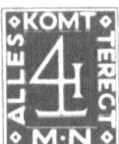

1981

MARTINUS NIJHOFF PUBLISHERS
THE HAGUE / BOSTON / LONDON

for

THE COMMISSION OF THE EUROPEAN COMMUNITIES

Symposium organized by The Coronary Research Group and the Computing Group, Clinical Physiology Institute, CNR, University of Pisa, Pisa, Italy, held 1-2 December 1978

Distributors

for the United States and Canada
Kluwer Boston, Inc.
190 Old Derby Street
Hingham, MA 02043

for all other countries
Kluwer Academic Publishers Group
Distribution Center
P.O.Box 322
3300 AH Dordrecht
The Netherlands

This volume is listed in the Library of Congress Cataloging in Publication Data

ISBN-13: 978-94-009-8249-9   e-ISBN-13: 978-94-009-8247-5
DOI: 10.1007/978-94-009-8247-5

Publication arranged by:
Commission of the European Communities,
Directorate-General Information Market and Innovation,
Luxembourg

EUR 7066

Copyright ECSC, EEC, EAEC, Brussels-Luxembourg, 1981

Softcover reprint of the hardcover 1st edition 1981

CONTENTS

VIII

APPENDIX A: SURVEY REPORT ON HEMODYNAMIC MONITORING IN CORO-
NARY CARE UNIT

A. Maseri, C. Marchesi, S. Chierchia, M.G. Trivella

FOREWORD

The dimensions of the socio-economic problem represented by ischemic heart disease require a concentration of effort for its treatment and prevention at least comparable to that in program for neoplastic disease. It appeared a logical conclusion of the work of the CMSI ad hoc group to organize a seminar on Perspectives of Coronary Care. Similar actions obviously are better undertaken at a supranational level because of: the dimension of the problem, the absence of expertises on all the different aspects in individual countries and the difference in patient population and in the phylosophy guiding the approach to coronary patients in different countries.

The review of the recent literature and the results of the survey report on hemodynamic monitoring in coronary care units in the member countries (document for the CMSI 1979 - Pisa) indicate that this field is in the process of rapid transience because of accumulating information which appears to modify substantially traditional concepts concerning patient management and prevention. While advanced technologies may potentially play a major role not only in diagnostic and therapeutic procedures but also in our understanding of disease processes, thus opening new lines for treatment and prevention, optimization of resources is a basic prerequisite in the attempt of containing the budget for medical care. Hence we aimed to identify the technologies of immediate benefit for extensive routine applications from those that should still be considered in the domain of research and development.

The conclusions of the seminar are in line with the document XII/201/74-E-F-N produced by the ad hoc group of the CMSI. There was unanimous agreement that CCU's have become a well established routine system of care of acute coronary patients fully justified by the experience collected over the years. It was emphasized that it was essential to separate clearly the problems of Research CCU's from those of Routine CCU's. It was stressed the fact that too often techniques and instrumentation, still in the domain of research and development, are distributed to routine CCU's before their usefulness had been convincingly proved. We believe that the papers presented by the invited experts and the stimulating discussion that followed provide a comprehensive evaluation of the technological developments for routine applications and pathophysiological studies. Finally the fundamental running theme throughout the seminar was the need for standardization of methods for joint, multicenter evaluation of new procedures and development of common protocols for classification of patients.

ACKNOWLEDGEMENTS

The seminar and the publication of these proceedings were made possible by the support from the Committee for Monitoring the seriously ill of the European Communities.
The success of the seminar was the result of the hard work of the Coronary and Computing Groups of the Institute of Clinical Physiology and of the organizational abilities of Hilda Biagini De Ruyter.
The editors are very grateful for the editorial assistance and typing skill rendered by Emanuela Campani and Daniela Banti in producing this manuscript.

CONTRIBUTORS

F.M. Antonini, Coronary Care Unit 'Carlo Fumagalli', Geriatric Department, University of Florence, Florence, Italy.

P. Attuel, Department of Cardiology, Lariboisière Hospital, Paris Cedex, France.

M.C. Aumont, Division of Cardiology, Beaujon Hospital, Clichy Cedex, France.

R. Balcon, Department of Clinical Measurement, National Heart & Chest Hospital and Cardiothoracic Institute, London, England.

M. Barthelemy, Division of Cardiology, Beaujon Hospital, Clichy Cedex, France.

Ph. Beaufils, Department of Cardiology, Lariboisière Hospital, Paris Cedex, France.

J.E.W. Beneken, Biomedical Engineering Group, Department of Electrical Engineering, Eindhoven University of Technology, Eindhoven, The Netherlands.

R. Bernard, University Hospital, Saint Pierre, Brussels, Belgium.

G. Bertini, Coronary Care Unit 'Carlo Fumagalli', Geriatric Department, University of Florence, Florence, Italy.

A. Biagini, Clinical Physiology Institute, National Research Council of Italy, and Department of Medicine, University of Pisa, Pisa, Italy.

M. Biella, Clinical Physiology Institute, National Research Council of Italy, and Department of Medicine, University of Pisa, Pisa, Italy.

J.A. Blom, Biomedical Engineering Group, Department of Electrical Engineering, Eindhoven University of Technology, Eindhoven, The Netherlands.

P. Bobba, Division of Cardiology, Policlinico S. Matteo, University of Pavia, Pavia, Italy.

N. Brooks, Department of Clinical Measurement, National Heart & Chest Hospital and Cardiothoracic Institute, London, England.

F. Camerini, Division of Cardiology, Ospedali Riuniti Trieste, Trieste, Italy.

C. Carpeggiani, Clinical Physiology Institute, National Research Council of Italy, and Department of Medicine, University of Pisa, Pisa, Italy.

M. Cattell, Department of Clinical Measurement, National Heart & Chest Hospital and Cardiothoracic Institute, London, England.

S. Chierchia, Clinical Physiology Institute, National Research Council of Italy, and Department of Medicine, University of Pisa, Pisa, Italy.

M. Chimienti, Division of Cardiology, Policlinico S. Matteo, University of Pavia, Pavia, Italy.

C. Contini, Clinical Physiology Institute, National Research Council of Italy, and Department of Medicine, University of Pisa, Pisa, Italy.

Ph. Coumel, Department of Cardiology, Lariboisière Hospital, Paris Cedex, France.

J.P. Delahaye, Cardiology Hospital, Lyon, France.

A. Distante, Clinical Physiology Institute, National Research Council of Italy, and Department of Medicine, University of Pisa, Pisa, Italy.

L. Donato, Clinical Physiology Institute, National Research Council of Italy, and Department of Medicine, University of Pisa, Pisa, Italy.

J.S. Duisterhout, Institute of Medical Physics TNO, Utrecht, The Netherlands.

W.A.H. Engelse, Thoraxcentre, Erasmus University, Rotterdam, The Netherlands.

F. Faletra, Centre of Cardiology 'A. De Gasperis', Ente Ospedaliero Niguarda, Milan, Italy.

G. Feruglio, Institute of Cardiology, Ospedale Civile Udine, Udine, Italy.

G. Frick, German Heart Center, Munich, Germany

K.L. Froer, German Heart Center, Munich, Germany.

P. Gaspard, Cardiology Hospital, Lyon, France.

L. Goppel, German Heart Center, Munich, Germany.

R. Gourgon, Division of Cardiology, Beaujon Hospital, Clichy Cedex, France.

D. Hall, German Heart Centre, Munich, Germany.

J. Heikkilä, Cardiovascular Laboratory and Intensive Care Unit,

First Department of Medicine, University Central Hospital, Helsinki, Finland.

N.M. Van Hemel, Antonius Hospital, Utrecht, The Netherlands.

S. Holmberg, Department of Cardiology, Sahlgrenska Hospital, Gothenburg, Sweden.

M.R. Hoare, Thoraxcentre, Erasmus University, Rotterdam, The Netherlands.

P.G. Hugenholtz, Thoraxcentre, Erasmus University, Rotterdam, The Netherlands.

I. Hutton, University Department of Medical Cardiology, Glasgow Royal Infirmary, Glasgow.

A. Janin, Cardiology Hospital , Lyon, France.

K. Jennings, Department of Clinical Measurement, National Heart & Chest Hospital and Cardiothoracic Institute, London, England.

F.F. Jorritsma, Biomedical Engineering Group, Department of Electrical Engineering, Eindhoven University of Technology, Eindhoven, The Netherlands.

D. Julian, Department of Cardiology, Freeman Hospital, Newcastle Upon Tyne University, Newcastle Upon Tyne, Great Britain.

R. Kraus, Cardiology Hospital, Lyon, France.

A. Irving, University Department of Medical Cardiology, Glasgow Royal Infirmary, Glasgow.

A. L'Abbate, Clinical Physiology Institute, National Research Council of Italy, and Department of Medicine, University of Pisa, Pisa, Italy.

L. Landucci, Clinical Physiology Institute, National Research Council of Italy, and Department of Medicine, University of Pisa, Pisa, Italy.

T.D.D. Lawrie, University Department of Medical Cardiology, Glasgow Royal Infirmary, Glasgow.

M. Lazzari, Clinical Physiology Institute, National Research Council of Italy, and Department of Medicine, University of Pisa, Pisa, Italy.

J.F. Leclercq, Department of Cardiology, Lariboisière Hospital, Paris Cedex, France.

A. Macerata, Clinical Physiology Institute, National Research Council of Italy, and Department of Medicine, University of Pisa, Pisa, Italy.

P.W. Macfarlane, University Department of Medical Cardiology, Glasgow Royal Infirmary, Glasgow.

P. Mancini, Clinical Physiology Institute, National Research Council of Italy, and Department of Medicine, University of Pisa, Pisa, Italy.

A. Mantero, Centre of Cardiology 'A. De Gasperis', Ente Ospedaliero Niguarda, Milan, Italy.

C. Marchesi, Clinical Physiology Institute, National Research Council of Italy, and Department of Medicine, University of Pisa, Pisa, Italy.

N. Marchionni, Coronary Care Unit 'Carlo Fumagalli', Geriatric Department, University of Florence, Florence, Italy.

P. Marzullo, Clinical Physiology Institute, National Research Council of Italy and Department of Medicine, University of Pisa, Pisa, Italy.

A. Maseri, Cardiovascular Research Unit, Royal Postgraduate Medical School, Hammersmith Hospital, Duncane Road, London W12 0 HS, United Kingdom.

F. Mauri, Centre of Cardiology 'A. De Gasperis', Ente Ospedaliero Niguarda, Milan, Italy.

M.G. Mazzei, Clinical Physiology Institute, National Research Council of Italy and Department of Medicine, University of Pisa, Pisa, Italy.

G.F. Mazzocca, Clinical Physiology Institute, National Research Council of Italy and Department of Medicine, University of Pisa, Pisa, Italy.

A. Medici, Division of Cardiology, Policlinico S. Matteo, University of Pavia, Pavia, Italy.

E. Moscarelli, Clinical Physiology Institute, National Research Council of Italy and Department of Medicine, University of Pisa, Pisa, Italy.

A. Nandorff, Department of Anesthesiology, University Hospital, University of Leiden, Leiden, The Netherlands.

S. Nieminen, Cardiovascular Laboratory and Intensive Care Unit, First Department of Medicine, University Central Hospital, Helsinki, Finland.

J.F. Pantridge, Regional Medical Cardiology Centre, Royal Victoria Hospital, Belfast, United Kingdom.

A. Pesola, I.N.R.C.A., Cosenza, Italy.

H. Petri, German Heart Center, Munich, Germany.

R. Pini, Coronary Care Unit 'Carlo Fumagalli', Geriatric Department, University of Florence, Florence, Italy.

R. Prasquier, Division of Cardiology, Beaujon Hospital, Clichy Cedex, France.

M. Previtali, Division of Cardiology, Policlinico S. Matteo, University of Pavia, Pavia, Italy.

M. Ray, Division of Cardiology, Policlinico S. Matteo, University of Pavia, Pavia, Italy.

R. Rocci, Centre of Cardiology 'A. De Gasperis', Ente Ospedaliero Niguarda, Milan, Italy.

D. Rovai, Clinical Physiology Institute, National Research Council of Italy and Department of Medicine, University of Pisa, Pisa, Italy.

F. Rovelli, Centre of Cardiology 'A. De Gasperis', Ente Ospedaliero Niguarda, Milan, Italy.

W. Rudolph, German Heart Center, Munich, Germany.

J.A. Salerno, Division of Cardiology, Policlinico S. Matteo, University of Pavia, Pavia, Italy.

S. Severi, Clinical Physiology Institute, National Research Council, of Italy and Department of Medicine, University of Pisa, Pisa, Italy.

I. Simonetti, Clinical Physiology Institute, National Research Council of Italy and Department of Medicine, University of Pisa, Pisa, Italy.

G. Specchia, Division of Cardiology, Policlinico S. Matteo, University of Pavia, Pavia, Italy.

J. Spierijk, Department of Anesthesiology, University Hospital, University of Leiden, Leiden, The Netherlands.

C.A. Swenne, Institute of Medical Physics TNO, Utrecht, The Netherlands.

T.P.M. Taylor, University Department of Medical Cardiology, Glasgow Royal Infirmary, Glasgow.

L. Tavazzi, Rehabilitation Medical Center, Veruno (Novara), Italy.

P. Touboul, Cardiology Hospital, Lyon, France.

T. Touche, Division of Cardiology, Beaujon Hospital, Clichy Cedex, France.

M.G. Trivella, Clinical Physiology Institute, National Research Council of Italy and Department of Medicine, University of Pisa, Pisa, Italy.

C. Valantin, Division of Cardiology, Beaujon Hospital, Clichy Cedex, France.

A. Vannucci, Coronary Care Unit 'Carlo Fumagalli', Geriatric Department, University of Florence, Florence, Italy.

H.W.A. Vennix, Institute of Medical Physics TNO, Utrecht, The Netherlands.

P. Vervin, Division of Cardiology, Beaujon Hospital, Clichy Cedex, France.

C. Warnes, Department of Clinical Measurement, National Heart & Chest Hospital and Cardiothoracic Institute, London, England.

M.P. Watts, Department of Clinical Physics and Bioengineering, West of Scotland Health Boeards, United Kingdom.

B. Wennerblom, Department of Cardiology, Sahlgrenska Hospital, Gothenburg, Sweden.

C. Zeelenberg, Thoraxcentre, Erasmus University, Rotterdam, The Netherlands.

B. Van Zoelen, Antonius Hospital, Utrecht, The Netherlands.

CHAPTER 1

PERSPECTIVES ON ARRHYTMHIA MONITORING IN CORONARY CARE
UNITS

1.1. INTRODUCTION
D. Julian

Dr. Maseri, Dr. Laurent, ladies and gentlemen. I think it is very appropriate that the first session should be related to arrhythmia monitoring in the coronary care unit because the coronary care unit at its initiation was essentially an arrhythmia monitoring unit although it has expanded into many other fields subsequently. I hope you will forgive me if I start talking a little bit about history of the CCU. Now history is something that the older members of the profession, like myself, like to use to impress our younger colleagues, and it usually succeeds in boring them. But it's important because our current practices are rooted in history rather than in reason or experience.

In about 1960 with the introduction of effective methods of external cardiac resuscitation, ECG monitoring was instituted and in 1961 the first attempts were made to start coronary care units. In about 1964 the first papers started to emerge on the frequency and characteristics of the arrhythmias in acute infarction. It was apparent at that time that there was a relationship between arrhythmias and ventricular fibrillation and further evidence was accumulated over the next few years so that by 1967 many physicians and cardiologists throughout the world were totally convinced of the importance of arrhythmias and their monitoring, and this was really enshrined in the articles of Bernard Lown at that time which impressed everyone and made us all practice the detection of ventricular arrhythmias in the belief that by detecting them we could treat them effectively and thereby prevent ventricular fibrillation. And it was at that time that Lown said that failure to prevent ventricular fibrillation was a serious, culpable fault and that one should not have ventricular fibrillation in the coronary care unit. Over the succeeding years many of us who tried to practice this found that we were not so successful as we would have hoped, and that ventricular fibrillation, although it was less common than it had been, still persisted.

One then started asking why this was so. Except in a very few units, monitoring has been left to highly trained nurses observing oscilloscripts. But nurses often fail to observe arrhythmias. If we had enough nurses and if we had nurses that were always fully awake then we would detect more of these. But one has to accept that there are such things, at least in our country, as nurse shortages. There are such things as unskilled nurses and there are such things as fatigue.

A number of units, including our own, have looked at the question of whether nurses really were as effective as we thought they were in detecting arrhythmias. We compared two adjacent rooms, one of which was monitored by nurses in the conventional way and one of which was monitored by an online arrhythmias computer. We found that the nurses were good, although not perfect, in detecting all the patients with ventricular tachycardia; that is, they detected 9 out of 11 patients who had ventricular tachycardia, whereas the computer detected all of them. But when it came to such things as pairs of ventricular ectopic beats or close-coupled ectopic beats, the nurses were extremely inefficient compared with the computer altough they were good at detecting frequent ectopic beats. Of course this has its inevitable clinical therapeutic implications in that if nurses don't detect the arrhythmias they don't treat the arrhythmias, or they treat them much later.

In our series there were 23 patients monitored by nurses who should have received immediate lidocaine treatment, according to the current criteria and 20 patients in the computer monitored room who should have received it. Only 4 of the 23 conventionally monitored patients received the treatment immediately. In many others it was delayed and in some they never received the treatment at all. In the computer monitored room virtually all the patients were treated immediately for the arrhythmia. The logical conclusion could be that either we train our nurses better, or we have more nurses, or that we go over to a computerized system of arrhythmia analysis. But a legitimate question is: are the things which we are looking for the things which we should be looking for? In other words, are the so-called warning arrhythmias that the computer was designed to detect really warning arrhythmias that require treatment? And there have now been a number of studies from Amsterdam and Miami and other places suggesting that the so-called warning arrhythmias are not of any significance and that they occur as often in those who do not go on to ventricular fibrillation as they do in those that do. Those of us who were involved in this business many years ago were worried about this because in our early experience there did seems to be a relationship between certain arrhythmias and ventricular fibrillation, and now there are those who say that there is no such relationship. It is difficult to explain this discrepancy. One explanation was that they are looking at something different.

We have been studying patients, none of whom have had any anti-arrhythmic therapy, and observing them in the natural course of the disease and seeing what happens before ventricular fibrillation occurs.

About one-quarter of patients who developed ventricular fibrillation do so without any warning arrhythmias at all. In other cases there are very sporadic warning arrhythmias, not giving any clear indication of proceeding to ventricular fibrillation one knows these occur

commonly in patients who do not go on to ventricular fibrillation.
But there are patients, in whom there does seem to be something new
occurring just before ventricular fibrillation occurred. In looking
at these cases in closer detail, there seems to be the very rapid
progression, both in frequency and in prematurity, of ventricular
ectopic beats. So we believe that there are many patients who have
no arrhythmias at all, there are many others who have the so-called
warning arrhythmias, but they are not really a warning, but there is
a small group of patients in whom there are phenomena that immediately precede ventricular fibrillation, which may be a warning.

What I hope will emerge from this afternoon's discussions is some
kind of agreement as to whether we should be monitoring for arrhythmias now, what arrhythmias we should be monitoring for, and how we
should do this. Do we select patients for monitoring? Do we monitor
them in any special way? Should we be using computer assisting
monitoring? Or should we look after all these patients at home and
give them some magic drug to prevent arrhythmias? And I hope that
this afternoon's discussion will help us to get nearer this decision.

1.2. METHODS FOR DETECTION OF ARRHYTHMIAS AND THEIR CLINICAL SIGNIFI-
CANCE
R. Bernard

The purpose of arrhythmia monitoring is detection of arrhythmias,
leading eventually to their treatment.

In acute myocardial infarction (AMI), ventricular fibrillation is
certainly the most fascinating arrhythmias: it kills the patient
within 3 minutes, but rapid and effective intervention may be
lifesaving (external electric stimulus, cardiac massage and simple
pulmonary ventilation). We are here concerned with primary ventricular fibrillation (PVF), occurring out of the clinical setting of
severe heart failure, shock or other severe clinical status. Let us
give a look to 18 cases of primary ventricular fibrillation (PVF),
we observed in a group of 747 AMI. The first table shows the higher
frequency of this complication in the younger age groups; this is a
common observation. There was no relation with a particular type of
necrosis.

Table 1. Frequency of primary ventricular fibrillation in different
age groups (acute myocardial infarction).

AGE	N of PVF	% of PVF/ N of patients
40 - 49	5	4.5
50 - 59	6	2.6
60 - 69	6	2.5
> 70	1	0.6

6

Table 2. Percentage of patients showing PVF in relation to the delay between the presumed onset of the disease and the hospitalization.

Delay: Onset of pain/hospitalization	% of patients + PVF
< 1 h	10
1 → < 2 h	6.2
2 → < 4 h	3.5
4 → < 24 h	1.7

The delay between the presumed onset of the disease and PVF is short (Table 2): patients hospitalized within 24 hours of the presumed onset of the AMI are divided into four groups in relation to the delay; 10% of the patients taken within one hour experienced PVF, 6,2% of those taken from one to two hours had PVF, 3.5% of those hospitalized within two to four hours had PVF; only 1.7% of those taken between four and twenty-four hours experienced PVF.

What is the future of these patients? If they have to die a few hours or days later, the benefit should be questionned. From these 18 cases of PVF, resuscitation succeeded in 17, two other patients died in the hospital. The 15 survivors leaving the hospital were followed; one died of sudden death two months after the AMI; a second died one year later from lung cancer. The thirteen others are alive with a follow-up of one year or more for twelve, and of more than two years for seven.

These results stress the interest of early hospitalization if we want to bring help to the patient and use our cardiac intensive care units in the most efficient way; the long-term survival offered to patients resuscitated from PVF is stimulating.

Regular arrhythmia monitoring on standard oscilloscopes being unable to offer a real, complete and continuous monitoring, led to research on computerized systems. The development of these arrhythmia computerized systems in cardiac intensive care units relies in several assumptions:

1. PVF is an important cause of death following AMI;
2. PVF may be suppressed by immediate and effective treatment;
3. Patients, resuscitated from PVF have a reasonable long-term prognosis.

4. PVF is heralded by warning arrhythmias, as ventricular premature beats (numerous, early ....);
5. Early detection (monitoring) of these warning arrhythmias is the clue to preventive action against PVF.

If points 1 to 3 are accepted, n° 4 and 5 are challenged:

A. Primary ventricular fibrillation may occur without warning arrhythmias (1-6).
B. Warning arrhythmias may be seen with the same frequency in two groups of patients: with and without PVF (5, 7); the specific "warning" value of these arrhythmias is thus questioned.

More studies are needed on the natural history (without any drug intervention) of PVF after AMI. Perhaps that special significance has to be given to really "warning" arrhythmias. But if the premonitory value of the ventricular premature beats was denied, we should review our attitude in the first hours of a myocardial infarction:

1. preventive antiarrhythmic drugs could be given systematically to all AMI patients during the first 12-24 hours, at least in the younger groups of patients (less than 70 years). But we are still waiting for a drug that could effectively protect the patient against PVF without harmfull iatrogenic manifestations.
2. we should direct technological developments in CCU, not in the search of all kinds of arrhythmias by computers, but on systems allowing the best possible detection of ventricular fibrillation.
3. first and second action combined.

REFERENCES

1. Dhurandar R, R McMillan, K Brown: Primary ventricular fibrillation complicating acute myocardial infarction. Am J Cardiol 27: 347, 1971.
2. Lie K, H Wellens, D Durrer: Characteristics and predictability of primary ventricular fibrillation. Europ J Cardiol 1: 379, 1974.
3. Wymans M, L. Hammersmith: Comprehensive treatment plan for the prevention of primary ventricular fibrillation in acute myocardial infarction. Am J Cardiol 33: 1327, 1974.
4. Pantridge J, A Adgey, J Geddes, S Webb: The acute coronary attack. Ed Pitman Medical, Tunbridge Wells, 1975.
5. El Sherif N, R Myerburg, B Scherlag et al: Electrocardiographic antecedents of primary ventricular fibrillation. Value to the R-on-T phenomenon in myocardial infarction. Br Heart J 38: 415, 1976.
6. Campbell P, A Murray, D Julian: Incidence, prevalence and significance of ventricular ectopic activity in acute myocardial infarction. In: "Management of ventricular tachycardia. Role of Mexiletine". Excerpta Medica, Amsterdam-Oxford, 35, 1978.

8

7. Lie K, H Wellens, F Van Cappelle, D Durrer: Lidocaine in the prevention of primary ventricular fibrillation. A double blind randomized study of 212 consecutive patients. N Engl J Med 291: 1324, 1974.

1.3. THE NATURAL COURSE OF VENTRICULAR ARRHYTHMIAS IN AMI
N.M. Van Hemel, B. Van Zoelen, C.A. Swenne, H.W.A. Vennix, J.S.
Duisterhout

1.3.1. INTRODUCTION

Nowadays, in coronary care units, computerized EKG monitoring is
generally accepted. However, in spite of improved EKG-anlysis (1,2),
the contribution to better care and shorter stay is questionable.
This is caused by the disputable prognostic value (3,4) of the
events to be detected by such systems. Research in order to determine valuable prognosyic parameters is therefore needed. Of course,
computerized EKG-analysis can be helpful in such studies.
    Doubting the prognostic value of the so-called 'warning arrhy-
thimas' (5), for this research we suggest a classification into
instantaneously threatening and non-threatening arrhythmias in a
hemodynamical sense, e.g.: in this philosophy, a pair of VPD's
should be considered as non-threatening. We intend studying characteristics of the 'non-threatening'-group in order to select features
with a prognostic value with respect to the 'threatening'-group.
Therefore we study the natural history of ventricular arrhythmias in
uncomplicated AMI up to either 48 hrs. after onset of MI, or when
threatening arrhythmias appear.

1.3.2. METHOD

Starting from September 1977 we recoreded on analog tape the EKG's
of all AMI-patients fulfilling the intake criteria. Selection criteria were: proven AMI and admission to the CCU within 12 hrs. after
onset of the MI. Exclusion criteria were: treatment with anti-
arrhythmics, beta-blocking and anti-hypertensive agents, digitalis
and vasopressors, hemodynamic complications, 'serious' ventricular
rhythms (e.g. VF, persistent VT), 2nd and 3rd degree AV-block, and
predominant supra-ventricular arrhythmias.
    As a pilot study, we observed the data of 14 patients with
respect to some of the properties of ventricular runs (VR). All
patients were male, age ranging from 39-73 years. All suffered from
first MI, localized: anterior 4, inferior 8, posterior 1 and non-
transmural 1. Figure 1 depicts the period of observation for each
patient. The study was not completed for patients 1, 4, 6, 8, 10 and
13. Patient 1 and 4 showed hemodynamic complications, the others
received anti-arrhythmic treatment because of threatening arrhy-

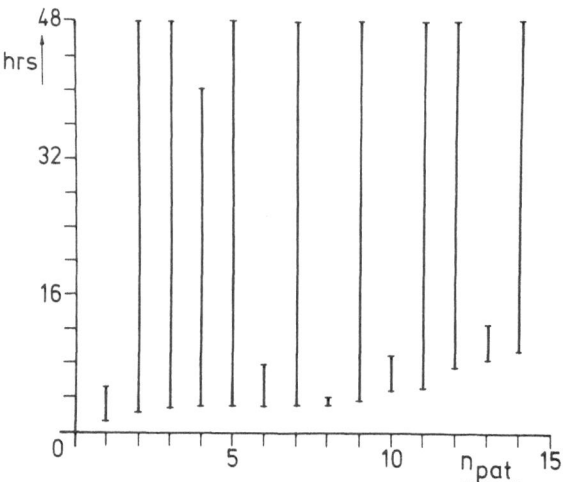

Fig. 1.

thmias.

EKG-recordings were made on an analog instrumentation tape-recorder, bandwidth 0-150 Hz. For each patient a 1-lead EKG (standard monitoring lead) was recorded together with a time - and event -code generated by a specifically devized micro-computer system (MINUTE) (6). For analysis, the tapes were fast replayed and analysed by specially developed computer system, called CENSOR (7) (CENSOR = Computerized ENumerative Scanning On Rhythm-disturbances). This computer processing is done in three phases. In phase 1 the EKG is digitized, QRS-complexes are detected and a preliminary classification into families takes place. In phase 2 the families are interactively typified by the cardiologist in an electrocardiographic sense. The QRSfamilies can be typified as S (supra-ventricular), V (ventricular), together with a corresponding focus, or A (artifact). Data (RR-intervals and correpsonding typification of the QRS-complexes) are stored on digital tape. In phase 3 any desired output based on these data can be produced. For this study we prepared output programs for extracting and plotting some of the properties of VR.

Patient data were scanned on VR, by searching for "patterns" minimally consisting of S-S-S-V-V-V without respect to the focus of the ventricular beats. In each VR the following parameters were measured:

RRSS (ms): average of the two preceding SS-intervals
RRSV (ms): coupling interval of the first ventricular beat
RRVV (ms): average VV-interval
NPVD (--): number of successive ventricular beats (NPVD $\geqslant$ 3)
ELAP (h) : time elapsed after onset of MI   ($0 < ELAP < 48$)

DURA (s) : duration of VR   (=NPVD*RRVV/1000)

1.3.3. RESULTS

In the following, all the data for all patients are summed. For better clustering of data, instead of intervals (RRSS, RRSV and RRVV) we used normalized intervals (RRSV/RRSS and RRSS/RRVV). In such a way, more general conclusions may be drawn from the data.

The incidence of VR as a function of time is shown in fig. 2, together with the number of patients studied (see also fig. 1). These data have been computed per hour. Considering the fact that these same patients have been observed from 13 up to 40 hours elapsed time, it can be concluded that in their case incidence of VR after 24 hours is strongly decreased.

Figure 3 represents the "prematurity" (= RRSV/RRSS) of the starting beats of all VR as a function of time. A decrease of VR's starting with a premature beat (RRSV/RRSS 100%) and VR's starting with a late beat (RRSV/RRSS 100%) can be noted. Late VR's start with a sligthly premature beat.

Figure 4 represents the "rhythm acceleration" (= RRSS/RRVV) of the VR. First VR's (ELAP 6 hrs) have about the same rate as the supra-ventricular rate (RRSS/RRSV 100%). Rhythms both faster and slower than the supra-ventricular rhythm may be seen between 6 and 24 hours. Later slower rhythms disappear as well as very fast rhythms (RRSS/RRSV 200%).

Figure 5 illustrates the relation between the rhythm acceleration (RRSS/RRVV) and the prematurity (RRSV/RRSS). No VR with a prematurity 100% and a faster than supra-ventricular rate was seen. Prematurities 100% do not have any relation to the rhythm acceleration. However, faster rates can be expected.

Figure 6 depicts the relation between the duration of the VR and the prematurity. All long-during VR started with the coupling interval the preceeding supra-ventricular interval.

Figure 7 represents the relation between the duration of the VR and the corresponding rhythm acceleration. All long-lasting VR but one showed a rate the supra-ventricular rate. One showed a rate 180% of the supra-ventricular rate with a duration of 23 s. This VR constituted the exclusion criterion for patient 10.

1.3.4. CONCLUSION

Within the limits of this pilot study, it may be concluded that:
A. the incidence of VR decreases after 24 hrs;
B. small and great prematurities decrease after 24 hrs;
C. slow and very fast VR's disappear after a 24 hrs;

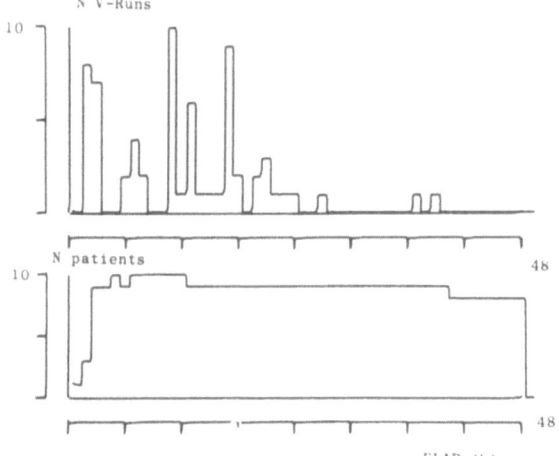

Fig. 2.

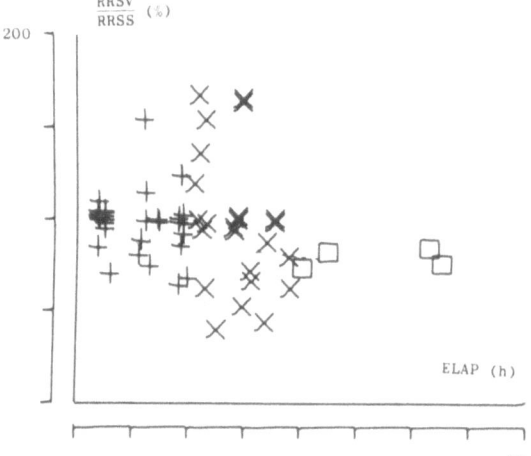

Fig. 3.

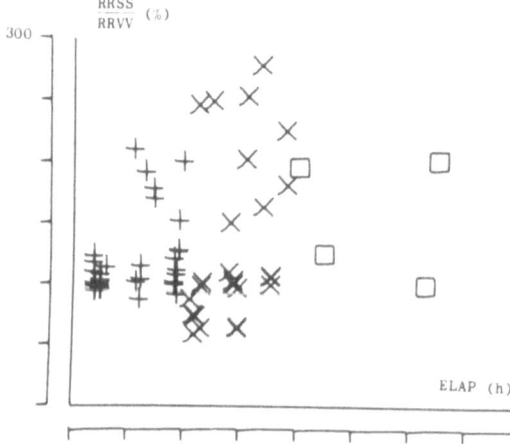

Fig. 4.

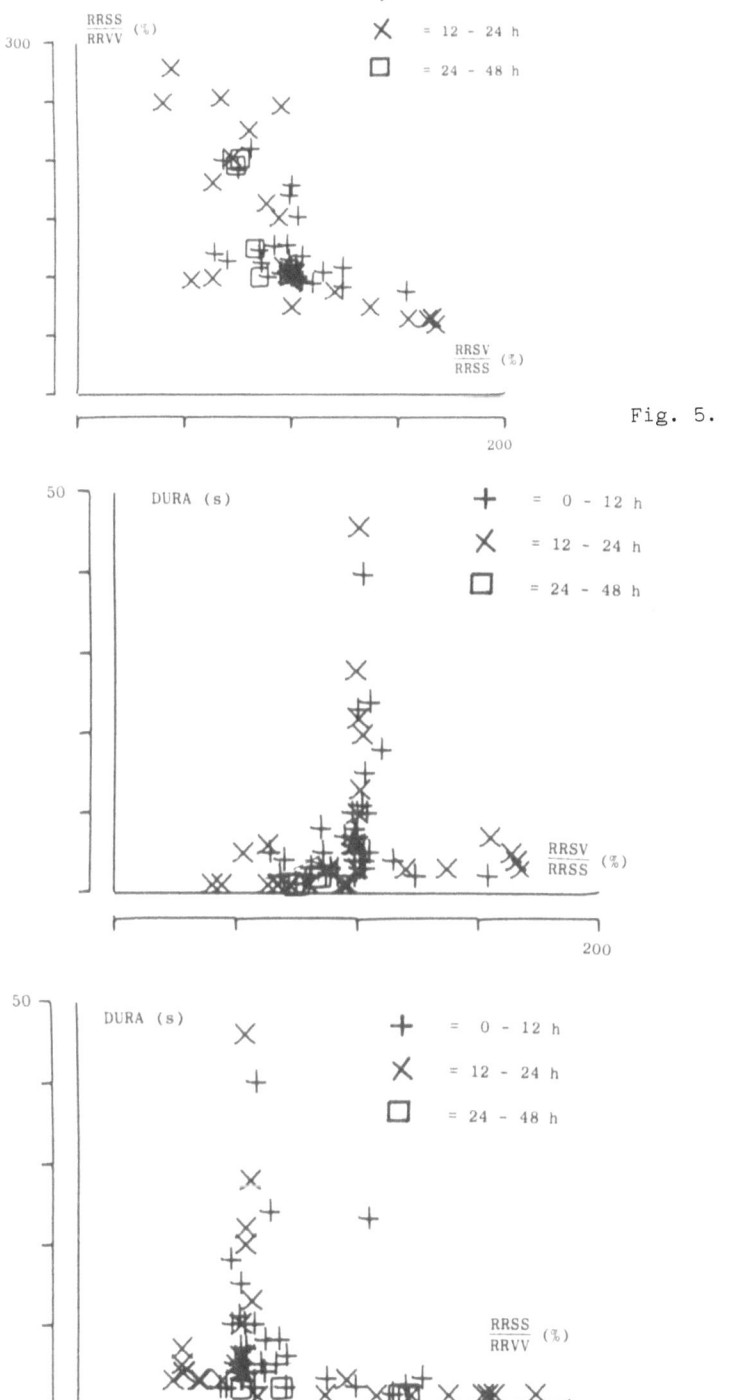

Fig. 5.

Fig. 6.

Fig. 7.

D. when the prematurity is more than 100%, no rhythm-acceleration is seen;

E. faster VR's have a prematurity 100%, the prematurity not being a predictor for the acceleration of the rate;

F. long-lasting VR's all start with a prematurity 100%;

G. for these Vr's the ventricular rate is about the same as the supra-ventricular rate (except in 1 patient).

The results of the pilot study are encouraging, revealing some lesser known aspects of VR (8,9).

This work will be continued in order to inspect the gathered data more extensively, in terms of the number of patients, as well as in different kinds of ventricular arrhythmias.

REFERENCES

1. Vetter NJ, DG Julian: Comparison of arrhythmia computer and conventional monitoring in coronary-care unit. Lancet 1: 1151, 1975.

2. Holmberg S, L Rijden, A Waldestrom: Efficiency of arrhythmia detection by nurses in a coroanry care unit using a decentralized monitoring system. Br Heart J 39: 1019, 1977.

3. Lie KI, HJ Wellens, D Durrer: Characteristics and predictability of primary ventricular fibrillation. Eur J Card 1: 379, 1974.

4. Harrison DC: Should Lidocaine be administrated routinely to all patients after myocardial infarction. Circ 58: 582, 1978.

5. Bigger JTh, RJ Dresdale, RH Heissembuttel, et al: Ventricular arrhythmias in ischemic heart disease: mechanism prevalence, significance and management. Prog Cardiovasc Dis 19: 255, 1977.

6. Vennix HWA, CA Swenne: MINUTE: a time and event code generator. In: Progress Report No PR6, 1978. (Eds: B van Eijnsbergen and FH Lopes da Silva). Institute of Medical Physics TNO, Utrecht.

7. Swenne CA, HWA Vennix, NM van Hemel, et al: CENSOR: A system for computerized enumerative scanning on rhythm disturbances. In: Progress Report No PR6, 1978. (Eds: B van Eijnsbergen and FH Lopes da Silva). Institute of Medical Physics TNO, Utrecht.

8. Rothefield EL, J Parsonnet, W McGorman, S Linden: Herbingers of paroxysmal ventricular techycardia in acute myocardial infarction. Chest 71: 142, 1977.

9. Roberts R, HD Ambos, CW Loh, BE Sobel: Initiation of repetitive ventricular depolarizations by relatively late premature complexes in patients with acute myocardial infarction. Am J Cardiol 41: 678, 1978.

1.4. A COMPUTER ASSISTED METHOD FOR A QUANTITATIVE EVALUATION OF
ARRHYTHMIAS

Ph. Beaufils, J.F. Leclercq, P. Attuel, Ph. Coumel

1.4.1. INTRODUCTION

The ATREC system (Analysis of the Troubles of rhythm of Electrocardiogram) has been developed to improve the semiquantitative analysis
presently given by the commercially available Holter monitoring
systems.

In principle computers can deliver an highly sophisticated ECG
diagnosis, provided that reliable data concerning both atrial and
ventricular activities be available. Practically, this cannot be
realized from magnetic tape recordings in ambulatory patients, because P wave abnormalities will never be distinguished accurately from
the artifacts. The automatic analysis achieved by current systems
does not include therefore atrial rhythm.

1.4.2. SYSTEM CONFIGURATION

The ATREC system consists of three basic units: analog recording and
playback units, analog pre-processing hardware and digital processing hardware.

As recording and playback units we are using the Avionics system
at sixty times real time reduction; any other system might be used
as well.

The pre-processing hardware accomplishes two functions, filtering
and wave recognition. A band pass filter, 3 to 30 hertz, combined
with a 50 hertz notch filter, eliminates both P and T waves, and a
substantial amount of baseline shift, muscle noise and power line
interferance. Therefore the processing unit furnishes the computer
signals related to the detection of R waves, the R-R intervals, the
QRS width and the QRS polarity. The reliability of this processing
unit is obviously essential and has been extensively tested. As it
is designed both to adapt the sensitivity of the detection of the
varying QRS amplitude, and to eliminate the majority of artifacts,
the proportion of false QRS detections or unrecognized QRS's is
extrémely low.

The key element of the digital processing hardware is a small
general purpose computer (Mitra 15-35 with 16 K words of core).
Approximately 4 K words of core are used by the arrhythmia program,
the remaining memory being used for trend data storage.

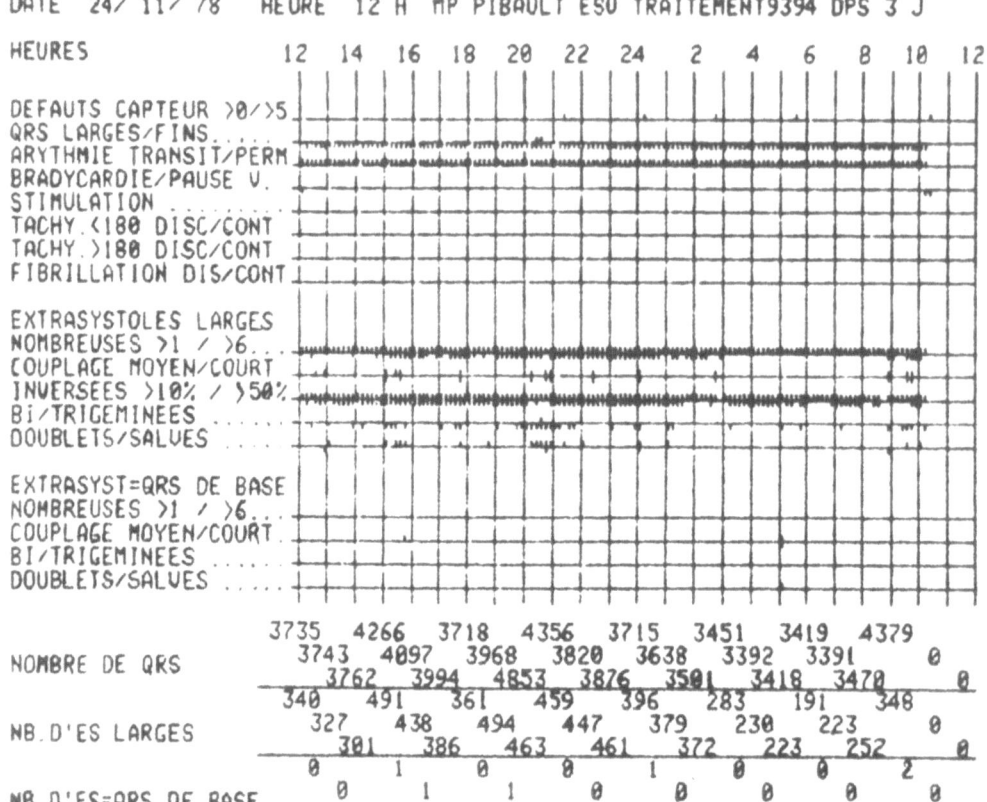

Fig. 1. First table; 24 hour magnetic tape recording. Many premature ventricular beats are present during the 24 hour, less numerous during sleep, with a varying coupling interval and distribution (bi and trigeminy, doublets). They are numbered in the lower part of the table.

The results of the analysis are displayed on the screen of a Tektronix 4060 and reproduced by a hard copy unit.

1.4.3. METHOD

The method of analysis is presented in three successive tables, first of which appears progressively on the screen as the magnetic tape is played back, the others being displayed after the end of the first one; the entire process takes about half an hour for a 24 hour recording.
   The first table (Fig. 1) presents the results concerning the monitoring of arrhythmias, the characteristics of the premature

beats (enlarged or not with respect to the basic QRS's) and the total numbers of QRS complexes. The table is divided into 144 periods of time, each corresponding to the 144th part of the total duration of the tracing.

If a 24 hour recording is processed, every period corresponds to 600 s. of real time. It is possible to examine the different scale tracings, so that, in 12, 6 or 3 hour recordings, the periods correspond to 300, 150 and 75 s. of real time respectively. Bars are progressively inscribed on the horizontal line which corresponds to the event which has been observed during the period.

The classification scheme follows a logical structure based on three groups of abnormalities. Three series of items on figure 1 correspond to these groups and the most significant are considered in detail.

A. The first serie of eight lines in the table relate to the arrhythmia detection.

QRS LARGES/FINS (= wide/narrow QRS's): classification in wide or narrow QRS complexes is given from the mean width of the 16 last beats compared to the threshold values of 90 and 110 ms. If the mean QRS duration (excluding the extrasystoles) is less than 90 ms, a bar is inscribed under the horizontal line. If it exceeds 110 ms the bar is inscribed above the line. As the mean value of QRS width may vary during the same period of time, the bar may appear on both sides; but to avoid too frequent changes in this evaluation (in case of complexes the duration of which is intermediate between 90 and 110 ms) an hysteresis system has been designed. In other words, in case of progressively enlarged R waves, complexes coming from the less-than-90 ms zone are considered narrow up to 110 ms. On the other hand, progressively narrowing R waves are considered wide until the threshold of 90 ms is reached.

BRADYCARDIE/PAUSE: a bar above the horizontal line signifies that the mean rate has been less that 40/min during at least 16 consecutive beats. A downward bar corresponds to either a pause of more than 2.1.s. or a pause of more than the mean cardiac cycle x 1.8.

The last possibility (relative pause) is forbidden by the existence of an arrhythmia or a tachycardia, and cannot follow immediately an extrasystole (compensatory pause). On the other hand, the beat following the R wave terminating the pause cannot be labelled extrasystole even though it is relatively premature.

TACHY <180 DISC/CONT (= Tachycardia <180; sustained/or not): tachycardias between 120 and 180/min are detected in this line. If the tachycardia coexists with the item of arrhythmia, it will be labelled as "sustained" (with a bar under the line) only if the frequency (from 16 beats) is more than 120/min during the whole period. But if the tachycardia is regular, a single R-R interval of more than 500 ms will be sufficient to make it labelled "not sustained" (with an upward bar).

TACHY > 180 DISC/CONT: the same mode of labelling applies to the tachycardias at more than 180/min.

FIBRILLATION DISC/CONT (= Transient/permanent ventricular fibrillation): the diagnosis of ventricular fibrillation implies the coexistence of three conditions: irregularity, cardiac rate above 220/min., and wide QRS. The fibrillation is labelled "transient" (DISCcontinue) if it does not last during the whole period (supposed 75 s. in this case), thus corresponding to some multiform ventricular tachycardias.

To summarize, in this first series of items, the computer does not formulate an electrocardiographic diagnosis in the medical meaning of the term. It only describes the events as far as the R waves are concerned. It is the physician's task to compare the different items: for example the coexistence of a sustained and regular tachycardia at a rate of more than 180/min with wide QRS complexes suggests the diagnosis of ventricular tachycardia, but it has to be confirmed by examining the tracing to rule out a supraventricular tachycardia with a functional bundle branch block.

   B. The second series of items (EXTRASYSTOLES LARGES) deals with the wide premature beats: in practice they may be either ventricular premature beats or supraventricular premature beats with a functional bundle branch block. The criteria needed for a QRS to be classified as such is to be premature by at least 10 percent with respect to the mean rate of the 16 preceding basic complexes, and to be enlarged with respect to the basic QRS.

NOMBREUSES: an upward bar is displayed if the number of extrasystoles is more than 1 and less than 6/min. The bar is displayed on both sides if the premature beats are more than 6/min.

COUPLAGE MOYEN/COURT (= mean/short coupling interval): no matter the frequency of the premature beats, no bar appears if their coupling interval is more than 220 ms + (mean RR interval)/5.

An upward bar is displayed if any extrasystole is coupled with an interval shorter than the preceeding value but longer than 180 ms + (mean RR interval)/5, and a complete bar appears if the coupling interval is less than this value.

BI/TRIGEMINEES (= by/trigeminy) bigeminated or trigeminated premature beats are signaled by an appropriate bar every time the arrhythmia appears durint a sequence of at least 12 and 15 consecutive cycles respectively.

DOUBLETS/SALVE: the presence of any doublet (basic QRS – extrasystole – extrasystole) or salvo (three to ten extrasystoles in a row) triggers the corresponding bar.

   C. The third series of items deals with premature beats which are not larger than the basic QRS complexes. As they may be either narrow with narrow basic QRS's (supraventricular premature beats), or wide but with wide basic QRS's (either supraventricular or ventricular premature beats with a pre-existing bundle branch block) they are labelled EXTRASYST. = QRS DE BASE, i.e. extrasystoles identical to the basic QRS instead of supraventricular premature beats. They must be premature by at least 20% with respect to the mean RR interval to be qualified as such, and the item of arrhythmia must not be triggered. Frequency of the premature beats, coupling interval, bi or trigeminy, doublets or slavos use the same criteria as in the preceding series.

The total number of QRS complexes for each hour, as well as that of both classes of extrasystoles are displayed in the lower part of the first table at the end of the process. Then the second table is called at that time.

The second table (Fig. 2) shows two diagrams related to the trends of cardiac rate and premature beat frequency. As for the first table, both are divided into 144 periods corresponding to either 600, 300, 150 and 75 s. according to the duration of the recording (24, 12, 6 and 3 hours, respectively).

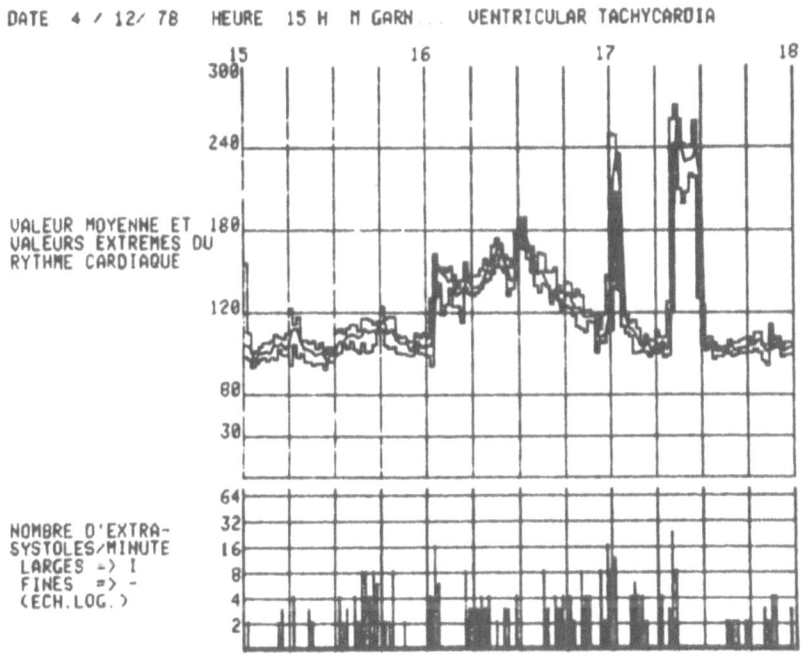

Fig. 2. Table II: ventricular tachycardia detection; upper diagram: trends of upper lower and mean cardiac rate corresponding to the events detected in table I.

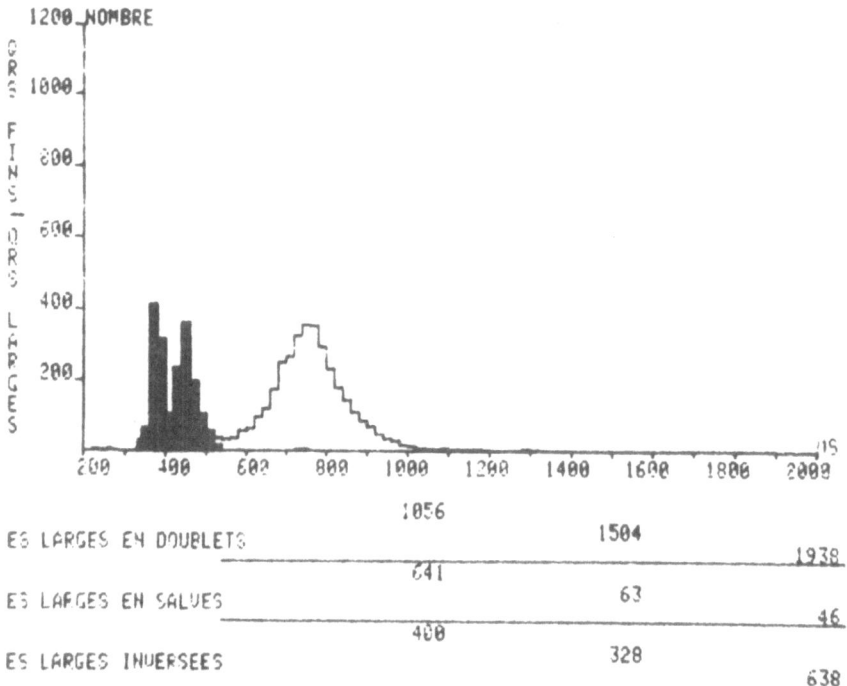

Fig. 3. Table III: the RR interval histogram distinguishes the wide QRS complexes (in block) from the narrow ones.

The upper diagram displays three curves concerning the mean cardiac rate and the extreme upper and lower values of the 16 cardiac cycles permanently taken as reference. The representation gives a very useful evaluation of the variations of the frequency but it does not correspond exactly to the maximal and minimal rates which should have been calculated from the shorter and the longer cycles of each period. On the other hand, a very short episode of tachycardia or bradycardia lasting only some seconds is clearly evidenced by this technique. The lower diagram represents the frequency per minute of the extrasystoles during each period of time. The wide premature beats are represented with vertical bars, and the non-enlarged by horizontal tracts. This diagram provides a more detailed approach to the distribution of events within each hours.

Figure 3 (third table) displays in its upper part the RR interval histogram of both narrow (open curve) and wide (in black) QRS complexes. Ninety classes of 20 ms from 200 to 2000 ms are represented on the abscissa. The number of R-R intervals in each class (ordinate) is averaged per hour, no matter the duration of the recording. This mode of representation allows us to study either long (24 hours) or even very short (some minutes) parts of the tracing if a particular phenomenon has to be evidenced. Finally, the lower part of the table provides additional quantitative information concerning particular categories of wide premature beats occuring in doublets or in salvos, or with inverted QRS polarity.

1.4.4. CONCLUSIONS

After 2 years of use, which represents more than 2000 days of electrocardiographic recordings in various situations, it appears that computer-analysis program is capable of identifying various arrhythmias and to differentiate them from many artifacts without physician's correction. The system has been used so far in playback at 60 times real time reduction. Its evaluation in real time, particularly interesting in coronary care units, is working out actually. Required transformations for ATREC real time version are:
A. incorporation of the pre-processor into a bed-side monitoring unit.
B. Use of a larger computer whose memory capacity will depend on the number of beds and on the wanted duration of the stored trend data.
C. Display of an alarm table on the screen giving three types of alarms and various artifacts;
    1. technical alarms relative to electrode faults and various artifacts;
    2. alarms relating arrhythmias, less than 2.5 sec pauses, tachy-cardias between 120 and 180 min, etc; both are auditive alarms and are not displayed with priority on the screen.
    3. urgency alarms, i.e. pauses larger than 2.5 sec and tachycardia above 180/min, which are presented immediately on the screen.

DISCUSSION: CHAPTER 1

Chairman: D. Julian

DISCUSSION CHAPTER 1

Paper 1: Methods for detection of arrhythmias and their clinical significance

PANTRIDGE: I think there is some electrophysiological evidence to support the proposition that there are two mechanisms of arrhythmias: ventricular arrhythmias that occurr early and those that occur somewhat later. The early ones are presumably due to re-entry phenomenons and the later ones to increased automaticity. It may well be that the later dysarrhythmias mean very little, and it wouldn't make very much difference whether you treat them with antiarrhythmic drugs. As far as the early ones are concerned, that may well be true as well, because we find it extremely difficult to prevent ventricular fibrillation in an individual within a few minutes or half an hour of the onset of his pain. It seems to us that the best way to prevent it is to correct the autonomic disturbance; in other words, to arrange that he has a proper heart rate.

PESOLA: Dr. Julian, did you make any correlation between QRS morphology of extrasystoles and subsequent onset of ventricular fibrillation? And before ventricular fibrillation, there was a changing pattern in QRS morphology of extrasystoles?

JULIAN: You are asking really whether, for example, they change from a right bundle or a left bundle configuration. Unfortunately, with single channel monitoring, even with two-channel monitoring, it can be extremely difficult to know whether this is the case. And we have in fact got records as to whether the same kind of ectopic beat initiated ventricular fibrillation, as we have seen previously, and in most cases where there is a premonitory ventricular arrhythmia the same kind of ectopic beat could be seen at an earlier stage as actually initiated the ventricular fibrillation. We have also looked to see whether there was a heart rate change, or whether there was a change in QT, or whether there was a change in coupling interval. And in fact there was no consistent change. Some cases show a prolongation of QT before ventricular fibrillation, others show a shortening of the coupling interval, others show a combination of the two. Some show an increase in heart rate; some do not. In our experience there seems to be no consistent pattern in the relationship between the arrhythmia one sees before the fibrillation, and that which actually initiates the fibrillation.

CAMERINI: Is there any data on different frequency of warning arrhythmia between ventricular fibrillation in the first hours of myocardial infarction, and ventricular fibrillation which appears later? We analysed recently about 70 cases of primary ventricular fibrillation and we found that in cases with anterior myocardial infarction about one-third of the primary ventricular fibrillations appeared after 48 hours, whereas in inferior myocardial infarction, the majority was concentrated in the first 24 hours. In the first group mortality was definitely higher during one year follow-up.

JULIAN: There must be some difference in the way we are defining primary ventricular fibrillation here because, as you pointed out, in the coronary care unit, particularly a coronary care unit that receives patients very quickly, nearly all primary ventricular fibrillations occur during the first 4 hours, or 6 hours. And therefore the cases to which you refer, I think, must be a different population, and not perhaps what we would call primary ventricular fibrillation. If one is talking about late ventricular fibrillation, occurring 5 or 10 or 15 or 20 days later, then I think you would probably agree that anterior infarction is a much commoner correlate than inferior infarction in such patients.

BALCON: I am very interested that nobody has mentioned the R on T phenomenon. I just wonder whether that is something we don't talk about anymore, because it doesn't happen, because your work has shown that it's not important. I suspect that's the case. I wonder if you'd answer.

JULIAN: Frequently there is a ventricular ectopic beat which is not R on T and the ventricular fibrillation occurs with another ectopic beat landing on the T wave, or that ectopic beat. Those are the group that a number of people have called 'late ectopic beats' although 'late' is a relative thing. All they mean it's after the end of the T wave. But about half our cases occur as initiated by an R on T occurring on a sinus beat. And I think some of the differences of opinion relate to something that Dr. Bernard said, that is, many of the series in the literature are about patients who were receiving antiarrhythmic drugs. And I think the ventricular fibrillation in that context is different from it occurring in the untreated patient. I don't know, would you like to comment on the R on T?

MASERI: How often do you see R on T which does not result in ventricular fibrillation?

JULIAN: I can't give you a precise figure but R on T is quite common in the first few hours after infarction. So it is not much a good predictor as we had thought. Now I think if you looked more carefully at R on Ts which were getting shorter then I think you would find that a better predictor. As you detect more and more R on Ts the correlation begins to disappear. So I think it is not an easy relationship, and I don't think one should regard R on T alone as a very good predictor.

Paper 2: The natural course of ventricular arrhythmias in AMI

JULIAN: If I understand you correctly, the long-runs were what most of us would call accelerated ventricular rhythm.
MARCHESI: Which method of evaluation did you use for testing your criteria?
VAN HEMEL: We had made a test for reliability in 20 patients with various rhythm disturbances and we have picked a random period of 30 minutes, looking by hand to the output of the program, and we found a good detection of abnormal beats of 73% and a specificity of 99%. Sometimes it is very difficult for the medical observer to make a differentiation between a normal and an abnormal beat. And I think it is necessary to have a special program so that we can put the fusion beats in a separate program.
JULIAN: Well, can we now enter on a more general discussion of the questions of the afternoon. In the first place, is anybody satisfied with the current usual system in coronary care units, that is, based essentially on the nurse observation of the monitors.

Paper 3: Computer assisted quantitative evaluation of arrhythmias

PANTRIDGE: I think the whole thing should be kept in perspective, particularly as people develop these enormous complicated hardware issues. With coronary care units we only succeed in reducing the mortality in the hospital by one-third, say from 30 % to 20 % or 25 % to 15 %, but whatever way it is you are only having an influence of 10 % of the overall issue. I am just suggesting that perhaps the whole business of developing this enormous complicated hardware, the enormous number of people who are doing these things and all this finance should be framed in the more general aspect of coronary care in particular to the precoronary care phase.
HUGENHOLTZ: All we are talking about today is one element of that whole chain, and in that chain there has to be a base, a home base. And that home base to me is the coronary care unit still, and I think it will remain that way. Perhaps tomorrow we can talk about the Nottingham and other experiences a bit in terms of total systems. But we are talking about coronary care systems and the reliability of the monitoring for rhythm disturbances in these units. And for your information, our coronary care death rates have been consistently below 10 % versus our ward rate which is about triple, and death from ventricular fibrillation or primary arrhythmias has disappeared. So I think the gain is a bit more than you wanted us to believe. Even so I concur with you. We shouldn't concentrate only on this aspect of the total battle. But since we are talking about it this afternoon, I'd like to, and this now the second part, state that I don't believe that we are at all at the end of the road of finding out the best rhythm detection system. I

would believe that the Italian nurses are better than the Dutch nurses, perhaps they are more devoted. We're dealing with current generations of nurses who aren't anymore the Florence Nightingales of the past. They do go away for coffee or something else. I fully concur with those here in the room who say that when you observe nurses carefully, even the best, they will be absent with their mind or with their eyes more than 50 % of the time. So, if we think it's relevant and now we come to what I think our Chairman said – if we think it's relevant to pick up all these arrhythmias, of which I am not sure, if we think it is relevant, then I think we must continue to talk about the best systems to detect them. And I think machines are there to help mankind, and I believe we continue to have a job in this committee and in these groups to continue to perfect the programs, to bring them down to much smaller size; obviously you don't need big things for that anymore. We have long entered the era of micro-computers and for very small dedicated systems. But they aren't perfect yet. Now, I'd like to go back to Desmond Julian: do you think it is necessary to really detect all arrythmias?

JULIAN: Perhaps I could give a personal experience on this as a way of challenging people to their views. As you know, some years ago we deliberately developed a computerized analysis system. And that is the system that we referred to already this afternoon. And, at least in our hands, we found it a very sensitive system, in the sense that we were picking up something like 98 % or so of ventricular arrythmias, of the so-called warning type, in our unit. And I may say that I am worried by many of the systems that are described, including I think the Argus system and the Hewlett-Packard system when the testing periods were extremely short. Our testing period was 90 days – continuous, on-line testing. And I think a lot of the systems are tested for half an hour, or an hour, and that's completely useless. And it also has to be done in a real-life situation, and not in a laboratory. However, I have to accept that such a system may be very sensitive, but it is not very specific. Usually, unlike a nurse monitoring system, with a computer system there are certain patients who are extremely difficult to monitor. And there are other patients who are easy to monitor, and you can identify these often quite quickly. There are problems of the configuration of their QRS; something like that makes it very difficult. So I think the nature of the problem is different in the two groups of patients. We used this for some time, and then we asked ourselves, well, that's very nice, but it is really doing anything? Are we justified in spending so much money, because this is expensive and it is always going to be expensive. So we went to the other extreme, and in the last 3 years have been having everybody recorded on tape continuously who comes into the coronary care unit, from the moment they arrive, and we have now about four or five hundred patients who are taped in this way, partially analysed, to see really whether this is something that we should be looking for. We don't have the answer to that yet. All I can say is using a system which is a conventional monitoring systems, with nurses who respond, we have had 18 ventricular fibrillations during this period of time, all of whom have been successfully defibrillated and survived. Now of course one could argue one is simply not looking for ventricular fibrillation. One is looking for lesser arrhythmias which have a hemodynamic importance which you may not be able to pick up without arrhythmia monitoring. That's a much more difficult question to answer, I think; whether we have lost something in that way. But I think in terms of simple ventricular arrhythmia detection, one could very well argue that we should be having simply a VF computer and not a general arrhythmic computer, which I think would be a much simpler approach. And to get back to your more specific point, and bearing in mind what Dr. Bernard said, one could very well say that, say for 4 or 6 hours, everybody ought to be under very intensive care because we don't know who is going to get ventricular fibrillation. After that period of time, by a whole variety of non invasive methods, even clinical examination, we may be able to differentiate those who require continued intensive care, and the rest can go to a general medical ward. That is my own view of the right approach, but I'd be very interested to know what people's attitudes are on such an approach.

BALCON: I believe that we should follow the line that you suggested, that's look for ventricular fibrillation monitor. But the question I'd like to ask is, we've been discussing the problems with nurses, outside of their appearance, and what do we think about, as a group, of closing the loop. In other words, once you've got ventricular fibrillation, having it dealt with without intervention of man or woman.

JULIAN: You mean automatic defibrillator? Okay. There seems to be general agreement that an automatic defibrillator would be a nice thing. Can we get down to the question is, have an answer to the question: do we think we should be monitoring for arrhythmias other than ventricular fibrillation? Can somebody answer that question?

MASERI: I think that you are just coming down to what the purposes of the meeting were I want to compliment you right away just before the scenery close. The problem is, that we are here asking this question, where to go in the next 5 years? I think that you are one of the persons that is likely to answer this question as soon as you have finished analysing the data of your 500 patients on continuous tapes. My feelings are that we should try to monitor just the most serious arrhythmias, VT, VF. I would be happy with that.

FERUGLIO: I'll try to answer the question of the moderator. Shall we monitor only the threatening arrhythmias or shall we be monitoring all the others, important ones? I think the answer is in graded system, we are using the HP system that you have thrown away, and we are very happy with the graded type of alarms.

JULIAN: I take your point. Again it comes back to the question: what you are wanting to be sensitive to? And if you take the kind of arrhythmias you are talking about then the system you describe I am sure is satisfactory. I think we have to differentiate between, the research use of computers and the routine use of computers. And I am sure that the system described by Dr. Beaufils, the system used by Prof. Hugenholtz and the kind of system we use and the kind of system, for example, that Dr. Hutton is going to describe from Glascow, are absolutely essential in understanding the natural history of these arrhythmias and I think one thing we must take from this meeting is the fact that this information is still very inadequate, and that the need for people to study these arrhythmias by computer system is obligatory. Anything other than a computer system is completely hopeless. So I think we need good computer systems and a lot of people making observations. I think many different centers need to do this because the patient populations are different. I think this has to be eventually get a consensus from different centers on this kind of approach. But if we are going to say that nursing systems are unsatisfactory, that we need to detect warning arrhythmias and that the only way of doing this is with computers, we are making a tremendous extrapolation with tremendous expense implications. An if we were to say to EEC this is the way that we should go; that's a very important recommendation. Now is this what we should be saying? Should we be trying to develop a computer for every coronary? Do you think so?

CHAPTER 2

NON INVASIVE HEMODYNAMIC MEASUREMENTS IN CORONARY CARE
UNITS

2.1. INTRODUCTION
P.G. Hugenholtz

We discussed this morning the problems of electrocardiographic monitoring for the detecting of arrhythmias. As our experience grows, we
are becoming more and more concerned with the evaluation of another
basic function of the heart: his function as a pump. This alley
appears now worthy pursuing in order to obtain a further reduction
of mortality in CCU. In particular we learned that pump function
alterations must be detected and dealt with as early as possible
even before clinical signs appear. We also learned that we wish to
be able to follow objectively in time the effects of our interventions on cardiac function. In critically ill patients, in centers
where adequate expertise is available, invasive monitoring is the
answer, as we will discuss tomorrow, but for less acute patiens and
for centers where invasive procedures are not available, non invasive techniques do represent a first line of attack.
We will consider this afternoon the use of ultrasounds in the CCU
setting: it nearly a novelty but I believe it might have a promising
future.

2.2. TWO-DIMENSIONAL ECHOCARDIOGRAPHY IN ACUTE MYOCARDIAL INFARCTION

R. Prasquier, M. Barthelemy, P. Vervin, C. Valantin, T. Touche, M.C. Aumont, R. Gourgon

2.2.1. INTRODUCTION

Since multiple segments of the left ventricle are displayed in a two dimensional echocardiographic examination, this method could hopefully obviate to the well known limitations of the M mode echocardiography in coronary artery disease (1, 2). The value of this technique would be further increased in acute myocardial infarction by the availability of sequential studies of left ventricular segmental wall motion, the size of the infarcted area being considered a major determinant of short term (3) and long term (4) prognosis.

In this study we attempted to determine the feasibility and sensibility of a wide angle 2 D equipment for detecting segmental wall motion abnormalities during the acute phase of myocardial infarction.

2.2.2. METHODS

Fifty consecutive patients without evidence of prior myocardial infarction admitted to the coronary care unit for acute myocardial infarction were studied with two dimensional echocardiography. These patients included 39 men and 11 women with an average age of 58 years (range 24-81 years). Myocardial infarction was defined by classical ECG and enzyme changes. There were 7 subendocardial (4 anterior and 3 posterior) and 43 transmural infarctions: 23 were anterior (including anteroseptal, anterolateral, lateral and circumferential MI) and 27 were posterior (including inferior and basal MI).

Patients had 3 cross-sectional echocardiographic studies: the first one (E1) within the first 4 days after the onset of chest pain, the second one (E2) between the 4th and 8th day and the third one (E3) during the 3rd week.

The real time two-dimensional echocardiographic instrument used in this study is an electronical phased array sector scanner with a 84° sector angle (Varian Inc. Salt Lake City USA; CGR France). The probe contains an array of 32 2.25 MHZ transducers, the emission of which is controlled trough a microprocessor unit; focalization is realized by an acoustical lens. The system operates at 30 frames/ second; the image is photographed through a vidicon tube by a video camera and recorded on 1/2 inch video cassettes using a Sanyo VTC-7100 cassette recorder.

The cross sectional study was performed in the left lateral position, the probe being placed in the third or fourth intercostal space to the left of the sternum (left sternal studies) and on the point of maximal cardiac impulse (apical studies). Four cardiac views (2 left sternal and 2 apical) were attempted in every patient. Seeing very slight movements of the probe can dramatically modify spatial orientation of the explored left ventricular segments, special care was taken to obtain in each of the four views one particular reproducible section, defined according to internal anatomical landmarks, and within these landmarks, selecting that section whice displayed the largest left ventricular area: these are termed standardized sections and are obtained in the following manner:

A. In the long axis sternal view, the beam plane is parallel to the walls of the aorta. To obtain the standardized longitudinal left sternal section (LS) the probe is angled medially until the posterior papillary muscle is visible on the screen.

B. The probe is rotated 90° in order to obtain the transverse or short axis view (TS). Two sections are selected: the mitral transverse section (TSm) at the tip of mitral leaflets and papillary muscle transverse section (TSp) which is visualised after a slight caudal angulation of the probe.

C. The horizontal apical views display the four cavities of the heart on the screen. The selected section (HA) is obtained by angling the beam direction immediately below the aortic valve plane: segmental left ventricular walls are thus recorded in their superior segments.

D. The probe still placed upon the PMI is then rotated counterclockwise until the right ventricular cavity disappears: this represents a vertical apical view where the standardized section (VA) is selected. It then shows the aortic valve plane and the upward diaphragmatic convexity of the inferior left ventricular wall.

The walls of the left ventricle were divided in to 13 different segments as represented in Fig. 1. The left ventricle is analysed as a pyramidal structure with three walls (septum S, inferior wall I and lateral wall L); the posterior segments (P) are adjacent to the base of the pyramid (plane of the aortic and mitral valve orifices), the anterior segments (A) are adjacent to the apex (Ap). Posterior and middle portions are divided in to superior and inferior segments. The apex is never seen in the long axis sternal section which foreshortens the left ventricular cavity.

Segmental wall motion was studied on the video cassette recordings by two separate observers, neither of whom had previous knowledge of the patient's medical history and ECG findings. Observer disagreements were resolved by a common reading. This was necessary in 10%

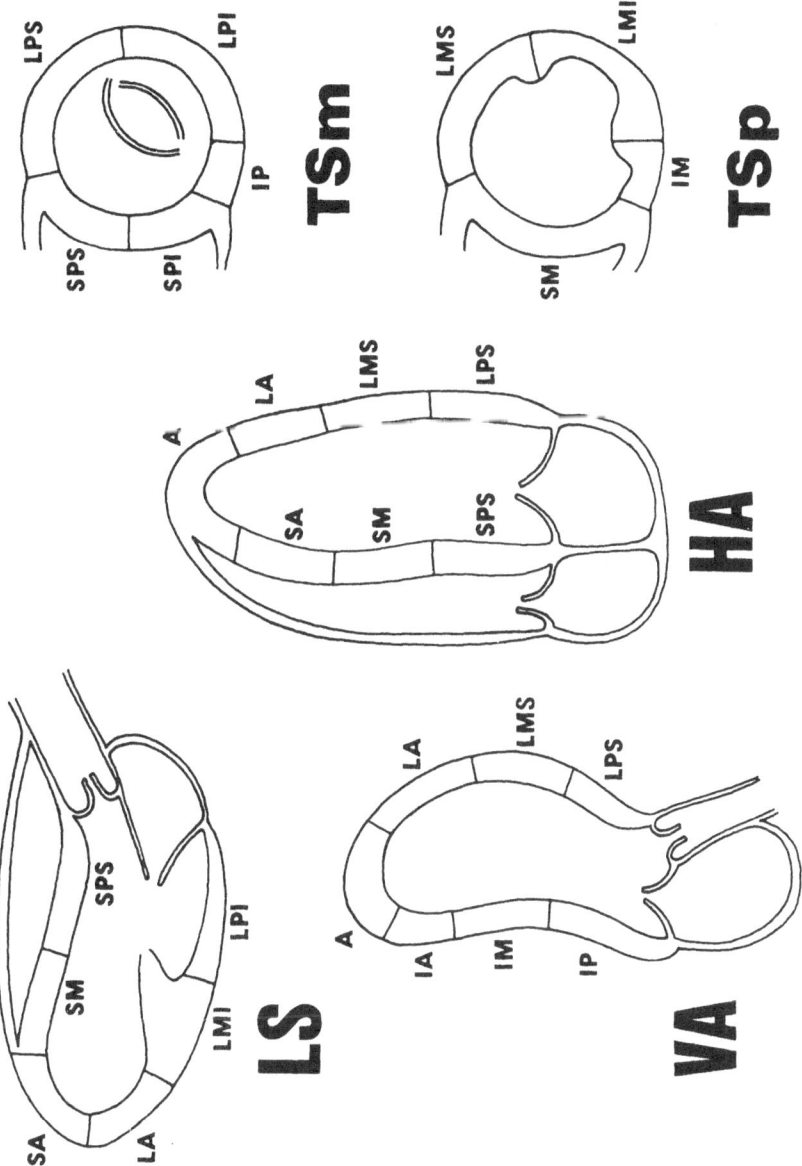

Fig. 1. Left ventricular echocardiographic sections and segments.
Sections: LS long axis sternal, TSm transverse sternal-mitral level,
TSp transverse sternal-papillary muscle level, HA horizontal apical,
VA vertical apical. Segments: IA inferior anterior, IM inferior
middle, IP inferior posterior, AP apical, SA septal anterior, SM
septal middle, SPS septal postero-superior, SPI septal posteroinferior, LA lateral anterior, LMS lateral middle superior, LMI
lateral middle inferior, LPS lateral postero-superior, LPI lateral
postero-inferior.

of the analysed segments.

A segment was defined as interpretable if either 50 % of the endocardium of this segment was seen throughout the cardiac cycle or, in the apical views, if 25 % of the endocardium was visible with a well delineated epicardium. Segmental motion was studied according to myocardial systolic thickening and epicardial motion of one segment in relation to the adjacent ones. Only akinetic, dyskinetic and definely hypokinetic areas were considered asynergic.

For ten patients with anterior transmural myocardial infarction who had their first cross sectional study within the first 24 hours after the onset of pain, the asynergic area in the HA section was measured as a percentage of diastolic left ventricular lenght and results were compared with those of the second and third cross sectional examination.

2.2.3. RESULTS

Two patients (4 %) had no interpretable segment on any of the echocardiographic examinations. The interpretability rate was very high in most of the explored segments except the inferior middle segment of the lateral wall (LMI) with 58 % of interpretability (Table 1). Apical, anteroseptal, anterolateral, postero superior lateral and postero inferior segments were adequately recorded in 48 patients (96 %). This is explained by the availability of the apical sections which yielded a very high percentage of adequate studies. Those of segments which could only be visualized through left sternal sections (LMI) had a much lower yield of interpretability. Short axis sections were the most difficult to record adequately.

Among 19 patients with anterior myocardial infarction, 18 had interpretable studies of anterior segments (Fig. 2). All these patients had at least apical (Ap) and anteroseptal (AS) asynergy. Eleven patients (61 %) had anterolateral akinesis; this was much more frequent when there was lateral Q waves in the ECG (9/10 vs 2/8). Asynergy extending to posterior segments was seen in each of the 3 circumferential infarctions and in 6/15 (40 %) anterior infarctions.

Among 24 patients with posterior transmural myocardial infarction, 23 had interpretable recordings of posterior segments (Fig. 3). Asynergy of one or several of these segments was found in every patient; the posterior inferior segment was nearly always (22/23) found to be asynergic. The inferior and posterior segment of the lateral wall (LPI) was asynergic in every patient in whom ECG disclosed basal extension (14/14); it was unconstantly akinetic (4/7) in isolated inferior infarction.

Mitral valve motion was frequently characteristic in these posterior transmural infarctions: in 14 pts. (58%) posterior leaflet had a

Table 1. Percentage of segmental Interpretability

	95 %	85-95 %	75-85 %	75 %
Apex	— apical (A)			
Septal	— ant. (SA)	— post. inf. (SPI)	— mid. (SM) — post. sup. (SPS)	
Lateral	— ant. (LA) — post. sup. (LPS)	— post. inf, (LPI)	— mid. sup. (LMS)	— mid. inf. (LMI)
Inferior	— post. (IP)	— mid. (IM)	— ant. (IA)	

very brisk backward motion toward the left atrium both at end diastole and at end systole. This motion was never seen in anterior infarction, and it was not related to the extent of akinesis, to clinical signs of mitral regurgitation nor to abnormal papillary muscle density.

Among the 4 anterior subendocardial infarctions, 3 had apical akinesis extending in one case to the anterior segments of the septum and lateral wall; 1 had a normal study.

Among the 3 posterior subendocardial infarction 2 had IP and LPI akinesis extending in one case to the middle segments of the inferior and lateral walls; 1 had a normal study.

Ten patients with anterior and 6 patients with posterior transmural infarction were studied within the first 24 hours after the onset of chest pain. The areas of the VA sections not being reproducible enough from E1 to E3, only the HA sections in anterior infarctions were measured to determine the percentage of akinesis (Fig. 4). No significant evolutionary change was found in this ratio.

There was 1 case of VSD during acute posterior myocardial infarction, the diagnosis of which was readily made by the cross sectional study which showed (Fig. 5), in the HA section, an echo free space within the septum with openings on the left and the right side. This corresponded to a dissecting hematoma of the septum. The patient was in cardiogenic shock during the cross sectional study, with a hyperkinetic LV on the M mode recording and died soon afterwards.

2.2.4. DISCUSSION

The potential usefulness of cross sectional echocardiography in

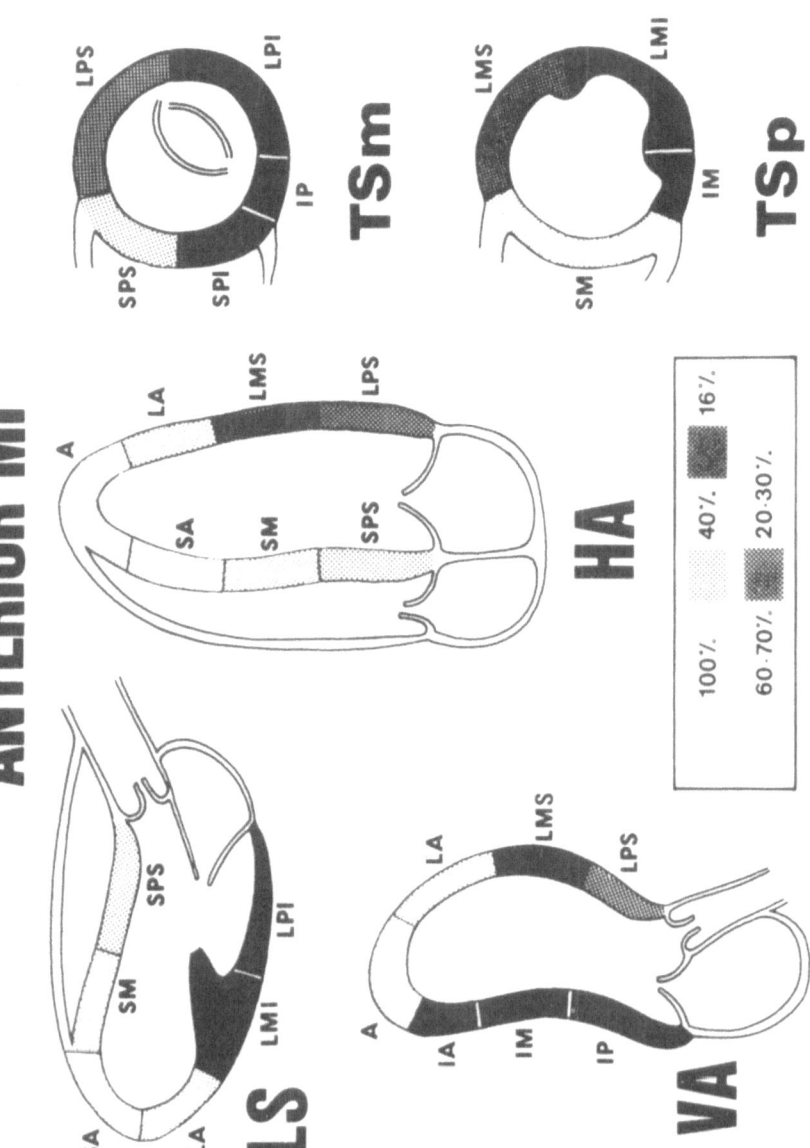

Fig. 2. Anterior transmural MI: segmental asynergy/segmental interpretability.

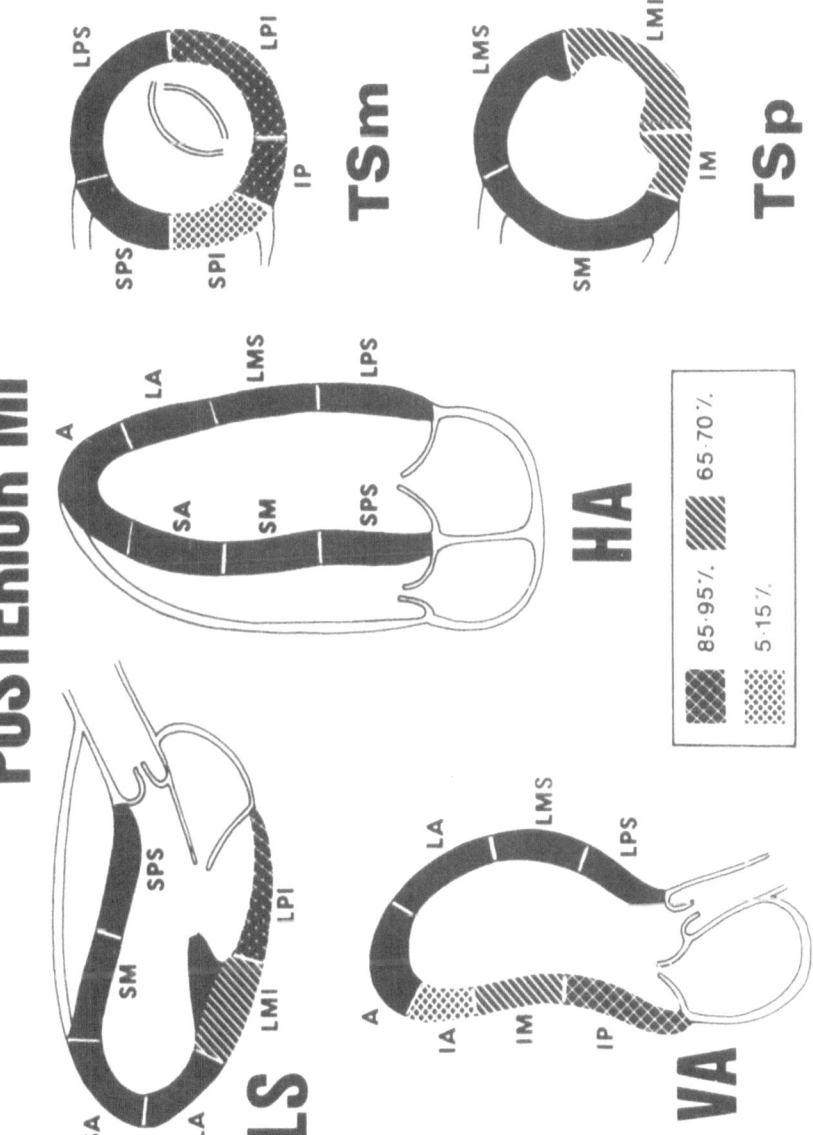

Fig. 3. Posterior transnural MI: segmental asynergy/segmental interpretability.

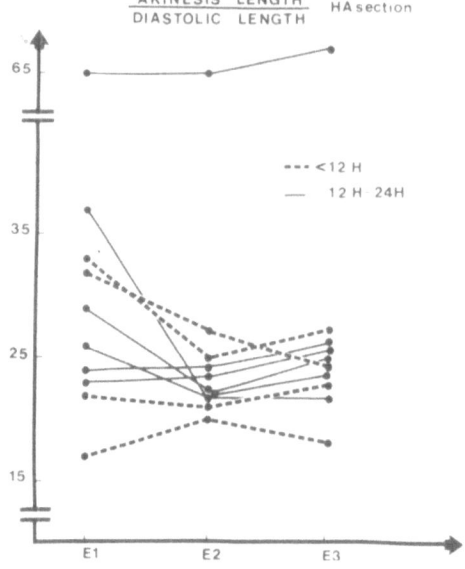

ANTERIOR MI

$$\frac{\text{AKINESIS LENGTH}}{\text{DIASTOLIC LENGTH}} \quad \text{HA section}$$

- - - <12 H
— 12 H · 24H

Fig. 4. Evolution of anterior akinesis.

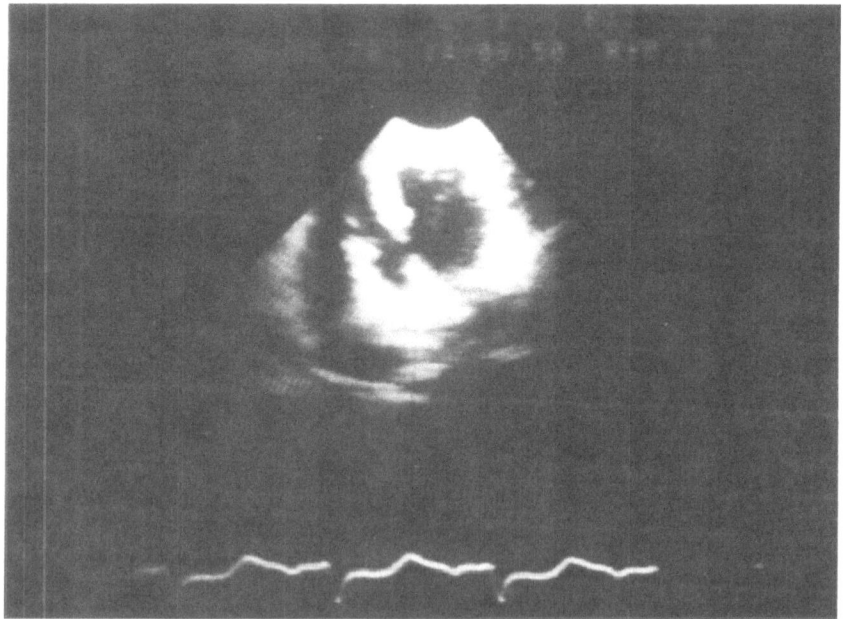

Fig. 5. HA section: ventricular septal rupture in posterior myocardial infarction.

chronic coronary artery disease has been suggested by Weyman et al.
(5) for detection of apical aneurysms, and by Kisslö et al (6) who
found a satisfactory sensibility in the analysis of segmental wall
motion abnormalities.

The present study amplifies the value of this method in the setting
of acute myocardial infarction, a period when left ventricular
angiography is usually not advisable, and in any case not repeata-
ble. In view of currently accepted concepts regarding the prognostic
value of the extent of infarcted area and the controversies about
salvaging the periinfarction twilight zone it would be extremely
useful to have a non invasive method of monitoring left ventricular
segmental wall motion.

The adequate visualization of segmental motion was realized in this
series in 95 % of a non-selected group of patients. In a previous
study of 45 acute myocardial infarctions there was a similar rate
(7 %) of complete echotomographic failures (7). Moreover, the
success rate in the adequate visualization of the inferior wall
segments was improved in the present series, increasing from 73 % to
90 %. This is probably due to a better selection of the vertical
apical section where it is mandatory to look for the diaphragmatic
convexity and to visualize the aortic valve.

The value of the apical views, as described by Schiller and col.
(8), cannot be overemphasized in the cross sectional study of
coronary patients. These views yield more topographical orientation
and are much easier to perform in these patients than classical left
sternal views. Thus, we feel that electronical phased array instruments offer a great advantage over the linear array echographs which
do not permit apical views, and over mechanical sector scanners with
which these views are difficult to realise because of the bulk of
the probe.

The fact that sternal views are less rewarding in coronary disease
could be forecast by the results of M mode echocardiography, which,
by standard technique, is successful in only about 60 % of these
patients.

In the present series, akinesis and/or dyskinesis was found in every
patient with transmural myocardial infarction and adequate cross
sectional study. Topographical accuracy is good, at least as judged
by the gross ECG criteria and the pyrophosphate and thallium scinti-
graphic studies which were performed in a limited number of
patients. The very high rate of septal involvement in anterior
infarctions, even when it was not suggested by the ECG, is unexplai-
ned, but might be due in part to the limited ECG sensitivity in this
topography. Thus, because of its simplicity and sensitivity, two
dimensional echocardiography may play an important role to play in
acute myocardial infarction when the diagnosis needs to be confirmed. It may also be valuable in the detection of mechanical complications of infarction as exemplified by our case of ventricular septal

42

defect but much more experience needs to be gained in this area.

Since we had no reliable index of extent of myocardial necrosis in this study and since most of the first echoes were performed relatively late, at least after the first six hours when presumably there is no hope for the reduction of infarct size, we cannot conclude from our serial studies to the value of this method in the sequential monitoring of left ventricular segmental dynamics. We were impressed by the fact that there is usually no detectable change from one study to another in the amount of left ventricular dysfunction, and in the very early distension that occurs in some of the more severe myocardial infarctions. These findings are in agreement with a recent isotopic wall motion study (9).

Some points of caution in the analysis of the two dimensional echocardiograms must be stressed:

1. Since this is a tomographical study one is never certain of having scanned the entire left ventricular area. For instance, the apical area, as defined by the most anterior portion of the apical views, may not correspond to the true apex, at least in some patients where the apex, mostly when akinetic and distended, is located well under the point of maximal impulse and hidden by the lung.
2. The definition of left ventricular segments remains somewhat arbitrary. Standardized sections are necessary to obtain a reproducible display of left ventricular cavity. Improvements in the geometrical determination of the probe motion would allow the study of the standardized sections and thus increase the precision of spatial analysis.
3. Improvements in lateral resolution of the echocardiographic equipment and in the recording system (where there is much loss of information) are necessary to perform a reliable quantitative study of the left ventricular segmental motion.
   Notwithstanding present technical limitation, two dimensional echocardiography is likely to soon become an useful clinical instrument in acute myocardial infarction.

REFERENCES

1. Sweet AL, RE Moraski, RO jr Russel et al: Relationship between echocardiography, cardiac output and abnormally contracting segments in patients with ischemic heart disease. Circulation 52: 634, 1975.
2. Teicholz LE, TH Kreulen, MV Herman et al: Problems in echocardiographic volume determinations: echocardiographic-angiographic correlations in the presence or absence of asynergy. Am J Cardiol 37: 7, 1976.

3. Page DL,JB Caulfield, JA Kastor, et al: Myocardial changes associated with cardiogenic shock. N Engl J Med 285: 133, 1971.
4. Chatterjee K, HJC Swan, VS Haushik, et al: Effects of vasodilator
   therapy for severe pump failure in acute myocardial infarction on
   short term and late prognosis. Circulation 58: 684, 1973.
5. Weyman A, H Feigenbaum, J. Dillon, et al: Evaluation of left
   ventricular apical aneurysms by real time cross sectional echocardiography. Circulation 54: 936, 1976.
6. Kisslö JA, D Robertson, BW Gilbert, et al: A comparison of real
   time, two dimensional echocardiography and cine-angiography in
   detecting left ventricular asynergy. Circulation 55: 134, 1977.
7. Prasquier R, T Touche, M Barthelemy: Echocardiographie bidimensio-
   nelle dans l'infarctus du myocarde. Trans Eur Soc Cardiol 1: 52,
   1978.
8. Silverman NH, NB Schiller: Apex echocardiography: a two dimensional technique for evaluating congenital heart disease. Circulation 57: 503, 1978.
9. Reduto LA, HJ Berger, LS Cohen, et al: Sequential radionuclide
   assessment of left and right ventricular performance after acute
   transmural myocardial infarction. Ann Int Med 89: 441, 1978.

2.3. ASSESSMENT OF VENTRICULAR FUNCTION IN ACUTE MYOCARDIAL INFAR-
CTION BY ECHOCARDIOGRAPHY: POSTMORTEM CORRELATIONS
J. Heikkilä, S. Nieminen

2.3.1. INTRODUCTION

Morphologic-echocardiographic comparison was carried out in 24 patients to determine the accuracy of the single-beam echocardiography
used with a multiaxis application in imaging the site and size of 22
acute fatal myocardial infarctions, and of 2 postinfarction ventricular aneurysms treated surgically. Echocardiography never missed
the infarction, whether the infarction was anterior or posterior
irrespectively. The correlation between the echocardiographic extent
of asynergy and pathologic-anatomic extent of infarct, as expressed
by a percentage of the left ventricular horizontal circumference,
was r = 0.88 (p<0.001) in 30 comparisons. Only the posterior septal
and the most lateral segments of the left ventricle remain out of
range of the single-beam echo method; in the other regions variation
remained within 1 cm (18 of the 24 patients). The regional asynergy
of the infarcted region was clear-cut: systolic thickening was never
seen (mean 0.06 ± 0.2 mm), and the wall motion was mainly paradoxical systolic outward motion at the infarct center (mean − 2.0 ± 2.0
mm). An old postinfarction scar was reliably differentiated from the
acute necrosis. Thus, segmental left ventricular wall akinesis, as
seen by the multidirectional echocardiography, permits a reliable
quantitative estimation of the actual size of acute myocardial
infarction in man.
The magnitude of the left ventricular muscle damage closely determines the development of heart failure, short-term and later prognosis
and even major ventricular arrhythmias following acute myocardial
infarction (1). It is now recognized that an evaluation of the
regional contractile function of the left ventricle provides very
rewarding information on a patient with acute or chronic ischemic
heart disease.
Abnormalities of the segmental wall motion are directly and accurately visualized by ultrasound in experimental studies (2, 3). In
patients with myocardial infarction, too, ventricular asynergy has
been described by echocardiography but usually only in rather restri-
cted segments in the left ventricle (4). We have used a multidirectional application of single-beam echocardiography (5). In this way
it is possible to image in detail the performance of multiple
segments around the entire left ventricle. The correlative study
reported here examines ·the capacity of echocardiography to locate

and quantify the size of myocardial infarction, when it is related
to pathologic-anatomic data either in autopsy or in cardiac surgery.

2.3.2. PATIENTS AND METHODS

Twenty-two patients were treated in the intensive care unit
because of serious acute myocardial infarction; 2 further patients
were operated on for postinfarction ventricular aneurysms. The patients comprised 21 men and 3 women, ranging in age from 31 to 71
years. The diagnosis of acute myocardial infarction was always
verified eventually in autopsy. Seventeen patients had their first
infarction while 7 patients had suffered from one or more previous
infarctions. The recent infarction was anterior in 14 patients
(including the 2 aneurysms) and posteroinferior in 7 patients; in 3
patients both the anterior and posterior walls were damaged. Death
was either from refractory pump failure due to an extensive myocardial damage in 18 of the 22 patients, or, in 4 patients caused by a
rupture of various cardiac structures.
The interval between the echocardiography and death was from 3 hours
to 12 days, except in the case of 2 patients who died 30 and 75 days
after echocardiography performed on admission. Echocardiography was
performed with a Picker Echoview II equipment (Cleveland, Ohio).

The ischemic region of the myocardium loses its mechanical contraction in a few seconds. This relationship has been repeatedly
documented experimentally by segment length and wall thickness measurements (2, 3). Mechanical alteration even precedes the appearance
of the ischemic ST-segment shifts, and precedes even more the onset
of measurable biochemical alterations. Our own experience nicely
demonstrated the ability of echocardiography to document rapidly a
marked mechanical dysfunction in human hearts when ischemia was
induced by atrial pacing (6). The functional aberration of myocardial contractility is thus obviously one of the most sensitive
markers of ischemia.

The regional function of the left ventricle in man can be
investigated rather comprehensively by echo using multiple beam
directions with careful gain and reject adjustments and utilizing
a 2:1 scale. Instead of the narrow 'icepick' pictures of only the
interventricular septum and the posterior wall obtained using the
conventional left ventricular echo axis, the multiaxis approach
(echoventriculography) provides a composite study of the upper and
lower halves of the septum, anterior, posteroinferior and often even
lateral left ventricular segments, though these must be recorded
sequentially. The echocardiographic precordial window is also larger
when the patient lies in a flat supine position. The technique has
been described earlier in detail (5, 6).

The anatomical orientation is performed in a standard way and

using four principal echo beam directions (5). Position 1 is the
same as the conventional position used to record the left ventricular transverse diameter. Left ventricular volumes and ejection fraction are usually calculated from these diameters using the cube function (5,7). The upper septal and posterolateral regions of the left
ventricle are reached from position 1. Position 2 is about 2 cm
lateral from the basic mitral valve point, i.e. positions 1 and 2
are about 5 cm apart. This beam axis traverses the upper posterior
and free anterior wall regions. Position 3 of the probe lies one
intercostal space below position 1; this axis scans the inferolate-
ral and septal regions in the lower half of the left ventricle. The
low free anterior and inferoposterior wall regions are recorded from
position 4, one intercostal space below position 2. These standardized scanning sites are necessary in order to obtain reproducible
data of the segmental wall motions in the sequential studies.
Additional positions (AW5-14) are used for more detailed estimation
of the anterior wall asynergy (5, 6).

The posterior wall segments are usually studied first. The same gain
and reject levels are used for each segment. The fine adjustments
are made by rotating the probe by slight movements according to the
A-mode control. The anterior wall regions are recorded in a similar
way, but a lower decibel gain is usually utilized. At each precordial position the probe is directed as perpendicularly as possible
towards the region desired. This is ascertained by rotating the
probe with small steps and finding a direction so that the echo
lines at the 2:1 scale from the myocardial layers move in a parallel
way in both the A-mode and M-mode display (5, 6).

The regional myocardial function is analysed quantitatively by measuring the amplitude of the systolic wall motions and the systolic
thickening at each site. The error of the axial accuracy in measuring wall motion amplitudes and thickening by the echocardiograph
used is less than 1 mm. In reproducibility studies of the same
variables the standard error of differences remained below 0.5 mm
both in healthy subjects and in infarction patients (6).

The regional function was assessed in detail from the sequential
individual segmental recordings from the upper and the middle thirds
of the left ventricle. The upper echocardiographic transverse slice
lies at the level of echo axes 1 and 2, i.e. at the junctional level
of the anatomical upper and middle thirds of the left ventricle. The
lower echo slice lies at a level between the anatomical middle and
lower thirds of the left ventricle.

The functional state of myocardial segments was recorded from 7
horizontal sectors of the left ventricle, and marked thereafter on a
schematic drawing (Fig. 1). A similar assessment during the autopsy
study was made with no knowledge of the echo recordings. Echocardiographically the sector borders are as follows: the junction of right
ventricle and free anterior wall divides the septum from the ante-

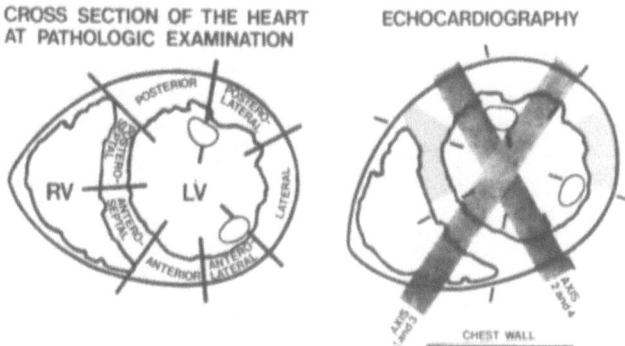

Fig. 1. At the postmortem examination the cross-sectional slice of the heart was divided into 7 segments. Respective segments using this framework and the echocardiographic landmarks described in the text were identified during sequential echocardiographic imaging. The stippled areas are not well reached with the single-beam echocardiography.

rior wall; the anterior commissure of the mitral valve and the anterior papillary muscle separates the anterior wall from the lateral left ventricular sector; the site estimated to be half-way between the above two landmarks separates the anterior and anterolateral segment; the segment medial to the posterior papillary muscle is the posteroinferior one; the segment lateral from the posterior papillary muscle the postero (infero)lateral segment. These landmarks permit an accurate orientation to the various horizontal sectors of the left ventricular circumference. Only the farthest lateral regions and the posterior parts of the interventricular septum are poorly, if at all, defined by the single beam technique. This is due to the oblique hit of the echo pulses on those segments. Recent myocardial ischemia or necrosis is recognized by segmental akinesis or paradoxical motion and by lack of systolic thickening. Echo lines from acute necrosis are softer than from the normal myocardium and tend to become broken. Myocardial scar tissue is identified echocardiographically on the basis of the high tissue density of the infarct scar. The wide echo lines of the high-amplitude myocardial echoes in the A mode are easily recorded by the adjustable wide-band radiofrequency signal processor of the present equipment.

At postmortem examination the site and size of the myocardial infarcts were observed by cutting the heart perpendicular to the long axis of the left ventricle into 5 or 6 transversal slices. Coronary artery obstructions were examined before slicing.

2.3.3. RESULTS

2.3.3.1. Regional dysfunction of the left ventricle by echo in fatal myocardial infarction.

Occurrence of asynergy at the inafarcted region: complete echocardiographic analysis of the left ventricular regional function was successful in all of the 24 patients with one exception, where pleural calcifications prevented a study of the anterolateral segments.

Regional loss of the left ventricular wall motion was observed by echocardiography in every patient with myocardial infarction (100%), irrespective of whether the site of the infarction was anterior, posterior, septal or lateral.

The amplitude of the systolic wall motion at the infarct center was reversed from the normal inward motion to a paradoxical (dyskinetic) outward motion; the mean amplitude was -2.0 ± 2.0 mm. Eighteen of the 24 patients (75 %) showed paradoxical systolic bulging, up to -6 mm at the infarcted region. The best motion amplitude was only of 1 mm (2 patients).

Systolic thickening of the infarcted region was completely absent. The mean thickening was 0.06 ± 0.2 mm.

The echoventriculographic contraction index (sigma regional amplitude of the left ventricle) is based on an analysis of the 8 standard segments located around the left ventricle, and expressed as a percentage of the sum of the means of the corresponding systolic amplitudes of the normal left ventricle (8, 9). It gives an 'overall' expression of the teamwork of infarcted and uninvolved segments of the whole left ventricle. The echoventriculographic contraction index was markedly reduced, the mean being 40.2 ± 21.1 % ($p < 0.0005$, normal = 100 %).

The wall thickening index was determined from the same 8 standard sites which are used for the echoventriculographic contraction index measuring the amplitudes of wall motions. Its mean value was 14.4 ± 6.7 % ($p < 0.0005$, normal 34.8 ± 2.1 %). These wall motion amplitudes and thickenings from multiple sites correlated well with each other ($r = 0.86$).

Fractional shortening and ejection fraction. The mean fractional shortening of the left ventricular transverse diameter during systole was 13.2 ± 6.7 % ($p < 0.001$, normal 29.5 ± 4.2 %). The ejection fraction was 33.5 ± 14.8 % ($p < 0.001$, normal 54.4 ± 8.5 %).

2.3.3.2. Site and size of acute myocardial infarction by echo: postmortem correlations.

The extent of the infarct as a percentage of the left ventricular horizontal circumference determined from the pathologic-anatomic specimens was plotted against the echocardiographically akinetic or parodoxical segments (Figs. 2 and 3). the correlation coefficient

ECHOCARDIOGRAPHY-AUTOPSY CORRELATIONS IN 24 HEARTS

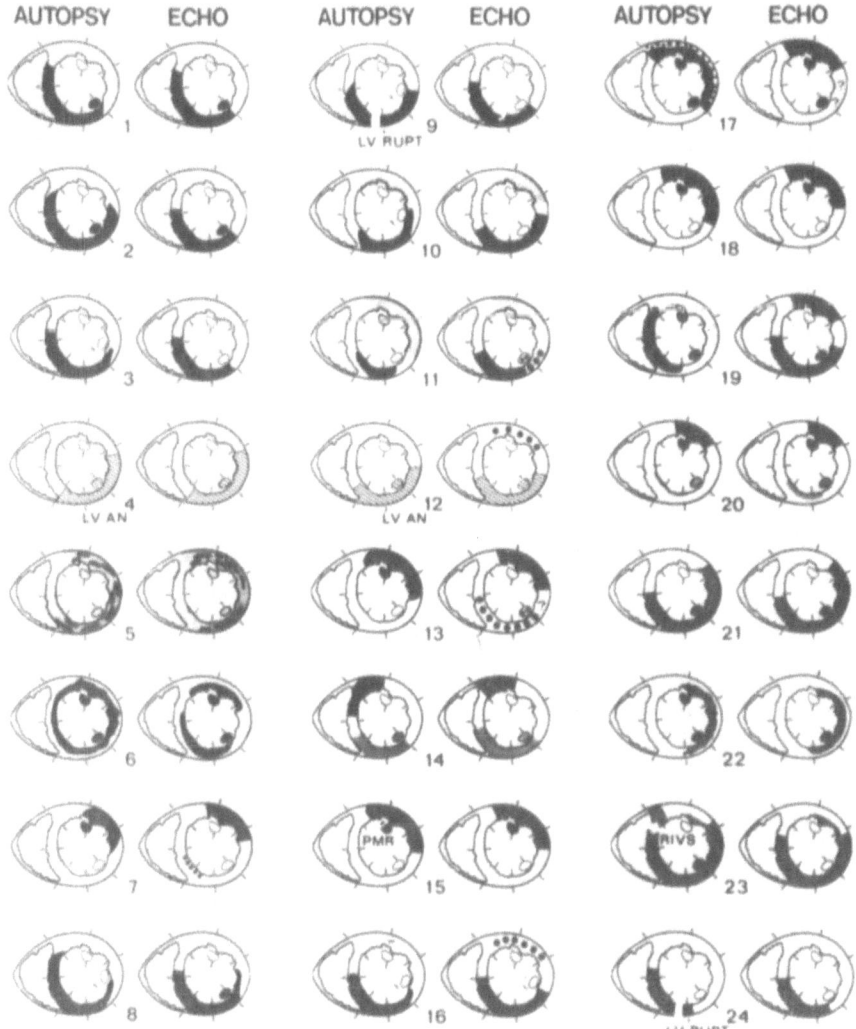

Fig. 2. Illustrations comparing myocardial damage in each of the 24 hearts as assessed by the postmortem study and the echoventriculographic imaging. The good correlation was influenced neither by the anterior or posterior site, nor by the size of the infarction. White – uninvolved myocardium, black – fresh necrosis, stippled – myocardial scar, lines (LV-AN) – ventricular aneurysm, asterisk – marked acute ischemia in echo but no macroscopic necrosis at autopsy, LV rupt – myocardial rupture, PMR – papillary muscle rupture, RIVS – ruptured interventricular septum.

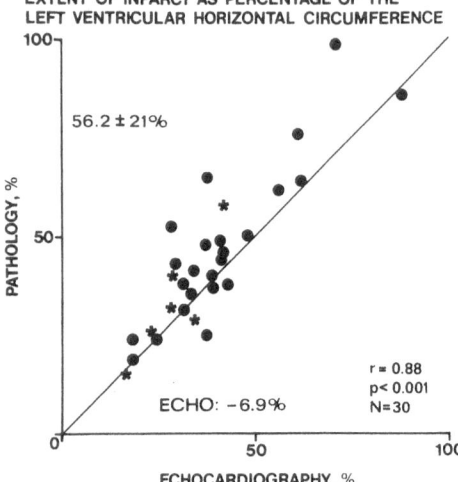

EXTENT OF INFARCT AS PERCENTAGE OF THE LEFT VENTRICULAR HORIZONTAL CIRCUMFERENCE

56.2 ± 21%

PATHOLOGY, %

r = 0.88
p < 0.001
N = 30

ECHO: −6.9%

ECHOCARDIOGRAPHY, %

Fig. 3. The correlation was good between the echocardiographic and the postmortem or surgical extent of infarct. Dots — fresh necrosis, stars — old scar.

was 0.88 for the circumferential extent of damage from the fresh infarctions and the old postinfarct scars analysed together (n = 30, p <0.001). From acute infarctions alone r was 0.87.

The difference between the echocardiographic and the postmortem extent of myocardial damage remained less than 15 percent of the circumference in 21 of the 24 patients (Fig. 3). The variation also remained within 1 cm in all but 6 cases (no. 2, 5, 6, 17, 19, 23) where infarcts extended to the lateral or posteroseptal segments, difficult or impossible to record by the single-beam technique. The anterior or posterior site of the infarct did not influence the accuracy of the estimation.

Myocardial infarcts were generally large, as the patients died mainly from severe left ventricular dysfunction. The mean horizontal circumference of the acute infarction at autopsy was 47.4 ± 20.0 % (echo 41.2 ± 16.5 %), and when the scars were included, 56.5 ± 21.2% (echo 49.6 ± 17.9 %) (Figs. 2 and 3).

Vertically, the infarcts extended in most patients from the base to the apex. In only 2 of the 24 patients all three levels (upper, middle, lower thirds) were not involved. No disagreement occurred in the echocardiographic estimation in the frame of the three vertical sections.

In 3 hearts (no. 7, 13, 16) echocardiography detected loss of function in segments where no gross myocardial pathology was found. However, during autopsy the major coronary artery branches supplying these asynergic segments were found to be completely occluded in 2 patients and 1 had a subtotal stenosis (> 75 %). The time from the

onset of symptoms and the echocardiographic examination to death was
a few hours in 2 patients, not yet inducing gross pathologic
changes. One patient (no. 12), operated on for an anterior ventricular aneurysm, had echocardiographic changes of fibrotic-ischemic
dysfunction at the posterior wall as well. Coronary angiography
showed a 90 % stenosis of the right coronary artery, and the left
anterior descending and circumflex coronary artery branches were
both completely occluded.

2.3.3.3. Old myocardial infarction.
The occurrence, site and size of scar tissue subsequent to the
previous infarction were detected with an accuracy similar to that
of the fresh myocardial necrosis (Figs. 2 and 3). The echocardiographic estimation of the site and size of postinfarction ventricular aneurysm in 2 patients (nos. 4 and 12) also agreed well with
the findings during cardiac surgery.

2.3.4. DISCUSSION

The local nature of myocardial damage resulting from ischemia or
infarction requires 'per se' examination of mechanical performance
in several regions of the left ventricle. This is not possible with
the conventional single-beam echo technique as it only displays
limited spots on the anterior and posterior walls (7), and thereby
only detects generalized changes in the left ventricle (7, 10).
Consequently, several other transducer positions such as the lateral, apical and subxiphoid sites have been developed (5, 11, 12). In
fact, our standardized multidirectional approach ('echoventriculography') made it possible to study the function and structure of most
wall segments around the entire left ventricle. Our previous excellent correlation of segmental asynergy by echo with the electrocardiographic site of acute myocardial infarction (13), and more
significantly, with asynergy documented by left ventricular cinean-
giographic analysis (8) have here been confirmed by the 'hard'
end-point of pathologic anatomic examination of the infarcted hearts.
So far, our data represent the first postmortem correlative study
on the application of echocardiography in man to detect, locate and
quantify the ischemic damage caused by acute myocardial infarction.
The echocardiographic and postmortem studies, each made with out
knowledge of the other, are in good agreement: no infarction was
missed in this unselected series by echo; anterior, posteroinferior,
septal or lateral infarctions were correctly located by echo; and
quantitatively rather close correlation was reached (r = 0.88;
differences of 1 cm or less at the horizontal borders, with only a
few exceptions. Echo never clearly overestimated the size of the
infarction. The trend towards an underestimation results from the

two blind sectors of the posterior septum and at the furthest
lateral wall, mainly due to the angulation problems. This documentation then provides a firm basis for the use of echocardiography to
study regional left ventricular dysfunction quantitatively, e.g.
myocardial infarction and its size, in addition to the established
information available from more diffuse heart alterations, e.g.
congestive cardiomiopathy (2, 14).

The detection of acute ischemic myocardial damage by echo is based
on the almost instantaneous loss of regional mechanical performance
of myocardium taking place after the onset of ischemia (3, 6). Such
regional wall motion abnormality was constantly (100 %) and conspi-
ciously recorded in this series of fatal myocardial infarction, as
noted earlier by us (in 100% of patients) (6, 9, 13) and by others
(in 84 % of patients) (4, 11) in less complicated infarctions, too.
For instance, systolic wall motions at the center of infarctions
were mostly paradoxical, and systolic thickening was never seen. The
latter finding is very valuable in differentiating infarction from
hypokinetic or even paradoxical regional wall motions caused by more
physiological phenomena, such as septal asynergy in the right ventricular volume overload (15), and physically highly-trained subjects,
from bundle-branch block, or simply due to the anterior mass motion
of the whole heart seen normally in systole.

Loss of systolic thickening together with reduced or absent systolic
motion amplitude is one of the characteristic forms of asynergy in
experimental myocardial ischemia or infarction (2, 3, 16). Experiments by Sasayama et al. (17) revealed a close correlation ($r =
0.97$) between wall motion amplitudes and wall thickening; in the
present clinical series this correlation from multiple left ventricular sites was also high, $r = 0.86$.

The advantages of the multiaxis echoventriculography method is
that it permits a simultaneous assessment of the size of the
myocardial damage and of the response of the uninvolved segments
(9). Of the other non invasive techniques available, only complicated radionuclide cardiography methods provide such information. These methods do, however, lack the resolution capacity of echo in
making a quantitative assessment of the segmental contractility
changes (1, 12).

The method of echoventriculographic analysis deserves certain comments in explaining the good accuracy obtained in assessing the myocardial infarction. In the horizontal plane particularly, orientation
demands a good conception of the left ventricular anatomy in the
space and not merely that of the interventricular septum and the
posterior wall, which are easily recorded by echo. For instance, the
7 sectors used in the present study must be correctly orientated
within the left ventricle and properly related to the mitral valve,
the papillary muscles and the right ventricle (Figs. 1 and 2).

The four basic axes of the present method, together with the cardiac landmarks mentioned, permit accurate orientation to these segments, as verified by the present postmortem correlations. However, this requires a persistent examination and considerable experience in echocardiography. The perpendicular direction of the echo beam against the segment under study is required to avoid false appearance of the asynergic motion. The 2:1 scale fundamentally facilitates this task by visualizing parallel motion of the myocardial echo lines. The equipment also plays a significant role. For the detailed study of regional myocardial segments the echo signal should be of high energy and have a short duration to reduce the disturbing noise echoes. Similarly, a wide-band radiofrequency signal processor markedly improves the clarity of the segmental pictures. The echocardiograph equipment on the market seems to vary greatly in this respect. More sophisticated techniques, such as the phased-array wideangle sector echocardiography (18) will probably avoid the presentday angulation and orientation limitations and in the future greatly facilitate assessment of the infarct size (see Prasquier in the Proceedings). Furthermore, echoventriculography provides a method for the rapid monitoring of the changes induced by acute ischemia in the contractile function of myocardium. The effects of pharmacologic therapy are seen directly when protection of acutely ischemic myocardium is attempted (6).

REFERENCES

1. Hillis LD, E Braunwald: Myocardial ischemia. New Engl J Med 296: 971, 1977.
2. Kerber RE, ML Marcus: Evaluation of regional myocardial function in ischemic heart disease by echocardiography. Progr Cardiovasc Dis 20: 441, 1978.
3. Ross J Jr, D Franklin: Analysis of regional myocardial function, dimensions, and wall thickness in the characterization of myocardial ischemia and infarction. Circulation 53: suppl 1: 88, 1976.
4. Corya BC, S Rasmussen, SB Knoebel, et al: Echocardiography in acute myocardial infarction. Amer J Cardiol 36: 1, 1975.
5. Nieminen MS: Applications of multidirectional echocardiography in myocardial infarction. Thesis, Helsinki 1977.
6. Heikkilä J, MS Nieminen: Rapid monitoring of regional myocardial ischemia with echocardiography and ST segment shifts in man: Modification of 'infarct size' and hemodynamics by dopamine and beta blockade. Acta Med Scand, suppl 623: 71, 1978.
7. Feigenbaum H: Echocardiography, 2nd ed. Lea & Febiger, Philadelphia, 1976.
8. Nieminen MS: Echoventriculography in chronic coronary heart disease. Correlations with single-plane cineangiography of the left ventricle. Eur J Cardiol 5: 343, 1977.

9. Nieminen MS, J Heikkilä: Echoventriculography in acute myocardial infarction: III. Clinical correlations, and implication of the non-infarcted myocardium. Amer J Cardiol 38: 1, 1976.

10. Fortuin NJ, CGK Pawsey: The evaluation of left ventricular function by echocardiography. Amer J Med 63: 1, 1977.

11. Corya BC: Echocardiography in ischemic heart disease. Amer J Med 63: 10, 1977.

12. Feigenbaum H, BC Corya, JC Dillon, et al.: Role of echocardiography in patients with coronary artery disease. Amer J Cardiol 37: 775, 1976.

13. Heikkilä J, M Nieminen: Echoventriculographic detection, localization and quantification of left ventricular asynergy in acute myocardial infarction. Brit Heart J 37: 46, 1975.

14. Corya BC, H Feigenbaum, S Rasmussen, et al.: Echocardiographic features of congestive cardiomiopathy compared with normal subjects and patients with coronary artery disease. Circulation 49: 1153, 1974.

15. Corya BC, S Rasmussen, H Feigenbaum, et al.: Systolic thickening and thinning of the septum and posterior wall in patients with coronary artery disease, congestive cardiomyopathy and atrial septum defect. Circulation 55: 109, 1977.

16. Heikkilä J, BS Tabakin, PG Hugenholtz: Quantification of function in normal and infarcted regions of the left ventricle. Cardiovasc Res 6: 516, 1972.

17. Sasayama S, D Franklin, J Jr Ross, et al.: Dynamic changes in left ventricular wall thickness and their use in analysing cardiac function in the conscious dog. Amer J Cardiol 38: 870, 1976.

18. Tajik AJ, JB Seward, DJ Hagler, et al.: Two-dimensional realtime ultrasonic imaging of the heart and great vessels. Technique, image orientation, structure identification, and validation. Mayo Clin Proc 53: 271, 1978.

2.4. PRELIMINARY EVALUATION OF TRANSCUTANEOUS AORTOVELOGRAPHY FOR MONITORING CHANGES IN CARDIAC OUTPUT

A. Distante, E. Moscarelli, D. Rovai, A. L'Abbate, A. Maseri

2.4.1. Introduction

The classification of patients with acute myocardial infarction into hemodynamic subsets appears to be helpful for selection of appropriate therapeutical interventions. Accordingly monitoring of hemodynamic parameters appears useful for an appropriate management of acutely ill patients.

Invasive techniques currently used (1-7) have some practical disadvantages:

1. disconfort and some risk to the patient
2. need for highly trained medical and nursing personel
3. difficulty in repeating the measurements for sequential studies in medium and long term follow-up.

Therefore non invasive techniques capable of providing information on the hemodynamic state of the patients and on its changes would ne highly desirable.

We have begun to evaluate transcutaneous aortovelography (TAV) a Doppler technique which was deviced by Light and Cross (8) with the purpose of providing information on serial changes in cardiac output (9-12) from estimates of aortic blood flow velocity. We decided to compare the parameters obtained by TAV with those given by standard techniques for measuring cardiac output in patients with low output state during the administration of an inotropic agent (13) infused at progressively higher doses to produce graded changes in heart function.

2.4.2. Material and Methods

Six patients (5 males and 1 female, aged from 30 to 55) entered consecutively the study because affected by low output state due to cardiomyopathy, either primitive (unknown etiology) or secondary to ischemic heart disease following multiple myocardial infarctions. All patients, informed that the possibility of trying a new agent was potentially useful for their clinical condition, gave the informed consent to the study.

A Swan-Ganz catheter was introduced under fluoroscopic control into the pulmonary artery and a short into a peripheral artery for continuous measurements of right atrial (RAP) pulmonary (PAP) and

systemic blood (BP) pressure. All tracings were recorded on Ana-Log
14 Philips analog tape recorder through P23dB Statham transducers,
played back on paper and analysed manually. Cardiac output measurements were obtained intermittently during each stage of the study
and at the same time of TAV measurements by a thermal dilution
instruments (Edwards mod. 9520). After a 30 min period of basal
recording, through a small needly placed in an antecubital vein a
stepwise infusion of dobutamine (2.5, 5.0 and 7.5 γ/Kg/min) was
undertaken, each stage lasting 30 min and being alternated with
equal periods of saline infusion. The total length of the study
consisted of seven 30 min periods, 4 basal with saline infusion and
3 with drug infusion.

A transducer (containing the emitting and the receiving cry-
stal) placed in the supersternal fossa emitts a continuous train of
ultrasonic waves. When appropriately oriented by the operator the
beam is directed toward the distal part of the aortic arch. According to the Doppler effect it estimates the velocity of blood flow,
which, in that part of the aortic arch, is directed nearly in line
with the beam and has a reasonably flat profile. Red blood cells act
as targets of the ultrasonic beam and backscatter the signal with a
frequency change (Doppler shift) proportional to their velocity
according to the following formula:

$$V = C\Delta f/(2f_o \cos \theta) \tag{1}$$

where: V = actual speed of the target (cm/sec); C = speed of propaga-
tion of ultrasound in the tissue (1540 m/sec); f_o = frequency of
emission (= 2 MHz); $\cos \theta$ = cosine of the angle   between the beam
and the direction of flow; Δf = frequency shift caused by .the
motion of the target and measured by the instrument.
The angle θ between the direction of the beam and that of the flow
must be less than 26 degrees, because when it is within this range
the absolute velocity (V) of mainstream flow can be determined with
$\pm$ 5 % accuracy. Since the factor $C/2 F_o$. $\cos \theta$ is a constant,
the Δf measured by the instrument is proportional to V, that is to
the velocity of red blood cells. It is worth of note that the
difference between the transmitted frequency and the frequency of
the backscattered signal is within the audible range (few KHz) and
can be of help in moving the probe toward the correct direction. The
beam is directed toward the aortic arch by the operator using as
criteria the pitch of the audial signal and the sharpness of outline
of the complexes simultaneously recorded on paper. The recording
represents the online spectral analysis of all the frequency shifts
present in the signal backscattered by the red blood cells at each
instant in time. Because all the constants in the Doppler formula
are known in this application, the outline of the spectrum indicates
the instantaneous velocity of the fastest moving particles of the

aortic flow (which can be refered to as mainstream blood flow velocity). With the TAV prototype instrument[1] the following measures can be derived:

1. Time-averaged (mean) flow velocity (cm/sec): is the total area of the flow complex divided by the duration of the cardiac cycle
2. Index of stroke volume (cm): is the area of the flow complex and corresponds to the column lenght of blood passing the site of measurement.
3. Index of systemic resistances (Units): is obtained by dividing mean blood pressure by mean (time-averaged) blood velocity.

For the calculation of the indices, the coordinates of the corner points of the triangular approximations to the actual velocity complexes, obtained on a digitizing tablet, were fed into a computer Average values over 10 beats were taken for each period (Fig. 1). The use of triangular approximation overestimates the area of the complexes by 10-25 %. However this error should be constant in each patient and thus it should not prevent the evaluation of sequential changes in the same patient, assuming the flow profile does not change.

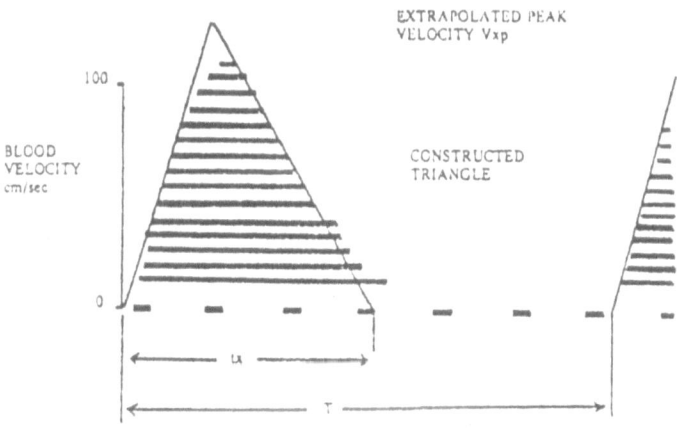

$$AREA = \frac{Vxp}{2} \times Lx$$

$$\text{TIME AVERAGED VELOCITY, } \bar{V} = \frac{A}{T} \text{ cm/sec}$$

Lx = EXTRAPOLATED EJECTION TIME
A = AREA
T = PERIOD OF CARDIAC CYCLE

Fig. 1.

[1] Kindly supplied by Mr. H. Light (Clinical Research Center MRC, Harrow, England) in a scheme of a collaborative study following a European Travelling Fellowship for the CMSI. Presently, produced by Muirhead Ltd., Beckenham, Kent, England.

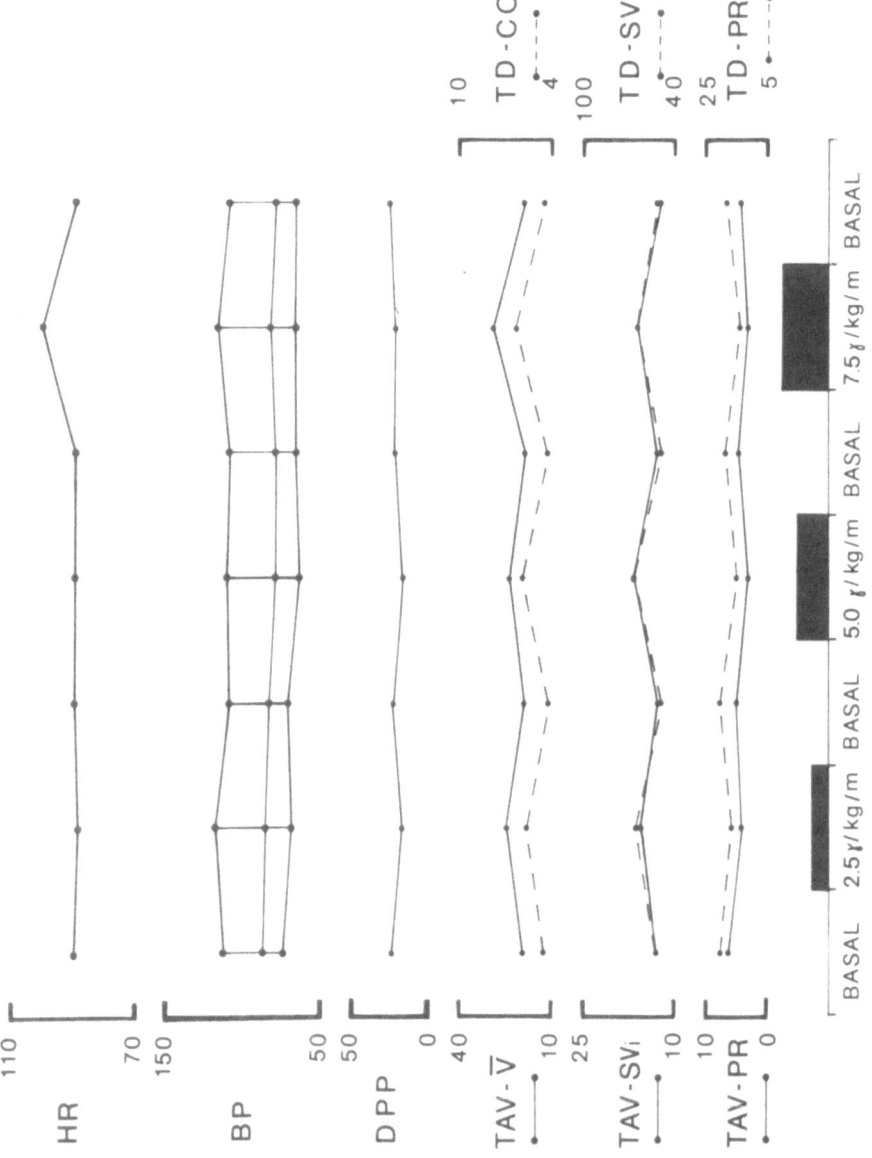

Fig. 2.

Statistical analysis has been performed according to classical methods. Moreover, with the purpose to compare the present results with those previously reported (9-11), we introduced also the measurement of the deviation from exact proportionality (standard deviation as % of the mean). Such a measurement expresses the deviation from strict proportionality of the observations obtained with the two techniques in each patient, and it has the advantage to give equal weight to each observation.

2.4.3. Results

Out of 6 patients who entered the study the TAV recordings were of good quality in 5. As far as the results obtained in these 5 patients the coefficient of variation of TAV mean velocity computed on 10 complexes for stage for all patients ranged from $\pm$ 5 % to $\pm$ 15 % (mean $\pm$ 10 %). For the 5 patients the mean values of TAV mean velocity average of 10 complexes, in each stage are reported in graphic form in Fig. 2.

Dobutamine infusion at the doses of 2.5 and 5.0 Υ/Kg/min caused a consistent increase of cardiac output estimated by thermodilution predominantly due to increase in stroke volume. At the same doses pulmonary diastolic pressure and systemic resistances decrease with increase in pulse aortic pressure. The highest infusion rate (7.5 Υ /Kg/min) caused a marked increase of heart rate which was responsable for the further increase of cardiac output. The changes of TAV mean (time-averaged) velocity and the TAV index of stroke volume reflected the corresponding changes of cardiac output and stroke volume respectively obtained by thermodilution method. Figs. 3-7 show the correlation between thermodilution cardiac output and TAV time-averaged flow velocity in the individual patients. The left size of each figure shows that the correlation coefficient (r) in the different patients varies from 0.872 to 0.964. On the right side of each figure is reported the deviation from exact proportionality (standard deviation as % of the mean) which varies from $\pm$ 5.7 % to $\pm$ 19.9 %. When considered as a group the mean value of deviation from exact proportionality in our patients is $\pm$ 11.8 %.

2.4.4. Discussion

Our study intended to evaluate the possibility of a Doppler non-invasive technique to follow serial changes in cardiac output in the same patient. We decided to study patients with low output state during stepwise increase of Dobutamine infusion, a new inotropic agent capable of increasing cardiac output. As a reference for measuring cardiac output we used thermodilution technique, a stan-

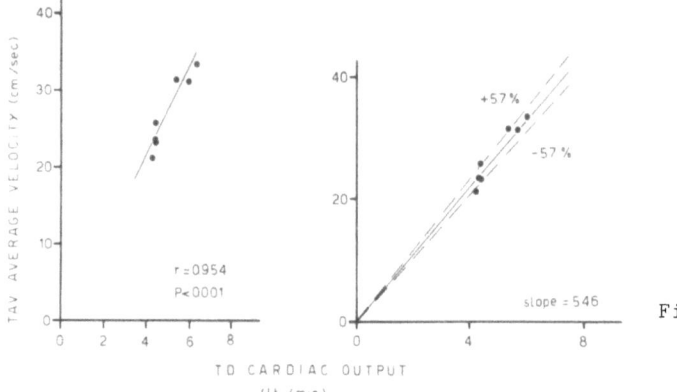

Fig. 3.

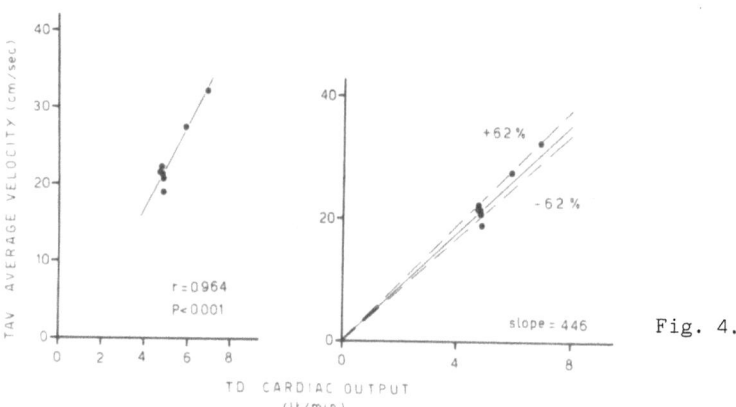

Fig. 4.

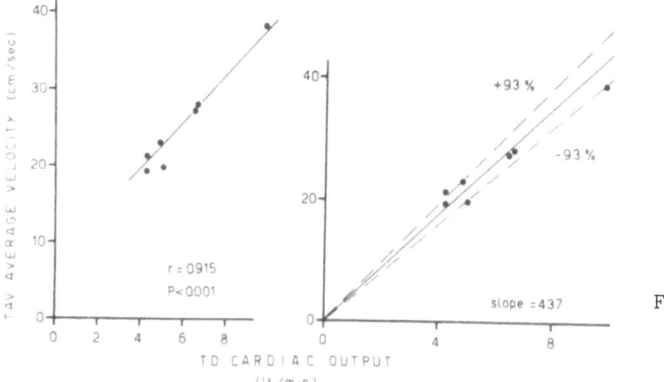

Fig. 5.

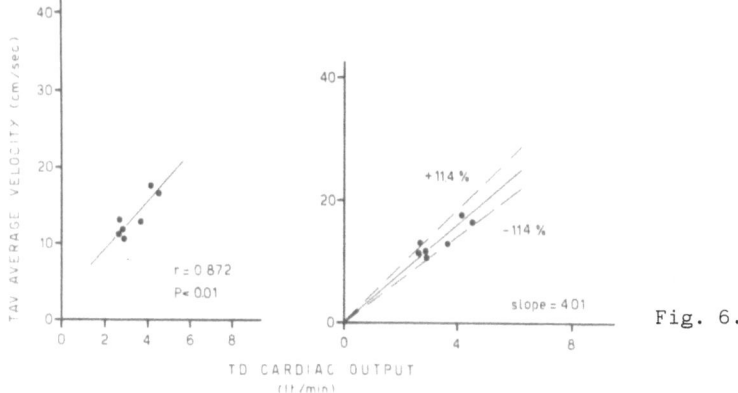

Fig. 6.

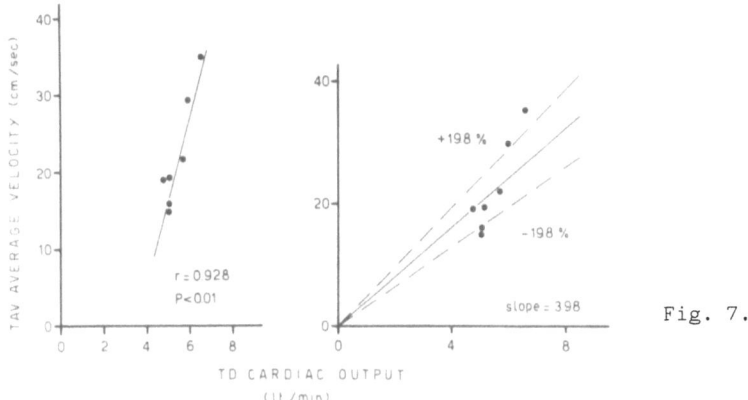

Fig. 7.

dard diffuse method for the measurement of cardiac output. The reference technique (thermodilution versus TAV) was used to verify the reliability of TAV to follow changes of cardiac output and not for comparing absolute values since attempts to derive actual values of cardiac output (lt/min) from measurements of TAV blood flow velocity, using aortic arch dimensions obtained independently by X-ray, did not prove to be accurate enough (9). Although other studies (14) have shown that abnormalities of the wave form of phasic blood flow velocity often convey diagnostic information we did not consider these aspects.

Our results, showing that TAV mean velocity reflects rather accurately serial changes of cardiac output over a considerably wide range of values, demonstrate that Dobutamine infusion at doses of 2.5 and 5.0 γ/Kg/min i.v. has an appearent beneficial effect both in increasing cardiac output and in lowering pulmonary pressures and systemic resistances. The correlation of changes in thermodilution cardiac output with TAV mean (time-averaged) flow velocity appears satisfactory although in some patient (Fig. 7) there is systemic overestimation of TAV values. Our results are in agreement with previous findings which indicated that in any one subject mean TAV velocity changes reflect proportional changes of cardiac output reasonably closely (9-11, 15-16). In those studies the deviation from exact proportionality (standard deviation as % of the mean) of TAV measurements against acetylene uptake, green dye and thermodilution was $\pm$ 11 % $\pm$ 13 % and $\pm$ 8.5 % respectively while in our study it is ranging ranging from $\pm$ 5.7 % to $\pm$ 19.9 % (mean $\pm$ 11.8 %). Our study extends the range of circumstances under which TAV has been shown to give non invasively an useful index of serial changes in cardiac output, in any one patient when applicable.

In conclusion, our preliminary data confirm and extend the results reported by other groups and suggest that TAV monitoring should be a useful non invasive technique for obtaining information on relative changes of cardiac output in coronary and intensive care units. Large scale trials are warranted to confirm the potentialities of this technique.

REFERENCES

1. Branthwaite MA, RD Bradley: Measurement of cardiac output by thermodilution in man. J Appl Physiol 24: 434, 1968.
2. Forrester JS, JA Diamond, HJC Swan: Bedside diagnosis of latent cardiac complications in acutely ill patients. JAMA 222: 59, 1972.
3. Russel RO, CE Rackley (Eds.): Hemodynamic monitoring in a Coronary Intensive Care Unit. Futura Publishing Co. 1974.
4. Ganz W, HJC Swan: Measurement of blood flow by thermodilution. Am J Cardiol 29: 241, 1972.
5. Forrester JS, W Ganz, G Diamond, et al: Thermodilution cardiac output determination with a single flow-directed catheter. Am Heart J 83: 306, 1972.
6. Jenkins BS, RD Bradley, MA Branthwaite: Evaluation of pulmonary arterial end-diastolic pressure as an indirect estimate of left atrial mean pressure. Circulation 42: 75, 1970.
7. Maseri A, A Pesola, C Contini, et al: Hémodinamique pulmonaire et coronarienne dans la phase aigue de l'infarctus du myocarde. Arch Mal Coeur 66: 401, 1973.
8. Light LH, G Cross: Cardiovascular data by transcutaneous aortovelography. In Blood flow measurements. Roberts C Ed, p 60, Sector Publishing, London, 1972.
9. Sequeira RC, LH Light, G Cross, et al: Transcutaneous aortovelography - a quantitative evaluation. Br Heart J 38: 443, 1976.
10. Bilton AH, J Brotherhood, G Cross, et al: Transcutaneous aortove-

lography as a measure of central blood flow. J Physiol 281: 4P, 1978.

11. Light LH: Transcutaneous aortovelography. A new window on the circulation? Br Heart J 38: 433, 1976.

12. Fraser CB, LH Light, EA Shinebourne, et al: Transcutaneous aortovelography reproducibility in adults and children. Eur J Cardiol 4: 181, 1976.

13. Sonnenblick EH, WH Frishman, TH LeJantel: Dobutamine: A New Synthetic Cardioactive Sympathetic Amine. N Engl J Med 300: 17, 1978.

14. Light LH: Aortic blood velocity measurement by transcutaneous aortovelography and its clinical applications. In Echocardiology N Bom Ed, p 233, Martinus Nijhoff Medical Division, The Hague, 1977.

15. Buchtal A, GC Hanson, AR Peisach: Transcutaneous aortovelography technique in management of critically ill patients. Br Heart J 38: 451, 1976.

16. Bilton AH, GC Hanson: Aortic velocity measurement in the care of the critically ill. In Doppler Ultrasound in the study of the central and peripheral circulation, Woodcock and Sequeira Eds, p 39, Bristol University Printing Unit, Bristol, 1978.

DISCUSSION: CHAPTER 2

Chairman: P.G. Hugenholtz

DISCUSSION CHAPTER 2

Paper 1: AMI and two dimensional echocardiography

HUGENHOLTZ: Our populations in the coronary care units are changing. That is to say, as we come to grips with the problems in the community it depends on the country in the European Community how the response is going to be. Some will like in Belfast, go on with the mobile coronary care units and are able, given that situation, to get at the patient very early. Other countries may not get there with their mobile systems early or may not even choose to go with the mobile systems and simply say we must bring the alertness of the community up. People who have once had warning signs or have had an infarct become self-referred, enter into the system quicker or even people may come when they think they have symptoms. We have started such a self-referral system and it turned out to be very little abused and very well used and there is a different type of arrhythmias you see in that type of patient: it is not the same patient that comes into the ambulance. And now we come to this graded approach that we talked about. I think we should continue in certain centers to spend money, on further acquiring knowledge because I think technology is still improving in terms of cost, in terms of efficacy, in terms of usefulness. We are going to get smaller and smaller units and as we pick out the proper jobs for the proper machine I don't think costs will ultimately be such a factor anymore.
MASERI: Talking about the perspectives, I would anticipate for the next few years the need to get understanding on the appropriate signals to be picked up by specialized microcomputers and microprocessors. Only when it will be proven that indeed the adequate detection of these signals allows the prevention of fibrillation and of dangerous arrhythmias, we should hand it over to the engineers to reduce the cost and then distribute adequate apparatus for routine use.
PANTRIDGE: I have a very simple question. You have said in conclusion there was no evolution after 24 hours. But as I understood it from the previous data, there is no evolution after 4 hours. Is that so? There is no change after 4 hours?
PRASQUIER: Well, I have no echos in the first 4 hours.
CAMERINI: If you study post mortem cases with inferior myocardial infarction, you usually find an involvement of the right ventricle in about 10 % of the cases. This is not an academic curiosity because some of these patients have a very peculiar hemodynamic pattern with a right atrial pressure higher than the left. These patients need a peculiar type of treatment. What is the pattern of

the right ventricle in cases with inferior myocardial infarction and possible involvement of the right ventricle? And, second question please, what about the assessment of ventricular function and of cardiac output. Is there any help from bidimensional echocardiography in this sense?

PRASQUIER: We observed only one of these patients with a typical pattern of right ventricular involvement. As to the second question, we hope that this technique should help us in this setting. We did study of left ventricular volumes and left ventricular cardiac output and ejection fraction in patients who were not coronary patients. We did find a reasonable correlation with angiography with an underestimation of the volumes by two-dimensional echocardiography of about one-fourth; this is understandable because in what we call the apical studies, actually we are not sure that we get the long axis. We underestimate this long axis.

HUGENHOLTZ: Even if you didn't have the correlation quantitatively because we are measuring different things, on can state, I think, that the echo permits you some measure of whether the heart behaves properly or improperly. And I think in the sense of monitoring, that is what the question is aimed at.

Paper 2: Assessment of myocardial infarction by echocardiography: post-mortem correlations.

HUGENHOLTZ: Well, you have two convincing bits of evidence on the table that the echo also can contribute to the assessment of myocardial function, and of the anatomical relationships. However, I am sure it brings out a lot of questioning about the transportability of this type of data from one laboratory to the other. It requires training, experience and an awfully good knowledge of patho-physiology. It isn't a matter of plugging down some electrode and getting a signal, and putting it somewhere. It is knowing where, knowing how. It is knowing the instrument and it clearly requires more from the doctor than any another technique does.

ROCCI: I would like to ask which is the place of traditional time motion in the coronary care unit? Our recent experience is favorable with this kind of method because we could find that with mitral valve stroke volume, we could define a high risk subgroup of patients with myocardial infarction.

PRASQUIER: We do not have as much experience with the M mode as Dr. Hejkkilä has and in our experience we weren't as successful as he was in the detection of left ventricular segmental disfunction. I think that with more experience in this very specific setting, one can get a lot more information. I don't have any experience with quantified indexes. The problem of quantified indexes is one of the major problems that we are also facing with two-dimensional echocardiography. We are still a little bit reluctant to give quantified indexes, for two major reasons. First, we feel that the resolutions of our equipment does not reach the resolution of the usual M mode equipment. This apparatus has a resolution of about 4 mm at the focal zone which means that you do not know exactly what is going on when you go much further than the focal zone. And this is one of the major problems - when you see the endocardium you don't know whether it's really endocardium or not. This is the first point. Second with this technique, we have a tomographic pictures: if you get a little bit on the side of a diseased region you can miss things. I think we need some kind of computerized device that would give us the precise position of our probe, and that could compute from the position of the probe some reconstruction of the left ventricle.

HUGENHOLTZ: I think you are quite correct in pointing out the restrictions. I think the technical restrictions, the varying specifications of our specific characteristics of each of the pieces of equipment, what nobody has mentioned yet, the fact that there are some patients who have no acoustical window. All of these, of course, will, in the practical terms, ultimately limit the value of this technique like any other, but we are only at the beginning of this. It's as if people were scared to touch the field of coronary artery disease with the echo. I think most people here would still have to get their feet wet. And whether or not ultimately we're getting there will depend on the usual things in medicine - diligence, perseverance, insistance, better equipment, cheaper tools, and a good model. And therefore your point that what we are looking at is really tomograms, to me is a very important model. I would like to have a tomographic section of that infarcted or not working heart.

HEJKKILÄ: Just because we are discussing echo in CCU, I want to tell about my experiences. Many times you must face acute cardiac surgery due to shock or some catastrophic hemodynamic situation: we have found echo extremely useful in screening if we should proceed to angio: if you find hypokinetic motion throughout, it's better not to proceed.

HUGENHOLTZ: Well, I am sure that's a very valid point. Perhaps, you also formulate what might well be an activity of those laboratories who get involved in the echo technique in the CCU in terms of developing something that has a prognostic value. It would be awfully nice if one could develop a form that we could hand out to those who work with it to be filled out at that very time that you make the observation or have the record at hand in order to really be used later in your interpretation of the prognostic value, because in your hands I am quite sure you know pretty well what you are going to get because you have looked so often at it. But for all the others to get convinced that the echo has prognostic information, we must make a very accurate record at that time and not later. Because then of course it is not really true prognosis anymore!

JULIAN: I am still not quite sure how you differentiate a dyskinetic change in contraction of the ventricle from infarcted behaviour. Can I ask a second question? There's a situation I would most like to have an echo in, is in a patient with electro-mechanical dissociation. This is an emergency decision, and maybe your machine is ideal for this situation. Has that in fact proved to be the case? I have a third question before I get this done. Your machine, you say, is going to get cheaper. Do we delay buying it until it's cheaper?

HUGENHOLTZ: Well, it's sort of like taking your first bath in spring. Those who delay that never end up taking a bath at all. So get your feet wet is my advice today, at current prices. I think echo will be a crucial element in the chain of steps of diagnostic information short of going to cath lab.

HEJKKILÄ: We can see with echo very well scar tissue from fresh myocardium, healthy myocardium and also fresh necrosis. Acute ischemia is manifesting itself with lack of motion. So we can't say if this is acute necrosis, at least today. But we can follow this border zone during drug studies.

PESOLA: Dr. Hejkkilä, how can you be sure that your transducers are always in the same point, with the same angulation? In different moments, using different drugs?

HEJKKILÄ: You can't make much error because we start from a basic axis where both mitral leaflets are seen. Thereafter you refer to other myocardial landmarks and we mark the transducer positions for sequential tracts.

Paper 3: Preliminary evaluation of transcutaneous aortovelography for monitoring changes in cardiac output.

BALCON: Can you tell me if the apparatus is now sensitive to the difference between forward and backward flow?

DISTANTE: This technique is able to sense both types of flow; forward flow is represented on paper above the zero line, while backward (receding) flow is below that line.

HUTTON: I'd be interested for you to repeat that experiment using a vasodilator or something that is unloading the ventricle, which has no inotropic effect and then see if you are still getting the same correlation with cardiac output.

DISTANTE: In other terms your question is how much this measurements are influenced by changing peripheral resistance. We do not have definite answer yet, but some preliminary results of ours obtained with prostacyclin infused in healthy volunteers show that time-averaged flow velocity and thermodilution cardiac output do correlate also when there is a marked reduction of peripheral vascular resistances.

HUGENHOLTZ: The point is well taken. Once you fiddle around with peripheral resistance and distribution of that flow and then see whether it holds up, you have a stronger feeling whether you should go on. So, in the next step in your study, that's a very good bit of advice to follow.

PRASQUIER: Does the aortic anatomy change the sensitivity of your method? When the flow gets rather perpendicular to the transducer, you may have troubles.

DISTANTE: The anatomy of the aorta in the last part of the arch, let's say the beginning of the descending part, is pretty constant, but if we have any kind of distortion of aorta due to mediastinal masses, we may be in trouble. If the beam is not in line with the blood stream, the signal is very poor and you can easily say, 'I cannot perform the test', which has been our case, for example, in a couple of patients with chronic obstructed pulmonary disease. As far as the direction of the beam, if you stay within plus-minus 25 degrees of the aorta axis you could stay easily within plus-minus 5% error of measurement.

MASERI: Professor Hugenholtz, I would like to ask you to summarize the second part of this afternoon. How do you see these applications that have been discussed? Are these techniques a reasonable field of common action in the Community?

HUGENHOLTZ: As I will say tomorrow morning, the attention in the coronary care unit, is shifting away from the management of the arrhythmias to the management of the acutely hemodynamic disturbed patient. I think we are seeing more and more early patients where hemodynamic state is severely disturbed, where patients who other-wise would have died in a community from their arrhythmia are temporarily kept alive by the Pantridge type of approach. You get there for patients who often are hemodynamically in instable states and I see a great future for non invasive monitoring of the status of the myocardium. I think Hejkkilä gave a good example of the decision making prior to acute surgery. I think this will be coming increasingly towards this. And so all efforts or all research that is continued to be put in that direction should be rewarding in either of two ways. Either it will tell us that 'sorry the signal is just not good enough. The method is just not suitable for this purpose', and then at least we have that answer because currently we cannot say that. Or we say the opposite 'yes, in this and this situation that and that tool does exactly what you'd hope it would do'. And in order to get to that point we need further research. There is no two ways about it.

MASERI: For the records, if I understood correctly, you believe that this has to be carried on in a number of research places, before it gets spread out.

HUGENHOLTZ: Yes, I would strongly urge that for the simple reason that one of the disappointments in my life has been the extent we doctors seem to mix up research with clinical practice. None of the

things that were discussed today, neither the echo nor the aortovelography is there; but this type of non invasive techniques should
come and I think we should work at it. And I think you should
perhaps at some later time formulate some things where one could
collaborate in. As far as that's concerned, let me end with one
final point of view. People often talk that cooperative things
should be along the same protocols, that the statisticians tell us
that this is important. I think you can find easily cooperation
among one another by at least telling each other what you're doing,
and perhaps making something of a coarse puzzle where the pieces
might somehow fit together. That is still some form of cooperation,
and it is often with these various countries that we have in Europe,
more practical to do that than to try to develop a common protocol.
That is not to say that, for example, if we are to use the echo in a
futuristic sense by M mode, which is by now ubiquitous, that a
common protocol in terms of recording plus the way you would put the
record on the table would not be useful either.

CHAPTER 3

HEMODYNAMIC MONITORING IN CORONARY CARE UNITS

3.1. WHY CORONARY CARE UNITS ARE BENEFICIAL AND COST-EFFECTIVE WHEN
THEY ARE USED WISELY

P.G. Hugenholtz

When in 1963 Day launched his concept (1) for intensive coronary
care, he probably was unaware that this was the only moment at which
a prospective comparative trial with random allocation to the 'new'
treatment and the 'old' could have been carried out with full
justification. It is sad that no one designed such a trial, but not
surprising, given the similar history of other medical innovations.
Yet the results of such a study might have prevented the current
unrest about the usefulness of the coronary care unit (CCU).

Where does this unrest originate? There are two sources, we believe,
which are often intermixed, but equally important. The first states
that CCU's despite their possible usefulness have not and cannot
really reduce the excessive mortality (including sudden death) in
the community. The second feels, and often justifiably so, that the
costly CCU is not appropriately used for those patients for whom it
was meant. Both sources agree that the CCU requires a disproportiona-
te amount of the health resources. So it is highly appropriate that
this WHO meeting is convened to assess current evidence in favour,
or against, the use of specialized coronary care units in hospitals.
In particular the recent publication by Hill of the Nottingham study
(2a) following earlier reports from Mather et al. (3) in Bristol,
both originating from the British Health Care system, has left the
impression that home care would be as effective as specialized
treatment in the by now virtually ubiquitous coronary care units in
the industrialized countries. But, are we really on the wrong track?
Not so, if one believes the ongoing discussion (2b-f) in recent
journals.

   In reading the extensive literature on the subject, there are
clearly two lines of evidence.

The first has proved impressive data of the benefits of specialized
coronary care units in terms of reduction in hospital mortality:
Lown (4), O'Rourke (5), Lie (6), Koch-Weser (7), Brown and MacMillan
in their textbook on coronary care (8), MacClean and co-workers (9)
and the Joint Working Party of the Royal College of Physicians of
London in 1975 (10), all have clearly indicated that in the period
from 1963 to 1976 a marked reduction of in hospital mortality of
myocardial infarction has been achieved compared to the previously
existing ward treatment. Our own data (Table 1A,B, Fig. 1) are in
keeping with these results. Although as A.B. Hill states in his book
Statistical Methods in Clinical and Preventive Medicine 'It is

TABLE 1A

ADMISSION FOR ACUTE CORONARY DISEASE

	TOTAL ADMISSIONS	CLASS I, II, III	%
1973	224	180	80
1974	660	493	75
1975	784	552	70
1976	907	710	78
1977	1000	740	74

Class   I   Definite acute myocardial infarction
         II Impending myocardial infarction
       III Primary cardiac arrhythmia

TABLE 1B

DEATHRATES FOR ACUTE CORONARY DISEASE

	ADMISSION CLASS I, II, III	DEATHS	%
1973	180	7	3,9
1974	493	21	4,3
1975	552	31	5,6
1976	710	42	5,9
1977	740	48	6,5

Class   I   Definite acute myocardial infarction
         II Impending myocardial infarction
       III Primary cardiac arrhythmia

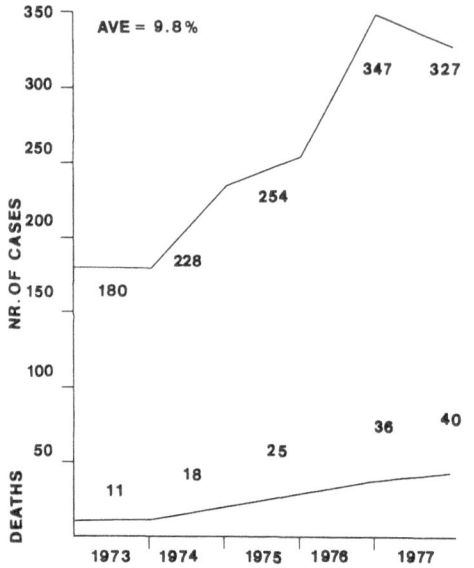

Fig. 1. Deathrates for acute myocardial infarction at the Thoraxcentre, Rotterdam.

rarely that one can feel wholly sure that these past observations do relate to a precisely similar group of patients. This is a most difficult thing to prove ..., yet it is the sine qua non if the comparison is to have any validity'., the time to carry out a randomized trial to deliver final proof is past. The other school of thought has raised the question of cost-effectiveness of such units. In particular Bloom and Peterson (11), as well as Sanders (12) have provided thoughtful insights. Still others have pointed out the psychological hazards of coronary (s) care (13) and the transport (14) phase. It is not surprising therefore that health authorities such as the WHO, currently request further evidence of coronary care efficacy and efficiency before acquiescing to demands for continued installation of such units throughout the hospitals of the world.

In a recent editorial (15) it is argued that the benefits of specialized coronary care in terms of the timely treatment of lifethreatening arrhythmias, are unquestionable. In fact, death from rhythm disturbances, primarily ventricular fibrillation, has become a rarity in the properly managed coronary care units. But the fight against death from second major complication of myocardial infarction, pump failure, has just begun (Fig. 2).

Current evidence suggests, but is not conclusive, that in cases with disturbances in hemodynamic function, adequate monitoring of pressures in the right and left side of the heart, early drug therapy, the support of respiratory function and the timely application of the intraaortic balloon pump, can lead to a further reduction of in hospital mortality. Particularly in certain, timely selected, patients the benefits are impressive (16). For this the continuous

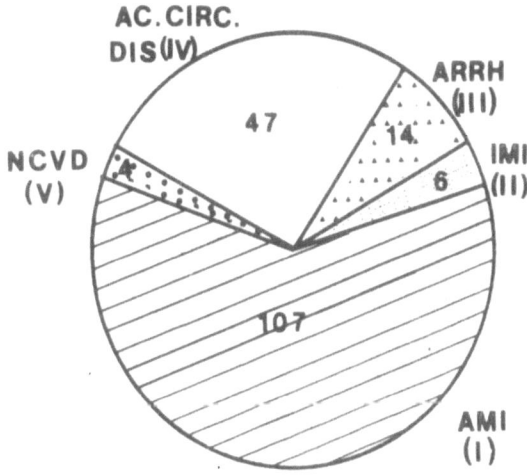

Fig. 2. Deaths as function of diagnosis of 3575 patients admitted to the CCU (class I to V) from 1973 to 1977; the average deathrate was 5 %.

assessment of the state of left ventricular function is mandatory. Radio nuclear methods (17) echo imaging of the left ventricle (18), and still other techniques currently in the research phase (19), may determine the localization and extent of infarction and permit us to follow the response to treatment.

Parallel to these developments the earlier surgical intervention in appropriate circumstances, will play an increasing role (20). Evidence has accrued that the progression in the impending infarction syndrome can be timely interrupted either through medical treatment with Beta-blockade or by pharmacological ventricular unloading with nitrites, aortic ballon pumping with or without additional surgery. What is even more exciting, recent data make it possible that appropriate and timely use of the intraaortic balloon pump and/or certain drugs will modify the course of early stages of cardiac infarction and reduce infarct size.

A major American trial is currently underway to elucidate the role of hyaluronidase and Beta-blockade (Braunwald, personal communication).

If these advances are of proven, or likely benefit to extend the life expectancy of the patients with acute cardiac events, what then is the real basis for worry?

It is most of all the evidence that these expensively equipped beds (which require a high nurse to bed ratio between 1-3 to 1-1) with their attendant high exploitation costs, are not always occupied by the patients for whom they are meant. Indeed, the nucleus of this problem lies in the fact that with the current emphasis on earlier

detection and treatment of acute coronary events within the community, patients are being referred to the CCU at a stage when the
existence of myocardial infarction is not yet proven, in fact only
suspected. Enhanced by increasing efforts at early cardiac resuscitation in the community, this development brings with it the nearly
unavoidable dilution of patient material offered for admission. It
is also evident from the literature, that the percentage of patients
ultimately discharged from the CCU with a proven myocardial infarction has gradually decreased (Table 1a). Lown indicates 70% in his
study in 1967 (4), Bloom and Peterson indicate 50% in 1973 (11) and
in our personal experience it was only 32% in 1975 (15) (Table 2).
That is not to say that another 47% with incompletely diagnosed
forms of cardiovascular dysfunction were not in equal need of
intensive care monitoring but the difficulty lies in exact definition of the actual state of risk to the individual when the
physician refers him for admission to the unit.

As long as he, in the community, cannot be certain of the prognosis
of the individual case which he is called to see, he will refer all
individuals, which he considers at risk, to the hospital. The
Nottingham study (2) has not provided us with a solution to that
dilemma. However attractive a scheme, who in the current setting,
can marshall a team which sits with the patients for 2 hours before
deciding whether to transport him or not? It is also noted that the
Nottingham study cannot be accepted as sufficient proof that patients can safely be selected for continuation of home treatment after 2
hours of coronary care at home. For the finding that the difference
in mortality between home and hospital care is statistically not
significant does not imply that both types of care are in fact
equivalent. It would take a much larger number of patients to
provide sufficient proof of equivalence. Evidence that one cannot
expect proper patient selections by the unassisted general practitioner can also be derived from the IMIR study (21) in Rotterdam
carried out in 1973-1975. Of 1343 patients (from over 25000 patients
in their practices) seen by 14 general practitioners for 'new or
worsening symptoms of possible cardiac origin' within 1 year 93
proved to have an acute myocardial infarction upon admission to the
study. Of these, less than half, 41 were recognized at that time by
the general practitioner as having, in fact, an infarct. On the
other hand among 1213 patients with the same signs in whom no
evidence of an MI could be found, 40 were diagnosed by the G.P. as
having an acute myocardial infarction. So, the accuracy of the
G.P.'s diagnosis is limited, when he is not assisted by laboratory
diagnostic aids (such as enzyme determinations and ECG), which
usually are found only in hospitals.

How then to combat the inappropriate use of expensive facilities?
How to define who can stay at home and who not? First of all, from
the excellent review of Bloom and Peterson (11), which may well be

TABLE 2

Comparison population pre-ccu 1976 with that of ccu 1975 and 1976, all from April through September.

Diagnosis at discharge	ccu 1975		ccu 1976		pre-ccu 1976		ccu+pre-ccu 1976	
	N	%	N	%	N	%	N	%
Myocardial infarction	127	31.6	197	44.6	17(13)	9.8	201	33.4
other cardio-vascular dis.	118	46.8	211	47.7	65(2)	36.7	274	45.6
non cardio-vascular dis.	87	21.6	34	7.7	92(0)	53.5	126	21.0
Total	402	100	442	100	174(15)	100	601	100
Case fatality*	18	4.5	25	5.7	0	0	25	4.2

ccu = coronary care unit; pre-ccu = pre-coronary care unit ( ) = of whom consequently were admitted to the ccu * case fatality in non-cardiovascular disease group: 1975: 0, 1976: 1.

the only critical study to analyse the cost-effectiveness of such units, one conclusion: 'Larger units, in teaching hospitals with full-time directors, showed lower mean case fatality rates from myocardial infarction, higher percentages of patients with infarction and greater productivity and efficiency. These important differences were often not statistically significant because of the great variation within hospital groups'. Yet, 'Intensive care for patients after myocardial infarction should be planned by region, not by individual hospitals, to assure effectiveness and economy. Intensive care of such patients presents an ideal model for regional planning'. So it is from the larger units (1-10) with regional activities that we must derive our information.

Let us look therefore at the data reported by Christiansen in Copenhagen (22) and by Hofvendahl in Stockholm (23). In a setting not much different from that in Bristol (3) or Nottingham (2), they come to different comclusions. Not only could Hofvendahl prove that the intensive care mortality was drastically reduced compared to the ward mortality when patients were allocated alternately, but Christiansen also proved that this gain could be maintained over the next five years of follow up of his patients. Their conclusion that the gain in reduced mortality is subsequently maintained also follows from the data collected from our unit. All these studies indicate that, while home treatment has a place, the decision making process, as to whether to hospitalize a patient suspected of having an acute coronary event or not, will vary widely between cities, regions and countries and therefore solutions will have to vary accordingly.

Now let us return to the matter of reduction of mortality in the community as a whole: It has been suggested that community mortality due to coronary events can be reduced by timely treatment of those individuals, who are recognized to be at increased immediate risk on the basis of prodromal symptoms. It was the primary objective of the IMIR study to elucidate this concept. It was shown that 19 of 62 sudden deaths, which occurred in the participating general practices, were preceded by prodromal symptoms, but these symptoms proved to be highly variable and unspecific. Their recognition could not form a basis for hospitalization in time to combat their ultimate outcome. In the same period there were 43 sudden deaths without any prodromata.

The conclusion presents itself that the total death rate is not likely to be reduced much by early detection and follow-up of suspected individuals, at least in the Rotterdam community setting. Nor is it likely that with a well organized ambulance service (in Rotterdam the median transit time home to hospital is 8 minutes) the death rate during the transport phase can be reduced much (there were 20 deaths after arrival of the ambulance team for 2907 transports and most of these were moribund as the transport began) (24).

TABLE 3

Complications within 3 weeks after leaving pre-coronary care unit for home

patient nr	sex and age M	W	hours in pre-ccu	diagnosis at discharge	days after discharge	complication
16	36		72	no abnormality found	10	sudden death
48	75		24	ischemic heart disease old M.I.	7	died after re-admission with pulmonary embolism and shock
68	60		72	upperabdominal symptoms permanent pacemaker old MI	7	died 2 days after re-admission with acute M.I. in cardiogenic shock
79		81	48	ischemic heart disease	?	MI (ECG changes) recovered at home
116	76		24	ischemic heart diseade emphisema	19	MI, recovered in hospital
176	43		16	hypertension hyperventilation	± 12	MI (ECG changes) recovered at home

MI = myocardial infarction

Rather the high death rate, indeed mostly at home, requires a different approach through a combination of effective secondary prevention by Beta-blockade such as shown in Göteborg (25), by anti-platelet aggregation drugs such as reported from Canada (26) and by a community wide cardiopulmonary resuscitation effort by laymen and family, the efficacy of which was demonstrated by Cobb in Seattle (27). As a consequence of all the above considerations we agree with Bloom and Peterson (11) when they state: 'Since it will be a long time before the question of effectiveness of coronary care units is settled, the best that can be done is to suggest second best solutions ... It is clear from recent history that if decisions about provision of coronary care units are left to individual hospitals, excess capacity and inefficiency will result. These decisions must be made by bodies that are more disinterested and have a broader view than that of the single institution'. Perhaps the WHO and this group of eminent scientists is such a body. Anyhow, particularly encouraged by the report by O'Rourke (5), in 1976 which showed that the 'new generation coronary care unit' should exist of a chain of facilities ranging from a well-run referral and transport service, via an adequately staffed and efficiently run intensive care unit to an associated intermediary care area for follow-up in the week following the intensive care period we have carried out a study into the efficacy of such a system to which was added a triage area consisting of a four bed pre-coronary care unit (28). In this triage area all patients which were admitted through the general practitioner for a suspected acute cardiac event were assigned to either: A = home care, B = CCU and C = pre-CCU. The 4 pre-CCU beds were operated during a test period in 1976 in conjunction with the 8 bed coronary care unit. The only extra equipment consisted of a single channel monitor for the continuous ECG and a defibrillator. There was 1 nurse for 4 beds. She was conversant with all resuscitation techniques. It could be shown that of 174 admissions to the pre-coronary care unit the hospitalization period was an average of 25 ½ hours only with a case fatality of 0% (Table 2). Two-thirds of these patients could be discharged within 24 hours, and most of them (78 %) went home. Eight percent required subsequent admission to the coronary care unit and could be proven to have serious acute coronary heart disease. The remaining 14 % were transferred to other divisions of the hospital since their cardiac symptoms were due to other disorders. Of the patients discharged directly home from the pre-coronary care unit, there were 5 deaths in the subsequent follow-up period. Detailed analysis (Table 3) indicated that the deaths were unavoidable, even if they had been kept in hospital. It was also found that during the same period the percentage of patients admitted to the CCU, with proven acute myocardial infarction at discharge, increased significantly (Table 1). Since most of the other patients in the CCU had either serious arrhythmias or

cardiac decompensation, their stay at the CCU was indicated equally.
It was our conclusion that the addition of a pre-coronary care area
of 4 beds to an 8 bed CCU increased the efficacy of the CCU.
These findings also provide a reasonable solution to the dilemma
which we have earlier posed. Given the fact that the recognition of
the seriousness of the coronary artery problem in the population
will mount and that there will be an increase in self-referred
individuals throughout the industrialized world in the next decade,
the development of such an integral concept must be encouraged if
the high case fatality in the community is to be effectively
reduced. Of this 'new generation coronary care unit' the creation of
a pre-coronary care area in connection with the existing coronary
care units with adequate subsequent follow-up in intermediary care
areas (28), provides the essential new ingredient. Surely such
integral units must be developed from existing facilities by improved management and by reorganization of smaller units in order to
achieve optimal utilization of the scarce health resources.
It is our firm belief that coronary care units are here to stay,
that they have proven their efficacy, as best as could be done after
1963 and that they do not have to be an unnecessary burden for the
health care system.
Furthermore there is still much to be learned about the genesis of
myocardial infarction (29).
A rationally designed integrated system between community and hospital will prove even the most critical health administrator with a
very high benefit to cost ratio. We also believe, with other authors
(30-37) that this reorganization is up to the medical profession. It
is they who must put their own house in order, so that the available
funds are optimally utilized for those patients who urgently need
them today as well as tomorrow.

REFERENCES

1. Day HW: An intensive coronary care area. Dis Chest 44: 423, 1963.
1b. Julian DG: Treatment of cardiac arrest in acute myocardial
    ischaemia and infarction. Lancet, October: 840, 1961.
2a. Hill JD, JR Hampton, JRA Mitchell: A randomized trial of home
    versus-hospital management for patients with suspected myocar-
    dial infarction. Lancet, April: 838, 1978.
2b. Letters to the Editor. Lancet, May: 1089, 1978.
2c. Letters to the Editor. Lancet, May: 1145, 1978.
2d. Letters to the Editor. Lancet, June: 1307, 1978.
2e. Letters to the Editor. Lancet, May: 1090, 1978.
2f. Medical controversies. Home or hospital care for coronary throm-
    bosis? Brit Med J 1: 1254, 1978.
2g. Annotations. Am Heart J 95 (4): 536, 1978.

3. Mather HG, NG Pearson, KLQ Read, et al: Acute myocardial infarction: Home and Hospital Treatment. Brit Med J 3: 334, 1971.

4. Lown B, AM Fakhro, WB Jr Hood, et al: Unresolved problems in coronary care. Am J Cardiol 20: 457, 1967.

5. O'Rourke MF, B Walsh, M Fletcher, et al: Impact of new generation coronary care unit. Brit Med J 837, 1976.

6. Lie KI, D Durrer: Moderne hartbewaking, een kostenbewuste benadering. Ned T Geneesk 120: 608, 1976.

7. Koch-Weser J: N Engl J Med 285: 1024, 1971.

8. Brown KWG, RL MacMillan, N Forbath, et al: An intensive care centre for acute myocardial infarction. Lancet 2: 349, 1963.

9. McLean KH, C Penington, JG Sloman. Med J Austr 1: 753, 1973.

10. Oliver MF: Report Joint Working Party. Journal Royal College of Physicians of London, 10: 5, 1975.

11. Bloom BS, OL Peterson: End results, cost and productivity of coronary care units. N Engl J Med 288: 72, 1973.

12. Sanders CA. N Engl J Med 288: 101, 1973.

13. Hackett TP, NH Cassem, HA Wishnie: The coronary care unit. An appraisal of its psychological hazards. N Engl J Med 279: 1365, 1972.

14. Hart HN: Hartbewaking in de prehospitale fase. Hart Bull 5: 127, 1978.

15. Hugenholtz PG, K Laird - Meeter, K Balakumaran, et al: Intensive Care. on AMI. Editorial: Reflections on Current Coronary Care. Intens Care Med 4: 1, 1978.

16. Hagemeijer F, JD Laird, MMP Haalebos, et al: Effectiveness of intraaortic balloon pumping without cardiac surgery for patients with severe hearth failure secondary to a recent myocardial infarction. Am J Cardiol 40: 951, 1977.

17. Wackers FJ Th, E Sokole - Busemann, G Samson, et al: Myocardscintigrafie bij patienten met acute en chronische coronaire insufficientie. Ned T Geneesk 120: 2151, 1976.

18. Heikkilä J, M Nieminen: Echoventriculographic detection, localization, and quantification of left ventricular asynergy in acute myocardial infarction. A correlative echo and electrocardiographic study. Br Heart J 37: 46, 1975.

19. Zeelenberg C, LS Deutsch, WAH Engelse, et al: Experiences with implementing argus in a cardiac surveillance unit. In: Trends in computer-processed electrocardiograms; p 31, Amsterdam: North-Holland, 1977.

20. Langou RA, AS Geha, GL Hammond, et al: Surgical approach for patients with unstable angina pectoris: Role of the response to initial medical therapy and intraaortic balloon pumping in perioperative complications after aortocoronary bypass grafting. Am. J Cardiol 42: 629, 1978.

21. Lubsen J, J Pool, E Does: Acute coronary events in general practice. Acute risk of myocardial infarction of sudden death in

a symptomatic patient. Hart Bull 7: 114, 1976.

22. Christiansen I, K Iversen, AP Skouby: Benefits obtained by the introduction of a coronary care unit. A comparative study. Acta Med Scand 189: 285, 1971.

22a. Christiansen I: Longterm prognosis after myocardial infarction. A comparative study. Abs, 7th Europ Congress Cardiol, p 55, 1976.

23. Hofvendahl S: Influence of treatment in a coronary care unit on prognosis in acute myocardial infarction: a controlled study in 271 cases. Acta Med Scand 519 (Suppl.): 9, 1971.

24. Hart HN: Hartbewaking in de pre-hospitale fase. Proefschrift, Rotterdam, 1978.

25. The anturane reinfarction trial research group: Sulfinpyrazone in the prevention of cardiac death after myocardial infarction. N Engl J Med 298: 289, 1978.

26. Wilhelmsson C, L Wilhelmsen, JA Vedin, et al: Reduction of sudden death after myocardial infarction by treatment with aprenol ranged 2. Lancet 1157, 1974.

27. Cobb LA, RS Baum, H Alvarez III, et al: Resuscitation from out-of-hospital ventricular fibrillation: 4 years follow- up. Circulation 51/52 (Suppl III): 223, 1975.

28. Laird - Meeter K, K Balakumaran, PG Hugenholtz: Ervaringen met een pre-coronary care unit. Hart Bull. 3: 76, 1977.

29. Baroldi G: Coronary stenosis: Ischemic or non - ischemic factor? Editorial Am Heart J 96: 139, 1978.

30. Oliver MF, DG Julian: Manual on intensive coronary care. World Health Organization, Copenhagen, 1970.

31. Gorfinkel HJ: Progressive coronary care. Luxury or necessity? Editorial, Arch Intern Med 138: 193, 1978.

32. Moss AJ, J De Camilla, H Davis, et al: The early post-hospital phase of myocardial infarction. Prognostic stratification. Circulation 54: 58, 1976.

33. Lie KI, YC Roels-van IJsseldijk, FJL van Capelle: Factoren die de prognose van het acute hartinfarct beinvloeden. Ned T Geneesk 119: 466, 1975.

34. Lindholm J, N Fabricius-Bjerre, K Astvad, et al: Coronary care units. Am Heart J 91: 673, 1976.

35. Rose G: The contribution of intensive coronary care. Br J Prev Soc Med 29: 147, 1975.

36. Moss AJ, S Goldstein: The pre-hospital phase of acute myocardial infarction. Circulation 41: 737, 1970.

37. Moss AJ, B Wynar, S Goldstein: Delay in hospitalization during the acute coronary period. Am J Cardiol 24: 659, 1969.

38. Oliver MF: The place of the coronary care unit. J Roy Coll Phycns Lond 3: 47, 1968.

39. Astvad K, N Fabricius-Bjerre, J Kjaerulff, et al: Mortality from acute myocardial infarction before and after establishment of a coronary care unit. Br Med J I: 567, 1974.

40. Resnekow L: University of Chicago Myocardial Infarction Research Unit. Comprehensive clinical and laboratory research. USPHS report PH-43-68-1334-A73, 1975.
41. Killip T, JT Kimball: Treatment of myocardial infarction in a coronary care unit: A two-year experience with 250 patients. Am J Cardiol 20: 457, 1967.
42. Mirowski M, W Israels, AG Antonopoulos, et al: Treatment of myocardial infarction in a community hospital coronary care unit. Arch Int Med 138: 210, 1978.
43. Oliver MF, DG Julian, KW Donald: Problems in evaluating coronary care units: Their responsibilities and their relation to the community. Am J Cardiol 20: 465, 1967.
44. Restieaux N, C Bray, H Bullard, et al: One hundred fifty patients with cardiac infarction treated in a coronary care unit. Lancet 1: 1285, 1967.
45. Sloman G, M Stannard, AJ Goble: Coronary care unit: A review of 300 patients monitored since 1963. Am Heart J 75: 140, 1968.
46. Isacsson SO, A Westerlund, H Wingstrand: A review of 191 patients with myocardial infarction treated in a Swedish coronary care unit. Acta Med Scand 185: 545, 1969.
47. Church G, RO Biern: Intensive coronary care - practical system for a small hospital without house-staff. N Engl J Med 281: 1155, 1969.
48. McGuire LB, MS Kroll: Evaluation of cardiac care units and myocardial infarction. Arch Intern Med 130: 677, 1972.
49. Astvad K, N Fabricius-Bjerre, J Kjaerulff, et al: Mortality from acute myocardial infarction before and after establishment of a coronary care unit. Br Med J 1: 567, 1974.
50. Lopes MG, AP Spivack, DC Harrison, et al: Prognosis in coronary care unit noninfarction cases. JAMA 228: 1558, 1974.
51. Reader R: Why the decreasing mortality from coronary heart disease in Australia? Presented as a communication at the American Heart Association Meeting, Dallas, 1978. Circulation Part II 58: II-32, 1978.
52. Dekker E: Hartbewakingseenheid. Acta Hospitalia, vol XIV, n 1, 1974.
53. Synopsis of Research Proposals presented by CMSI's ad Hoc Groups on Coronary Care Systems. Postsurgical and Respiratory Intensive Care and Standardization of Electronic Equipments in Intensive Care Units European Communities: Committee on Medical Research and Public Health (CMR) and Committee Monitoring the Seriously Ill (CMSI).
54. Colling A: Coronary care in the community. Croom Helm Ltd, 1977, London.

3.2. HEMODYNAMIC MONITORING IN ACUTE MYOCARDIAL INFARCTION FOR PRO-
GNOSTIC ASSESSMENT OF SURVIVAL AND INCIDENCE OF REINFARCTION
W. Rudolph, K.L. Froer, D. Hall, L. Goppel, H. Petri, G. Frick

This study was carried out to investigate the value of hemodynamic
monitoring for assessment of changes incurred during the acute phase
of myocardial infarction and a subsequent observation period, as
well as the value of these measurements as compared with respect to
the 6-month rate of reinfarction and the 6-month survival.

3.2.1. MATERIAL AND METHODS

Studies were performed in a total of 128 patients documented to have
acute myocardial infarction (77 anterior wall and 51 posterior
wall). There were 99 men with a mean age of 56 years and 29 women
with a mean age of 58 years. After admission to the Coronary Care
Unit, a triple-lumen semi-floating catheter was passed, via the
cubital vein, into the pulmonary artery for determinations of pulmonary artery and pulmonary capillary wedge pressures, as well as
cardiac output by means of thermodilution. Blood pressure was determined by cuff or radial artery cannulation. The initial measurements
were obtained between the first and 10th hour after onset of
symptoms and these parameters were then registered through continuous monitoring over a period of up to six days. For further comparison, hemodynamic parameters were redetermined in 44 of these patients through complete cardiac catheterization 2 to 4 months after
infarction. After a subsequent observation period of 6 months,
survival rate and incidence of reinfarction were evaluated. Statistical analysis was carried out by grouping the patients according to
normal, intermediate or markedly abnormal initial values of pulmonary capillary wedge pressure (PCP), cardiac index (CI), systolic
arterial blood pressure (SBP), heart rate (HR) and stroke work index
(SWI). Intercurrent medical treatment was standardized and administered when necessary for the underlying disease and its complications.

3.2.2. RESULTS

Classification of the patients into 3 groups according to their
initial values of PCP demonstrated that those with pressures less
than 12 mmHg (n = 48) consistently had normal values of CI, SBP, HR
and SWI and that these values remained unchanged throughout the
observation period in those subsequently reinvestigated (n=19). In
this group there were no reinfarctions and the 6-month survival was

100%. In those with moderate elevations of PCP from 13 to 18 mmHg (n = 45), SBP, HR and SWI were generally similar to the values found in the preceding group and in those restudied (n = 19) while on no medication, there was a modest decrease in PCP and no significant changes in SWI. This group had a 7 % rate of reinfarction and an 89% 6-month survival with all deaths occurring suddenly in the late phase. In the group with markedly elevated PCP to more than 18 mmHg (n = 35), CI, SBP, HR and SWI were moderately to markedly abnormal; there was a 17 % rate of reinfarction and only 49 % survival with all but one death due to pump failure in the early phase. Cardiac catheterization data obtained during temporary cessation of medication in 8 of the survivors showed no significant changes from initial values.

Normal CI of more than 2.5 $l/min/m^2$ at the initial measurement (n = 82) remained so throughout the entire observation period (n = 35) and was associated with a low rate of reinfarction of 4.5% and good survival of 97.5 % where both the non-survivors and those with reinfarction were found in the group with intermediate elevation of PCP. Moderately decreased CI to values between 2.0 and 2.5 $l/min/m^2$ (n = 27) remained constant (n = 12) and were associated with a 37 % rate of reinfarction and 78 % survival where, again, the mortality was confined to the groups with moderate to marked elevation of PCP. CI values of less than 2.0 $l/min/m^2$ (n = 19) were invariably associated with marked elevations of PCP which were found unchanged in the survivors who underwent subsequent catheterization (n = 2). There were no reinfarction in this group but the 6-month survival rate was reduced to 21 %, with all deaths due to intractable heart failure during the hospital phase.

In a display of the respective values of PCP plotted against CI (Fig. 1), it can be seen that the most favorable prognosis was found in those with normal PCP which was uniformly associated with normal CI. In the presence of normal CI, moderately elevated PCP implied a notable increase in morbidity and mortality. Prognosis worsened progressively with increasingly abnormal values of each parameter.

Classification according to the initial level of systolic blood pressure showed that those with pressures in excess of 130 mmHg (n = 61) had a 15 % rate of reinfarction and 90 % survival with all deaths occurring suddenly in the late phase. Those with SP between 90 and 130 mmHg (n = 47) had a 7 % rate of reinfarction and one early death due to congestive heart failure as well as one late sudden death, accounting for a 6-month survival of 95 %. SBP of less than 90 mmHg (n = 19), which essentially represents the group with marked elevation of PCP and markedly decreased CI, was associated with a poor survival rate of 21 %, with all early deaths due to pump failure. There were no reinfarctions in the survivors of the latter group.

Analysis according to initial heart rates showed that those with

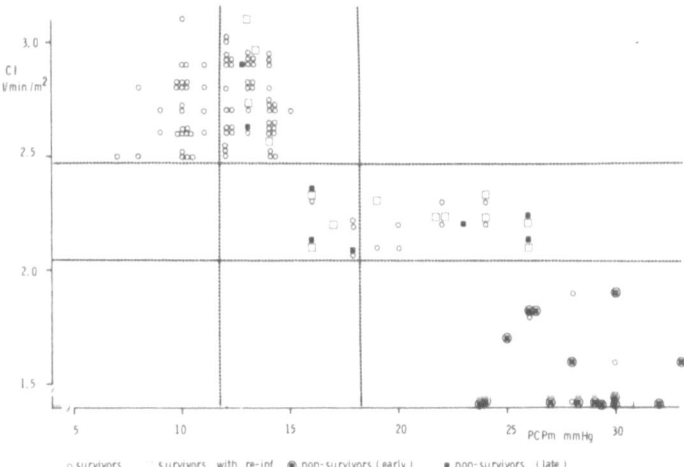

Fig. 1. Prognosis of the patients relatively to CI and PCP ratio.
For description see text.

less than 80 beats/min (n = 31) had a 13 % rate of reinfarction and
a 90 % 6-month survival with deaths occurring late and suddenly.
Those with initial HR between 80 and 100 beats/min (n = 81) had a
10% rate of reinfarction and a 89 % survival with an even distribution of early deaths due to intractable heart failure and late sudden
deaths. Those with HR in excess of 100 beats/min (n = 15) again
represented, primarily, the group with markedly abnormal values of
PCP and CI; there were no reinfarctions, but the survival rate was
only 27 % where, again, heart failure in the hospital phase was the
cause of death.
In consideration of SWI, those with values greater than 30 g.m/m^2 (n
= 94) demonstrated a 17 % rate of reinfarction and a 93 % survival
rate with all deaths occurring late and suddenly. Values between 20
and 30 g.m/m^2 (n = 13) were associated with a 23 % rate of reinfarction and one late sudden death accounting for a 6-month survival
rate of 92 %. Those with SWI values of less than 20 g.m/m^2 (n = 20)
had only a 20 % survival rate with all deaths occurring in the
hospital phase due to heart failure and there were no reinfarctions
among the survivors.

3.2.3. DISCUSSION

The results of this study show that normal filling pressures could
be regarded as indicative of normal cardiac output and that these
patients have an excellent prognosis with no reinfarction and 100%
survival in the first 6 months after infarction. Single initial
measurements were representative of their hemodynamic status and,

thus, permit consideration for early discharge from the hospital. Patients with moderate elevations of PCP may have a normal CI but were found to be at moderate risk of reinfarction and mortality. Markedly elevated wedge pressures associated with only moderate decreases in CI also carried substantial risk of mortality and, in particular, reinfarction. With or without therapy, those in the latter 2 groups may demonstrate alterations in hemodynamic parameters and, in consideration of the relatively small number of these patients who underwent subsequent catheterization, their initial measurements could not be considered necessarily representative of hemodynamic status. The relatively high risk of complications implies the necessity of early catheterization, preferably prior to discharge from the hospital, as a guide to specific management.

In all patients with markedly lowered values of CI, markedly elevated PCP was found. The majority of these patients were obviously in shock and the ominous prognosis of this hemodynamic constellation at initial measurements demands immediate and aggressive treatment. SBP and HR rendered prognostically useful information only if they were markedly abnormal in which case they were consistently associated with marked abnormalities of PCP and CI. As could be expected, SWI considered on its own furnished no additional information to that provided by PCP and CI since this value also reflects the HR and SBP.

Thus, PCP appears to be the decisive parameter with regard to prognostic implications. In the acute phase of myocardial infarction, a single initial measurement is adequate for providing prognostic assessment in those with normal pressures. With increasingly abnormal values of PCP, prognosis steadily worsens, in particular, if adequate CI cannot be maintained. The value of hemodynamic monitoring in these patients provides not only prognostic information but also guides management.

3.3. SIGNIFICANCE OF PROGNOSTIC INDEXES DERIVED FROM HEMODYNAMIC MONITORING IN ACUTE MYOCARDIAL INFARCTION

G. Bertini, N. Marchionni, R. Pini, A. Vannucci, F. M. Antonini

The purpose of this study was to obtain a prognostic index based on hemodynamic and anamnestic data in a series of patients with acute myocardial infarction (AMI).

3.3.1. MATERIALS AND METHODS

Two hundred twenty five consecutive patients, admitted to the coronary care unit (CCU) within 24 hours of the onset of an AMI, underwent a right heart catheterization and hemodynamic monitoring without previous selection on clinical basis. The diagnosis of AMI was established according to the MIRU protocol.

The sample consisted of 181 men (average age 60.7 ± 9.8 years) and 46 women (average age 71.4 ± 9.8 years). Hospital mortality was 16.7 percent. The higher mortality observed in the group of females (26.1 percent) compared to that of the males (14.4 percent) can probably be attributed to the significant difference of average age ($P<0.01$). No significant difference of incidence of anterior and inferior infarctions between survivors and non-survivors was found.

Before admission all the patients had been given only analgesics; during the hospitalization the basic treatment consisted of sodium heparin 6000 U sc twice daily, oral dipyridamole 300 mg daily and oral diazepam 20 mg daily. No significant difference in the pharmacological treatment of hemodynamic complications between survivors and non-survivors was found.

The hemodynamic monitoring and the elaboration of the derived parameters were performed in real time by a CII 10020 32 Kbytes dedicated digital computer.

Differences between quantitative data were compared by student's t test; distribution differences were analysed by the chi-square test. Linear discriminant function analysis according to Fisher (1) were used to calculate equations for predicting mortality rates.

3.3.2. RESULTS

The patients were grouped in to 6 hemodynamic classes according to the pulmonary artery mean pressure (PMP) and the left ventricular stroke work index (LVSWI) values measured at the onset of monitoring

Table 1. Hemodynamic classes

Class	Patients no.	Patients %	Mortality %
1. Normal PMP 19 SWI 45 – 85	39	17.1	2.6
2. Hyperdynamic PMP 19 SWI 85	4	1.8	0
3. Heart failure PMP 19 SWI 20 – 45	89	39.0	27.0
4. Cardiogenic shock PMP 19 SWI 20	8	3.5	100
5. Hypovolemia PMP 19 SWI 45	49	21.6	8.0
6. Reduced left ventricular compliance PMP 19 SWI 45	38	16.7	2.6

Number of patients with percentage incidence rate and mortality rate are reported for each hemodynamic class. PMP = pulmonary artery mean pressure (mmHg); SWI = left ventricular stroke work index $(g.m/m^2)$.

(Table 1). PMP was employed as an index of left ventricular filling pressure because it can be easily obtained as an integrated value from analogic circuits, and this form is particularly useful for the continuous monitoring by the computer. The use of PMP does not seem to alter substantially the validity of hemodynamic classes except for the 6th one, in which pulmonary hypertension might also be a consequence of high pulmonary vascular resistances.

A comparison of hemodynamic data for survivors and non-survivors is reported in Table 2. A seven variable discriminant analysis of parameters reported in Table 2 was developed for all the 227 patients.

The resultant equation may be given as:

Table 2. Comparison of hemodynamic data for survivors and nonsurvivors

	Lived	Died	t	P
Patients (no.)	189	38		
HR	84 ± 17	99 ± 20	- 5.035	0.001
SI	33 ± 13	22 ± 8	5.175	0.001
SAP	140 ± 29	128 ± 29	2.329	0.05
DAP	85 ± 17	79 ± 17	2.115	0.05
PMP	22 ± 8	29 ± 9	- 5.229	0.001
TRP	1863 ± 601	2198 ± 700	- 3.052	0.01
SWI	46 ± 19	28 ± 11	5.711	0.001

Reported hemodynamic data have been measured at the onset of monitoring. Statistically different pairings are identified by the P values. DAP = diastolic arterial pressure (mmHg); HR = heart rate
(beats/min); PMP = pulmonary artery mean pressure (mmHg); SAP = systolic arterial pressure (mmHg); SI = stroke index (ml/m^2); SWI = left
ventricular stroke work index (g.m/m^2); TPR = total peripheral systemic resistance (dyne.sec.cm^{-5}).

DF (Discriminant function) = -0.4235 - 0.0301HR +
+0.0593SI - 0.0014SAP + 0.0536DAP - 0.0845PMP -   (1)
-0.00003LVSWI - 0.0006TPR.

(where: HR = heart rate, SI = stroke index, SAP = systolic arterial
pressure, DAP = diastolic arterial pressure, TPR = total peripheral
systemic resistances).
In spite of the high statistical significance (F=2778.45; P< 0.005)
many errors in prediction were noticed: 72 survivors out of 189 were
erroneously predicted dead while 5 deceased out of 38 were predicted
alive. The causes of death of the 5 patients erroneously predicted
alive seem to be indipendent of their initial hemodynamic conditions
(2 cases of ventricular fibrillation on the 8th and 20th day
respectively; 1 massive pulmonary embolism on the 15th day; 1
rupture of the free wall of the left ventricle on the 2nd day; 1
rupture of the papillary muscle on the 4th day). The 72 errors

observed in the group of survivors are all in the 3rd and 5th hemodynamic classes, while the equation provided prognostic indications with a 97.8 percent accuracy rate in the 1st, 2nd, 4th, and 6th classes; this accuracy rate concerned 89 patients (39.2 percent). Thus, two further discriminant function analysis of PMP and LVSWI only (the parameters employed for the initial hemodynamic classification) were developed, for the 3rd and 5th classes, between the survivors correctly predicted as such and the survivors erroneously predicted as dead.
The calculated equations are as follows:

$$DF_3 = -5.05 - 0.23PMP + 0.28LVSWI \quad (F= 883.24; \ P<0.005) \qquad (2)$$

$$DF_5 = -18.29 + 0.003PMP + 0.53LVSWI \quad (F= 1544.23; \ P<0.005) \qquad (3)$$

They subdivided the 3rd and 5th classes in two areas respectively. In the two groups of patients with a positive discriminant score (DF> 0 = survival; 3a and 5a classes) we obtained a good accuracy rate of prediction, while in the groups with a negative discriminant score (DF <0 = nonsurvival; 3b and 5b classes) we still found a very low accuracy rate.
Thus, anamnestic data from the patients of these last groups (3b and 5b) were analised. Only mean age showed a significant difference between survivors and non-survivors (64 ± 12 and 70 ± 10 years respectively; P< 0.05). A history of previous hypertension, diabetes and coronary artery disease was present with an incidence rate of 18.8, 17.2 and 29.7 percent respectively in the group of the survivors, while incidence rates of 28.0, 32.0 and 32.0 percent respectively were found in the group of the non-survivors. None of these differences was statistically significant.
A further three variable discriminant analysis of age and previous history of hypertension and diabetes was developed for all the patients in the 3b and 5b classes, assuming hypertension and diabetes as binary categorical variables.
This last equation:

$$DF_A = 3.60 - 0.05 \ AGE - 0.61 \ HYPERTENSION - 0.51 \ DIABETES$$
$$(F = 236.79; \ P<0.005) \qquad (4)$$

correctly discriminates 43 survivors from 19 deceased out of 89 patients. Thus, the residual error of prediction in these two classes was reduced to 21 live patients predicted dead and 6 dead predicted alive. Combining age together with previous history of hypertension and diabetes improved prognostic accuracy compared with that of age only; no further improvement was reached by adding the history of previous coronary artery disease.
After the three discriminant steps, a final 85 percent accuracy rate

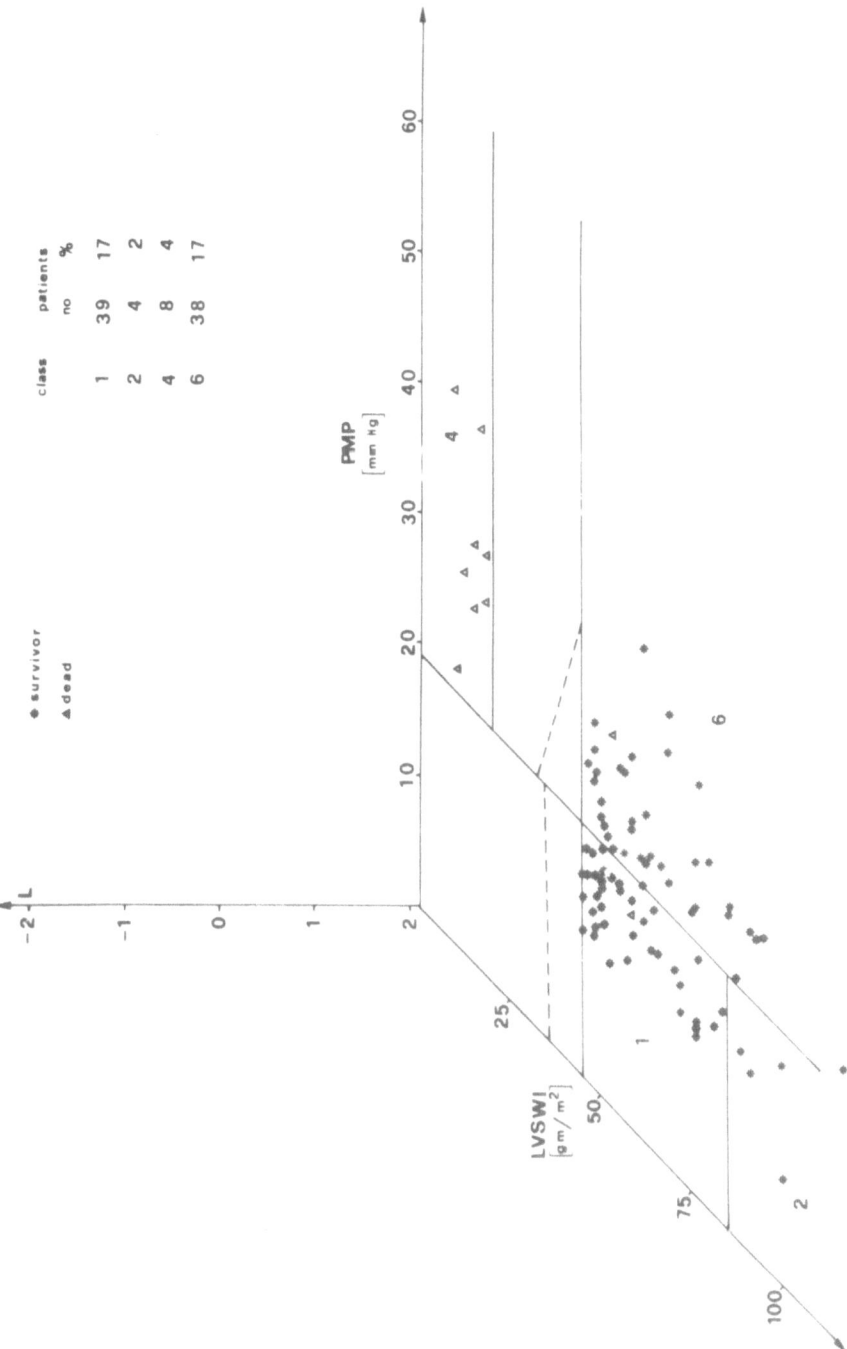

Fig. 1. Distribution of patients in the 1st, 2nd, 4th and 6th classes. Each area is identified on the plane by the PMP - LVSWI relationship. L values reported on the third axis are derived from the discriminant function performed for age, hypertension and diabetes (DF$_A$, see text), unnecessary for predicting prognosis in these hemodynamic classes.

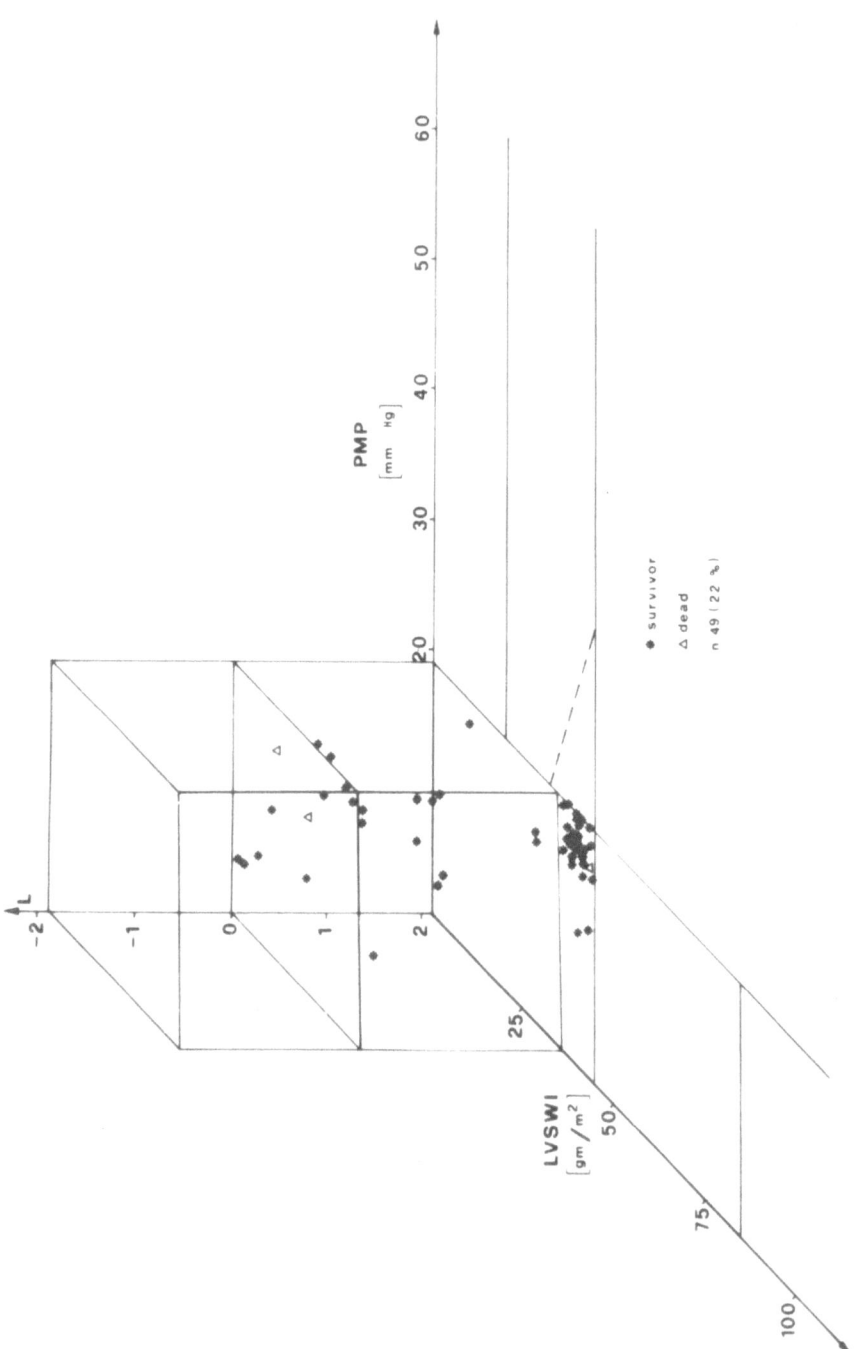

Fig. 2. Distribution of patients in the 5th class (hypovolemia). DF_5 and L values derived from DF_A are employed to separate patients with three different prognoses in the same hemodynamic class.

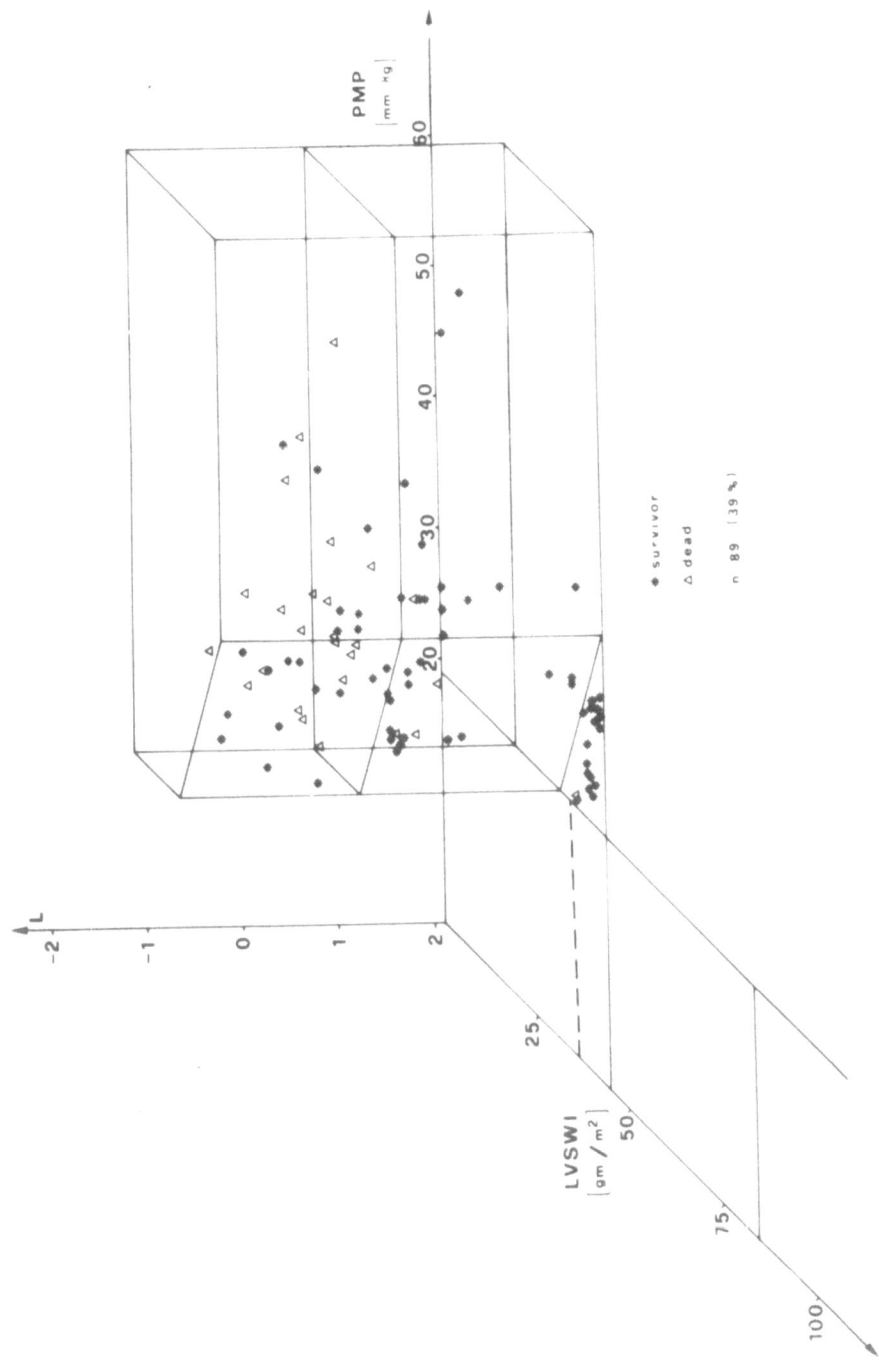

Fig. 3. Distribution of patients in the 3rd class (heart failure). DF_3 and L values derived from DF_A are employed to separate patients with three different prognoses in the same hemodynamic class.

was obtained in the whole group of 227 patients who, from the six hemodynamic classes (Figs. 1, 2, 3), were distributed in ten hemody- namic and historical prognostic groups. The entire stepwise process for predicting prognosis can be easily computerized (Fig. 4).

We want to point out that in class 5b1, in spite of lower values of LVSWI, there was an inferior mortality rate than in class 5a. This atypical behaviour of the group of patients with hypovolemia can probably be attributed to the presence of factors not directly correlated with left ventricular function in determining this parti- cular physiopathological condition.

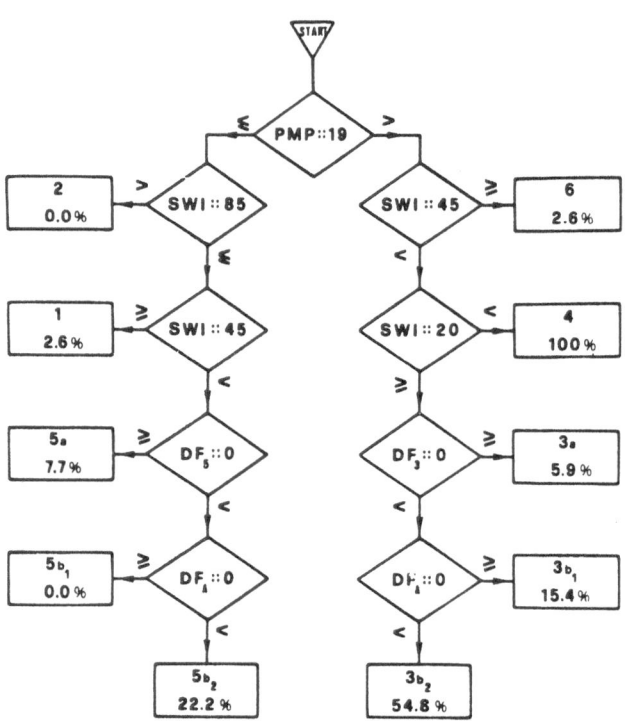

Fig. 4. Algorithm derived from analysis of hemodynamic and anamne- stic data to identify ten prognostic classes for patients with AMI. In the rectangles the number and the correspondent observed mortali- ty are reported for each class.
:: = comparison operation; PMP = pulmonary artery mean pressure; SWI = left ventricular stroke work index; for DF_3, DF_5 and DF_A see text.

3.3.3. DISCUSSION

The distribution of the patients in the six hemodynamic classes and
their percentage mortality rate observed in this study both agree
with previous observations (2). Several authors (3, 4) reported
that, according to clinical evaluation alone, 50 percent of cases of
AMI are usually considered as uncomplicated, while on hemodynamic
evaluation only 15-20 percent of patients show normal cardiac performance.
In the present study the incidence rate of normal hemodynamic
conditions was only 17.1 percent (mortality rate 2.6 percent). These
data confirm an unsatisfactory correlation between clinical and
hemodynamic evaluation.
In their studies, Peel et al. (5), Norris et al. (6) and Hughes et
al. (7) identified several clinical and historical data such as age,
infarct location, previous coronary heart disease, hypotension,
radiological and physical signs of failure which correlated with a
poor prognosis. Yet the importance of these clinical criteria -
semiquantitative and not clearly objective - for predicting prognosis has still to be proved. For the same reasons our opinion is that
these prognostic indexes cannot be applied to series of patients
different from the original one and are not useful for comparison of
results from different CCU.
More recently Weber et al. (8) subdivided 400 patients with AMI in 4
classes according to the clinical criteria of Killip (9); hemodynamic data were examined in order to develop discriminant function
analysis to identify high risk subsets within each clinical class.
For the 1st, 2nd and 3rd classes a two variable discriminant
function analysis of heart rate and pulmonary capillary wedge pressure provided an estimate of survival with a 72 percent accuracy rate;
a three variable discriminant analysis (left ventricular stroke work
index, cardiac index and pulmonary capillary wedge pressure) provided an 83 percent accuracy rate in predicting mortality in the 4th
class. The authors reported a fairly good agreement between hemodynamic and clinical methods, when applied to a large group, in
separating patients with different degrees of impairment of cardiac
function, but they observed that, in the individual patients, the
clinical examination could not accurately reflect the degree of left
ventricular dysfunction. Lorente et al. (10) proposed a hemodynamic
prognostic index based on a discriminant function analysis of LVSWI
and TPR and they obtained a 90 percent accuracy rate in predicting
mortality; this analysis was performed on data from 71 patients with
clinical evidence of congestive heart failure and therefore it
cannot be applied to all cases of AMI.
   The goal of our investigation was to realize a prognostic index
derived from objective data only. The three discriminant functions
seem to provide a reliable prediction of prognosis for patients with

AMI on the first hemodynamic evaluation soon after the admission. The use of only quantitative and objective parameters makes it possible to eliminate errors peculiar to the clinical evaluation and enables a more consistent comparison between groups of patients from different medical centers. An 85 percent accuracy rate in predicting prognosis was obtained for the whole group after the three steps of analysis. Furthermore, we identified a subset with a mortality rate of about 50 percent (3b2 class; Fig. 4); it is possible that these patients at high risk might benefit by the application of mechanical cardiac assistance, like intra-aortic balloon counterpulsation, with perhaps much more successful results than those achieved up till now by medical treatment of cardiogenic shock. The availability of a reliable prognostic index might provide a more exact indication to this aggressive management program of severe heart failure complicating an acute myocardial infarction.

REFERENCES

1. Lison L: Statistica applicata alla biologia sperimentale. Milano, Casa Editrice Ambrosiana, p. 313, 1961.
2. Chatterjee K, HJC Swan: Hemodynamic profile of acute myocardial infarction, chap 6. In, Myocardial Infarction (Corday E., Swan H.J.C., ed.). Baltimore, Williams & Wilkins, p. 51, 1973.
3. Ramo B, N Miers, AG Wallace, et al: Hemodynamic findings in 123 patients with acute myocardial infarction on admission. Circulation 42: 567, 1970.
4. Saadjian A, JL Arnould, JA Trigano, et al: La pression télédiastolique ventriculaire gauche à la phase aigue de l'infarctus du myocarde. Arch Mal Coeur 8: 869, 1974.
5. Peel AAF, T Semple, I Wang, et al: A coronary prognostic index for grading the severity of infarction. Br Heart J 24: 745, 1962.
6. Norris RM, PWT Brandt, DE Caughey, et al: A new coronary prognostic index. Lancet 1: 274, 1969.
7. Hughes WL, JM Kalbfleisch, EN Jr Brandt, et al: Myocardial infarction. Prognosis by discriminant analysis. Arch Int Med 111: 338, 1963.
8. Weber KT, JS Janicki, RD Russel, et al: Identification of high risk subset of acute myocardial infarction. Am J Cardiol 41: 197, 1978.
9. Killip T, JT Kimball: Treatment of myocardial infarction in a coronary care unit. A two years experience with 250 patients. Am J Cardiol 20: 457, 1969.
10. Lorente P, M Delabre: Use of correspondance analysis in processing hemodynamic data from acute myocardial infarction. Comput Biomed Res 10: 213, 1977.

3.4. A SYSTEM FOR REAL TIME HEMODYNAMIC MONITORING IN A RESEARCH
ENVIRONMENT
S. Chierchia, L. Landucci, M. Lazzari, A. Macerata, C. Marchesi, A.
Maseri, I. Simonetti

3.4.1. INTRODUCTION

It should be recognized that one of the relevant roles of research
CCU's is that of improving patient care by expanding our understanding of the disease processes. Commercially available computer
systems are essentially designed for routine clinical applications.
Therefore with the aim of investigating the pathogenetic mechanisms
of transient recurrent anginal attacks occurring at rest, we developed a computer system for continuous beat by beat analysis of
intravascular pressures and ECG. With this system we have analyzed
the data collected during continuous hemodynamic monitoring in a
group of patients with frequent anginal attacks.
The large amount of collected data and the high temporal resolution
necessary to detect the very rapid trends we were interested in,
required:
1. continuous beat by beat acquisition and analysis of ECG and
   hemodynamic signals (included ventricular waveforms);
2. rational data presentation.

3.4.2. MATERIAL AND METHOD

We studied 26 anginal patients admitted to our CCU for transient,
recurrent anginal attacks occurring at rest. Pressures were sampled
by standard, fluid filled catheters connected to Statham P23dB
transducers continuously flushed by saline under constant pressure.
In the early version of the system the computer analysis was performed on a 'off-line' basis. Pressure waves and one or more ECG leads
were continuously recorded on a 14 channels analog magnetic tape and
analysed, at the end of the study, both manually and by the computer
programs. For the manual analysis low (0.5 to 2.5 mm/m) and high
speed (25 mm/sec) play-backs of selected parameters (Fig. 1) were
obtained on a photographic recorder according to the previously
described technique (1-2). For the computer analysis the ECG was
sampled at 200 s/sec and pressure waves at 100 s/sec. The algorithms
for feature extraction of each signal have been described in detail
in our previous contributions (3-4). A systematic comparison was
performed between the results obtained by manual and computer

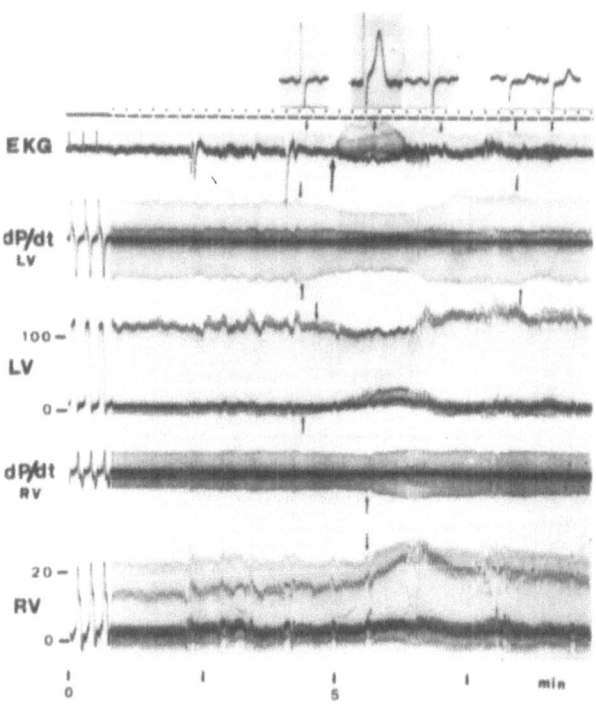

Fig. 1. Low speed recording for manual analysis.

analysis over a total period of about 100 hours of recording, obtained in 9 consecutive patients.

Following the evaluation of the algorithms, a real time version (SOTER) of the system has been developed (5), also oriented to research purposes, particularly for increasing the temporal resolution of the system and for speeding-up the signal analysis. The system has been developed on a minicomputer in satellite position of a small 3 mini's network. The values of each derived parameter calculated on a beat by beat basis, are stored on a disk and displayed on a console. Filing on mag-tape and hard copies are obtained during and at the end of the monitoring period. The ECG and hemodynamic derived parameters calculated by the computer program are listed in Table 1.

In the play-back version of the system, values of the various derived parameters, calculated on a beat by beat basis, are averaged over ten second periods and represented with the mean standard deviation in numerical form by a line printer or in graphic form by an incremental plotter.

Table 1. List of parameters measured by SOTER.

ECG		
Heart Rate		HR
QRS Duration		QRSD
ST-T deflections area		STAT
LV/RV		
Pressure at beginning of diastole		LVPD
End Diastolic Pressure		LVED
Systolic Pressure		LVS
Peak Contraction Dp/Dt		LDPC
Peak Relaxation Dp/Dt		LDPR
AO		
Systolic Pressure		AOS
Diastolic Pressure		AOD
Stroke Volume		STV
Cardiac Output		CO
Mean pressure		AOM
PA		
Systolic Pressure		PAS
Diastolic Pressure		PAD
Mean Pressure		PAM
O_2 SAT		
O_2 Saturation (fiber optic cath)		SO

Two formats of data display are available in the real time version. The first is a simple display on a screen of the waveforms, used mainly to control the quality of the data and the accuracy of the thresholds used; the second allows the display of selected parameters plotted against time with variable time resolution (Fig. 2). The real time process can be interrupted from the keyboard to adjust the configuration of the programs or to obtain retrospective displays. The data stored on the disk are saved on mag-tape and are available for hard copies on a printer/plotter (Fig. 3).

3.4.3. RESULTS

During over 300 hours of continuous recording of several electrocardiographic and hemodynamic signals a total of 350 transient ischemic episodes was collected. In none of them an increase in the hemodynamic determinants of myocardial metabolic demands was observed preceding the onset of ST-T changes. By contrast a sudden drop of left ventricular contraction and relaxation dp/dt was detected preceding or accompanying the onset of ST changes. The evaluation of the hemodynamic patterns typical of transient ischemic episodes indicated the changes of left ventricular contractility as the most

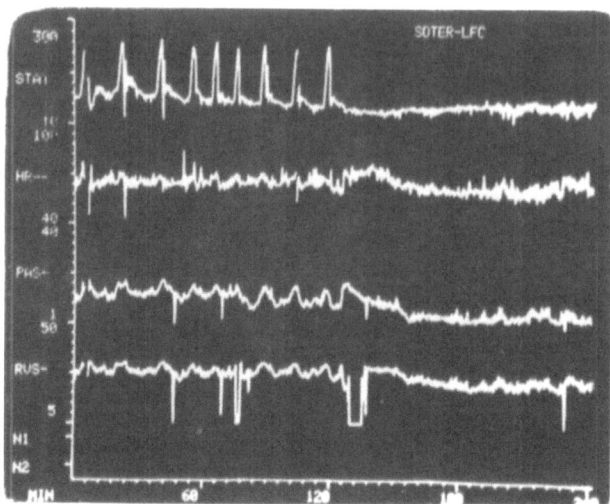

Fig. 2. Plots of parameters on the terminal screen.

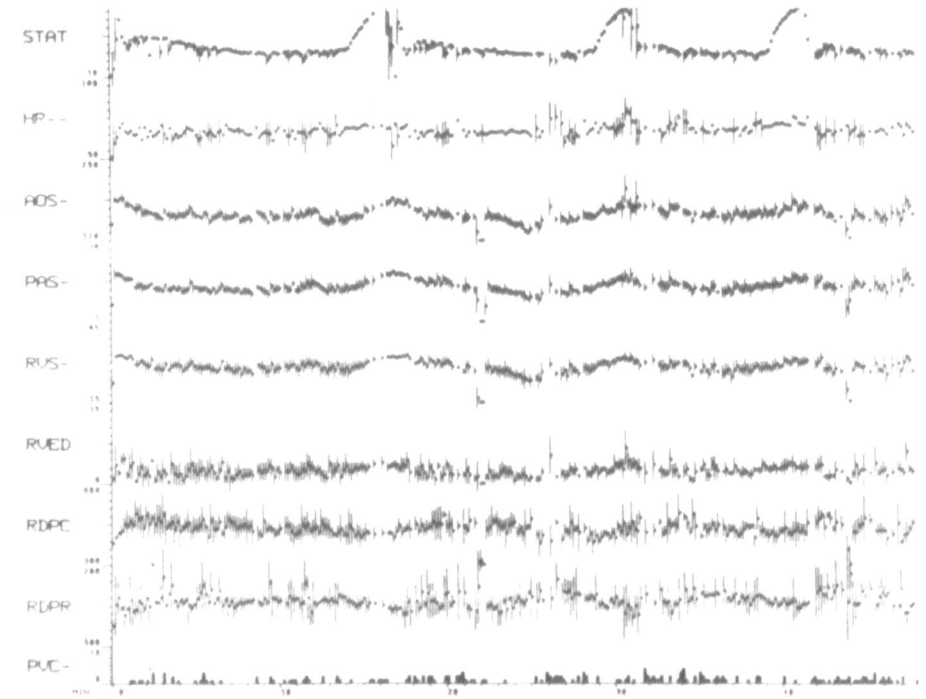

Fig. 3. Plots of parameters on the printer/plotter.

sensitive feature of the transient ischemic attacks, even in the presence of minor ST-T changes (1-3).
The ability of the computer system of recognizing the ECG and the hemodynamic patterns during transient ischemic attacks was evaluated by a systematic comparison of the data obtained by manual and automatic measurements performed in 130 episodes recorded in 9 patients. This comparison showed a total agreement between the manual and automatic episode detection.

3.4.4. DISCUSSION

The use of this system allowed to achieve remarkable information concerning the pathophysiological mechanisms of angina pectoris, as well as it allowed to test algorithms in an extremely variable set of conditions. It has provided the demonstration that the spontaneous attacks of angina at rest are not caused by an increase in myocardial demands as traditionally assumed. Furthermore, it showed severe alterations of the left ventricular function even in the presence of minor and short lasting ST-T changes unaccompanied by anginal pain, traditionally considered unrelated to acute myocardial ischemia. The collection of this information was made possible by the beat to beat resolution used for the analysis of the recorded data. The large amount of ischemic episodes of variable severity, collected during long periods of continuous recording in a rather large population of patients provides a large data base for statistical evaluation of the specificity of ST-T segment changes in detecting acute myocardial ischemia, by systematic comparison with the typical hemodynamic changes.
The versatility of this home made computer system is particularly suitable for studying rapid transient and for developing rational forms of data presentation.

REFERENCES

1. Maseri A, R Mimmo, S Chierchia, et al: Coronary artery spasm as a cause of acute myocardial ischemia in man. Chest 68: 625, 1975.
2. Chierchia S, C Marchesi, A Maseri: Evidence of angina not caused by increased myocardial metabolic demand and patterns of electrocardiographic and hemodynamic alterations during 'primary' angina. In 'Primary and Secondary Angina Pectoris'. Edited by A. Maseri, GA Klassen and M Lesch, Grune and Stratton, New York, p 145, 1978.
3. Marchesi C, S Chierchia, A Maseri: Left and right ventricular pressures monitoring in CCU: methods and significance. Proceedings of Computers in Cardiology, Rotterdam. Edited by IEEE

Computers Society, Long Beach California, p 579, 1977.

4. Chierchia S, A Maseri, C Marchesi, et al: Computerized continuous beat-by-beat analysis and rational plots of ECG ventricular and arterial pressure waves during transient ischemic episodes. Proceedings of Computers in Cardiology, Stanford. Edited by IEEE Computers Society, Long Beach California, p 105, 1978.

5. Landucci L, A Macerata, C Marchesi, et al: Real time computer based Electrocardiographic and Hemodynamic monitoring in CCU. Proceedings on Medical Informatics, Berlin. Published by Springer, p 325, 1979.

3.5. PROGNOSTIC INDICES, TREND DETECTION AND PREDICTION TECHNIQUES

J.E.W. Beneken, J.A., Blom, F.F. Jorritsma, A. Nandorff, J. Spierdijk

3.5.1. INTRODUCTION.

In patient care, measurements are, in general, obtained at considerable cost. This cost is composed of different elements: discomfort and risk for the patient, time of physicians and nursing staff, depreciation of expensive equipment and facilities, and the expenses for maintenance and disposables. Thus it is our responsibility to make full use of the results obtained.

Why are these measurements performed? They serve, in general, one of the following purposes: diagnosis, confirmation of an earlier diagnosis or evaluation of the effect of therapy. Population screening in another important class, which, however, will not be discussed here.

Before measurements can be interpreted considerable data processing is necessary, this means feature analysis, reduction of data, and determination of derived quantities. This results in a set of independent patient variables upon which proper patient management can be based. This management sometimes requires a notion about the future course of the patient's state.

Among such reasons are:

A. informing the patient and his relatives
B. selection of the best therapy
C. planning the adaptation of housing for a disabled patient
D. planning the occupation of intensive care units of the basis of expected discharge of patients.

Such forecasting can be performed using methods of different hierarchical level: prognosis, trend detection and model based prediction.

Prognosis is the prediction of the duration, course and outcome of disease in an individual patient. In some studies just one of these topics is considered. Although generally used in a qualitative, descriptive sense, here the term prognosis will only be considered in the sense of quantitative predictions based on measurements of physiological variables. Variables that have prognostic value are called prognostic variables. Several prognostic variables, each individually giving predictions with a low accuracy, may be combined in some way to obtain one variable with a higher accuracy. Such a variable is called a prognostic index. A prognostic index combines in one number all prognostic information, that is available and deemed relevant. Prognosis in a quantitative sense is usually expressed in what is called a response variable. This is a measure

of the future health or illness of the patient. Its value is usually
dependent on several prognostic variables (1), and can be considered
a transformation of the prognostic index.

The functional relationship is usually found by some form of discriminant analysis based on data obtained from a large data base. Thus
while a prognosis may have an average certainty of say 80%, there is
no guarantee of the same accuracy for any individual patient.
Particularly common response variables include lenght of survival,
lenght of disease-free interval and death or survival (one or the
other). Afifi et al (2) trasform the response variable, which
classifies a patient as a survivor or non-survivor, into a probability of survival.

One of the aims of a prognostic study is to identify the available
variables which have substantial prognostic value. This is important, since it provides insight into the mechanism of a disease by
revealing which of a number of variables are most significant for
the course and outcome of a disease. It is evident, that the
prognostic variables are strongly related to the primary cause of
the disease. Thus, a variable may have a large prognostic value in
one disease, while it may not have any prognostic value in another.
A prognosis, in general, is established on the basis of momentary
patient data, because this may be the only information available
about the patient in an emergency situation. The relation between
prognostic variable and derived response variables need not be
causative.

A trend may be defined as a slow but consistent, unidirectional
change. Trends may be observed or calculated from:

A. directly measured signals, if they are smooth and noisefree (e.g.
   temperature)

B. time averages of signals, if they are periodic and/or noisy (e.g.
   central venous pessure)

C. properties of signals, especially from periodic signals (e.g.
   heart rate from ECG)

D. relations between signals or properties of signals (e.g. difference between systolic and diastolic arterial pressure).

For the determination of a trend a series of measurements must be
performed. Trend analysis is therefore possible only if patients are
under surveillance for some time, either continuously or intermittently. Slowly developing processes can be monitored at intervals. To
establish a trend in signals it is necessary to observe the accuracy
and reproducibility of the measurements and the possible influence
of different factors on this variable. For this reason, trend
analysis of more than one variable is much more meaningful. The
coincidence in time of the onset or termination of certain trends
may give clues to relations between variables and to underlying
common causes. Analysis of sequential cardio-respiratory observations has provided descriptions of the common history of various shock

syndromes and some insight into underlying patho-physiological mechanisms (3). Trend analysis will, in general, give more insight into (patho-) physiological phenomena than prognostic indices, which of necessity give a static picture of the patient's state. However, it is also possible to consider trends of a prognostic index.

Trend prediction is extrapolation toward the future of the momentary state of a patient. Reliable predictions, i.e. predictions which are accurate enough to be meaningful, are possible only, if sufficient information is available about the patient's past and present state. This information is available in two ways:

1. much is known about general physiological principles that govern the dynamics of the patient's state
2. observations of a particular patient are or will be available to estimate the dynamics of the patient's physiological system.

Thus for trend prediction there are two necessary conditions:

A. the patient's state must be measured over a period of time; all relevant signals must be measurable. If this condition is fulfilled, trends may be calculated of measured and derived variables.
B. A mechanism (model, transfer function or mathematical rule) must exist to extrapolate these trends into the future with sufficient accuracy, including the effects of all possible therapies on the trends.

Both conditions are difficult to fulfill. Some of the relevant signals may only be measurable with discomfort or increased risk, or may not be measurable at all. It may not even be clear what the most relevant signals are. Also, accurate models that give reliable long term predictions may not exist, or even be possible. Yet the great attraction of trend prediction is, that it could develop into a basis for optimal therapy. Given the possibility of evaluating beforehand the effect of any therapy, it will be possible to calculate the best therapy.

Another attractive side of model-based trend prediction is the possibility to obtain an integrative view of the patho-physiological mechanisms. The importance of this is stressed by Shoemaker (3). He states that normal values may not be the most desirable goals of therapy, since compensatory protective mechanisms of the body in response to stress also produce departures from the normal values. The case of the critically ill patient requires indicators for the performance of biological key systems which can be continuously monitored and constitute a reliable and sensitive basis for diagnostic, therapeutic and prognostic decisions, even in conditions of emergency (4).

3.5.2. METHODS

Response variables for prognosis are determined from dichotomous prognostic variables by correlation techniques counting occurrences. The cases are subdivided on the basis of the most significant prognostic variable and within each half a search is made for the next most significant variable (1).

A second approach is multiple regression in which the response variable is regarded as being normally distributed with a mean value which is a linear function of the prognostic variables. If y is the response variable, and x_1, x_2, ..., x_k are prognostic variables, the model postulates that

$$y = a_o + a_1 x_1 + a_2 x_2 + \ldots + a_k x_k + e \qquad (1)$$

where e is an "error term". This error term is often assumed to have a normal distribution with a mean value equal to zero and an unknown variance. It is extremely important to test the normality (or at least the symmetry) of the distribution. If such conditions are not fulfilled it may lead to large errors in the regression coefficients. The a's are regression coefficients to be estimated, usually by least squares. If one of the a's is zero, this means that the corresponding variable has no effect on the response variable, and can be deleted. Standard methods are available to test whether the estimated a's are significantly different from zero. The easiest method of trenddetection is the so called 'trend- recording'. In fact, this is only a manner of presentation of a variable in such a way that either a nurse or a physician has a quick overview over the course of that variable in the past. In this way changes in the variable can be detected easily. For this purpose one can use a 'trendrecorder' or, if using a computer aided monitoring system, a graphical display.

For the automatic detection of trends, trendrecording is not sufficient. A further data processing is necessary. This can be either the exponentially weighted time average method or the autoregressive technique. Two further extensions are described in the literature. One can take the difference of two averages, each with a different time constant (5). By using different time constants the two averages have different delays in following the signal. This means that the difference is unequal to zero as long as a trend in the variable is present. The method, most commonly used for automatic trenddetection, is the time weighted average (6, 7) with an exponential function as weighting function. The importance of a measured value is decreasing in time for the calculation of the average.

A more general method is an autoregressive model. This model states that at moment k y_k is determined by a number of preceding values of the same variable

$$y_k = c + a_1 y_{k-1} + a_2 y_{k-2} + \ldots + e_k \qquad (2)$$

with e_k a noise term with zero mean value. The coefficients a_1, ..., a_n must be estimated from a number of measured values. When the coefficients a are estimated the next value y_k can be predicted. This means that this method gives the possibility for prediction. Besides that, a difference between the estimated y_k and its realisation gives information about the presence of a trend (or a change in trend) of one variable only.

A more integrative approach is followed in model based trendprediction. Such models generally are input-output models, or iso-cybernetic models; this means that they are mathematical in nature and that the parameters not necessarily correlate uniquely with the physiological properties of the patient. A possible mathematical formulation is

$$\underline{y}_k = \underline{c} + A(\underline{y}_{k-1} - \underline{c}) + B\underline{u}_{k-1} + \underline{e}_k \tag{3}$$

Where $\underline{y}_k$ is the complete set of independent variables that represent the state of the patient at instant k; $\underline{u}_{k-1}$ the set of input or control quantities (therapy) applied to the patient at instant k-1, $\underline{c}$ represents the mean value of the variables. A is the system matrix which reflects the interrelationships between the state variables and B is the distribution matrix which describes the influence of the various inputs $\underline{u}$ applied to the patient on the state variables. It is clear that when A, B and $\underline{c}$ are determined for a particular patient during a learning period, a future value of $\underline{y}$ can be calculated on the basis of the present value of $\underline{y}$ and $\underline{u}$. That is prediction on an integrative basis: all variables and a complete model are present. If an optimal state of the patient is known in terms of the variables: $\underline{y}_{opt}$. Then equation 3 can be used to calculate the set of $\underline{u}$ values which minimizes the difference between $\underline{y}_{opt}$ and $\underline{y}_k$. This set of $\underline{u}$ values is the optimal therapy (8-10).

3.5.3. APPLICATION.

In many coronary units prognostic indices are used to assess the severity of a myocardial infarction, to predict a recurrency, an expected period of survival, a probability of survival or some similar measure (11, 12, 14). Different indices are more or less standard now (15). Emergency therapy may be indicated by the value of a prognostic index (16). In a cardiovascular intensive care unit a prognostic index may be used to assess the patient's condition after open heart surgery (17).
The trend method described by Taylor (5) which uses the difference between two averages of the same signals, as calculated with two different time-constants has been compared with the 'normal' type of

alarming (the value of the variable is exceeding a set minimum or maximum) for blood pressure and heart rate (5). There was both a considerable decrease in false positive and false negative alarms.

The other possibility is to use the statistics that are available in the signal.

Besides the time weighted average, one calculates an estimator of the variance; as long as new values fall within predetermined tolerances, the situation is considered stable. This method is used to detect arrhythmias (18).

Haywood et al. (19) described arrhythmia detection using an autoregressive model and Uhley (20) uses trendrecording for the same purpose.

Model based trend prediction is relatively new and complex and sofar very few results have been published. The model for human respiration as developed by Dickinson (21) probably comes closest; optimal therapy is found by trial and error, and the adaptation of the model to the patient is possible to a limited extent.

The results are promising and further improvement of the adaptation and optimization procedures are in progress.

3.5.4. DISCUSSION

It is clear that all three methods operate at a different level of sophistication and that a certain hierarchy can be distinguished. Prognosis is certainly the oldest technique amongst the three. Yet, relatively few methods are in clinical use. The concept of trend is gaining popularity. Experimental and commercial equipment is becoming available for displaying trends in one signal, or more signals simultaneously. Yet each time-plot represents the development of one single signal and no information is extracted from coincidence of changes or other signal properties. The use of prognostic indices seems very useful for patient management in general. For the more limited application in the intensive care unit, the combination of instantaneously measured quantities, with easy availability of information about the past values in terms of trends seems to hold promises for the future in patient monitoring.

Another possibility in this area is a combination: i.e. develop a method that looks at trends in prognostic indices. This seems logical, since the prognostic index is a weighted combination of a number of variables relevant for the patient's condition. The development with time of such an index must show information about the development of the patient's state.

Trendprediction is a sophisticated method which has not yet found much clinical application. However it is felt that this is the most promising approach. It opens up the possibility for an integrated view of the patient in which the relative importance of certain

patient variables is automatically taken into account.
This model based approach forces the user to think in quantitative
terms. Compressing all the available information in a patient model
is the best way of data reduction.
This patient model is the basis for finding the optimal therapy.

REFERENCES

1. Armitage P, EA Gehan: Statistical methods for the identification
   and use of prognostic factors. Int J Cancer 13: 16, 1974.
2. Afifi AA, ST Sacks, VY Liu, et al: Accumulative prognostic index
   for patients with barbiturate gluthemide and meprobate intoxica-
   tion. N Engl J Med 285: 1497, 1971.
3. Shoemaker WC: Pathophysiology and therapy of shock in: Proc. 8th
   Pfizer Symposium. Eds. Wolker and Taylor. Churchill - Livingsto-
   ne Edinburgh Chapter 6 p 51, 1975.
4. Attinger EO: Computer models using monitored physiological variables in an intensive care unit. Automedica 1: 3, 1973.
5. Taylor DEM: Probabilistic trend detection: implementation theo-
   ry. Chartridge Symposium Seried: Realtime computing in patient
   monitoring. Ed. by J.P. Payne & D.W. Hill, Peter Peregrinus Ltd.
   p 175, 1976.
6. Hitchings DJ, MJ Campbell, DEM Taylor: Trend detection of pseu-
   do-random variables using an exponentially mapped past statistical approach: an adjunct to computer assisted monitoring. Int
   J Biomed Comp 6: 73, 1975a.
7. Hope CE, CD Leurs, IR Perry et al: Computed trend analysis in
   automated patient monitoring systems. Brit J Anaesth 45: 440,
   1973.
8. Beneken JEW, M Sluyter, JA Blom: Computer models of halothane
   anaesthesia: application leading to Servo-anesthesia. In: Measurement in Anaesthesia, Leiden University Press, p 183, 1974.
9. Blom JA: Automatic control applied to patient intensive care.
   27th ACEMB, Philadelphia, p 261, 1974.
10. Blom JA: Trendprediction and automated therapy in patient inten-
    sive care. In: Computers in Cardiology, Rotterdam, p 213, 1975.
11. Gallitz T, P Sandel, M Haider et al: Zur prognostischen Bertei-
    lung beim akuten Myokardinfarkt. Verh Dtsch Ges Inn Med 80:
    1048, 1974.
12. Peel AAF, T Semple, I Wang, et al: A coronary prognostic index
    for grading the severity of infarction. Br Heart J 24: 745, 1962.
13. Arnould JL, A Saajian, JA Fonderai, et al: Les Données hemodyna-
    miques dans l'appréciation du prognostic de l'infarctus de myo-
    carde. Acta Card. 30: 181, 1975.
14. De Rhomatis M, G Oddone : Indici prognostici immediati nell'in-
    farto miocardico. Min Cardioang 19: 513, 1971.

15. Gallitz T, P Sandel, M Haider, et al: Zur prognostischen Bertei-
    lung beim akuten Miokardinfarkt. Deuts Med Wochenschrift 49:
    2517, 1975.
16. Michat L, C Cabrol, I Brdowski, et al: Prognostic assisté sur
    ordinateur. La Nouvelle Presse Med 3: 679, 1974.
17. Boothroyd MA, M Demeester, A Swietochowski, et al: Implemen-
    tation aspects of a CCU arrhythmia monitoring system. Proc IEEE
    Comp Soc, Computers in Cardiology, p 175, 1975.
18. Haywood LJ, SA Saltzberg, VK Murthy, et al: Clinical use of R-R
    interval prediction of ECG monitoring: time series analysis by
    autoregressive models. J Assn Advan Med Instrum 6: 111, 1972.

3.6. PROBLEMS WITH INSTRUMENTATION FOR MONITORING
A.H. Engelse, C. Zeelenberg, M.R. Hoare

3.6.1. INTRODUCTION

The last decade has seen some significant advances in the management
and care of the critically ill patient. One major advance was the
introduction of highly specialised units dedicated to the care of
such specific conditions as coronary incident or shock. While the
medical problems encountered in these units vary widely, the manage-
rial and technical aspects exhibit many common elements. The patients require constant surveillance from the clinical staff; for
optimal therapy they also need frequent, accurate detailed measurement of many physiological parameters and signals. This means that
modern technology in general, and computers in particular, have come
to play an increasingly important role and today form an integral ,
not to say intrinsic, part of the concept of 'Intensive Care'.
Computer analysis of physiological signals was initially largely an
offline process on the large central digital computers of University
Hospitals. By the mid-1960's, the advent of the early minicomputers
made online, and even real-time, signal analysis feasible and several institutions explored the possibilities (1-2) while, at the same
time, various research teams looked at ways to improve and extend
the by now traditional methods of signal monitoring with 'hard-
wired' analog and digital logic (3). By this time the users of large
systems were also experimenting more with online analysis, although
the stringent requirements of 'hard' real-time usually meant that
some degree of compromise was necessary in terms of front-end
preprocessing. The latter was also true of the mini-based systems
handling large numbers of beds. Most of these systems, large or
small, used terminals with special purpose keyboards at bedside
and/or nurse station to provide the necessary communication between
clinical staff and computer. Most of these early developments were
specifically directed towards either Coronary Care applications (4,
5) or else towards Post-operative (6, 7), Respiratory monitoring
(8), or other specialist fields of Intensive Care. A few institutions combined two or more of these applications in a single system
(9).
The different fields of Intensive care monitoring varied both in
approach and in typical applications. The 'CCU system', for example,
in general concentrated heavily on detailed ECG monitoring, in
particular on the detection of PVC's and other ventricular dysrhythmias. Post-operative monitoring, on the other hand, was largely

concerned with stabilisation of the patient after open heart surgery, and thus with the continuous or intermittent monitoring of a large number of different signals: pressure, temperature, ECG and, perhaps above all in terms of time, fluid balance. Closed loop operation, non existent in Coronary Care, was here used with great effect by a couple of institutions (10).

By the middle of the next decade, however, the online digital computer system had extended its range and become a fairly common feature in large scale ICU's. The typical system at this time was a dedicated minicomputer servicing a number of beds simultaneously. The traditional analog system, the bedside monitor, was usually used in parallel and, in practice, most systems used the bedside monitors to condition and sometimes to preprocess the signals for input to the analog-digital converters of the computer system. Most of these systems were in fact essentially the same as the ones designed five years earlier. The hardware was, of course, somewhat changed and applications had been extended and improved, although review papers of the period (11) show that reliability in daily clinical use was still far from optimal, and operation often inconvenient for the clinical staff.

The one constant factor in all these systems, and certainly one of the main sources of difficulty, was the analog front-end equipment. Its existence caused many problems, not least because its output often differed from that of the usually more exact digital equipment. Signal calibration and connection were not simplified by the dual apparatus. Heavy filtering and often pre-processing in the analog equipment might have unforeseeable repercussions in the digital programs. A profusion of different types of plugs, sockets, dials, meters and keys, some relating to the computer and some to the analog monitor caused further confusion, particularly during training, and the ability to affect the characteristics of the signal being monitored digitally by merely altering settings on the front-end could obviously adversely impact system operation. Finally, the necessary cabling and the physical duplication of much equipment helped to make the digital computer systems barely economic. However, the analog front-end was far from being the only problem area in the by now 'typical' dedicated ICU monitoring system of the 1970's. The application programs themselves needed constant improvement, often necessitating considerable research, and of course highly trained staff. Many of the systems were essentially 'one of a kind', limited to the large University Centres and their satellites. The minicomputers themselves, although small, cheap and flexible in comparison to the large central main-frames were still physically large and fairly expensive, and were limited in both memory size and speed with few systems able to handle more than six to eight beds simultaneously. Hardware reliability was generally quite good, though many institutions preferred to have a complete back-up system as well. Price considerations meant that such systems were usually obliged to handle multiple beds, thus still retaining some of the features and disadvantages common to centralised systems. Data transmission caused many problems since the computer was still unsuited for use within the clinical area (temperature, noise, safety considerations). Both cabling and telemetry had many drawbacks, with the most important being installation cost and maintenance for the former, artifact and unreliability for the latter. Finally, these systems required highly skilled specialised people to run them. In-house system needed a development and maintenance staff in addition, while commercial systems either allowed few or no modifications or else again required specialised personnel. Modifications to the front-end equipment were usually impossible. Hardware maintenance was normally carried out by the manufacturer and consequently mean response time for repairs was, and is, an important factor both in selecting system components and in customer satisfaction. Some in-house systems contained specially designed hardware, often necessitating more skilled personnel for its development and maintenance.

3.6.2. DESCRIPTION OF THE SYSTEM

In the mid-1970's a new phenomenon, the microprocessor - the now ubiquitous 'chip' - made its first appearance. One or two research teams were already experimenting with attempts to simplify or even eliminate tha analog front-end and the cabling which were the source of so many problems. The advent of the microprocessor stimulated this research, resulting in a number of different 'computer per bed' systems becoming available (12). The term 'microprocessor' covers almost as many different types of equipment as does the term 'computer' and many different ones were applied to monitoring. The approaches taken varied almost as widely from straightforward replacement of analog or digital logic in the front-end, through connecting the result to an intelligent microcomputer (or minicomputer) for data storage to the fully integrated design in which the whole structure, analog front-end and central computer, was replaced by a hierarchical network of microcomputers with 'intellingence' distributed over the network. It is the latter approach which will now be considered in more detail.

3.6.3. MATERIAL AND METHODS

The Thoraxcentre in Rotterdam has been working with computer-aided patient monitoring since the end of the 1960's. Two in-house systems were developed, a 'large' system for general ICU monitoring (13) and

a 'small' system, for ECG monitoring only for pre-Coronary Care
(14). Experience with these systems had involved many of the problems previously described, and had led to considerable dissati-
sfaction with the centralised approach. The system now operational
at the Thoraxcentre incorporates many points intended to reduce or
eliminate the difficulties encountered with the previous generation.
The system was designed as a hierarchical network of microcomputers
(15). The base level is made up of a single type of unit, the Unibed
(16). Each Unibed combines the functions of front-end and signal
processor and can be used completely stand-alone (Fig.1). In practice, however, one or more Unibeds are usually coupled via a standard
serial link to another microcomputer at the nurse station to provide
time-trend graphics, strip recording, alarm setting and other centralised functions. Should a Unibed cease to work it may be replaced
without affecting the rest of the network while failure of the nurse
station will cut out the nurse station functions (graphics, strip
recorder etc.) without endangering the bedside Unibed operation. In
this way the system attempts to provide one of the primary requisi-
tes for this type of equipment, 'fail-soft'. The nurse stations in
their turn may be linked to a higher level, say for database and
long term statistics.

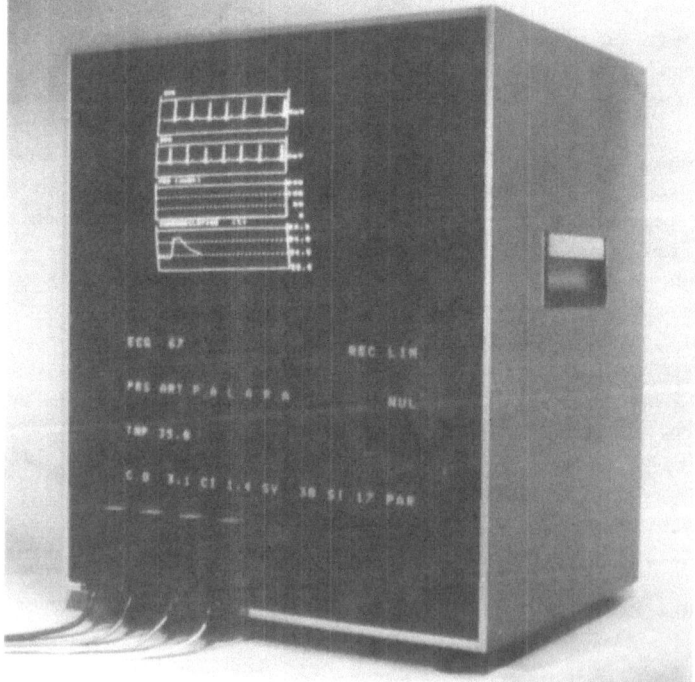

Fig. 1. The Unibed.

Each Unibed is made up of four basic elements: the command modules, the LSI-11 microcomputer, the video display and the Unibox with its power supply, mounting rack for LSI-11 and command modules and sockets for the transducer plugs.

To the user, the command module appears as the intelligent component of the Unibed, although it is infact operating as a computer peripheral. A Unibox can contain a number of identical and completely interchangeable command modules (typically four or six). A command module has two identifiable tasks the patient and the user interface. The patient interface consists of a very versatile four channel amplifier, analog multiplex, analog to digital converter, a 16 bit digital interface and all the required patient isolation circuitry. Because of its unique structure, the analog subsystem is capable of handling signals from many different physiological transducers. The signal dependent characteristics such as gain, input impedance and frequency response are determined by circuitry in the actual signal plug. Fig. 2 illustrates this structure whereby, for example, an ECG plug, plugged into any command module, form together a complete ECG amplifier. Plugs are designed for handling signals from a single

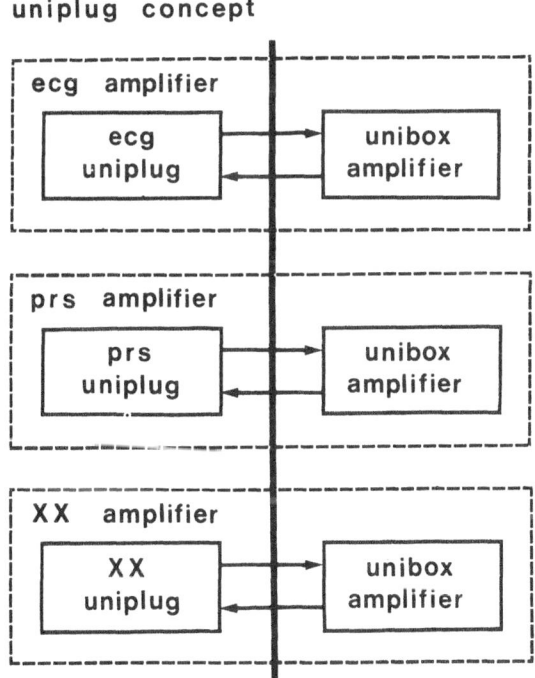

Fig. 2.

lead ECG (with defibrillation protection and electrodes loose detection), a pressure transducer, a dual temperature probe, and a thermodilution cardiac output catheter. The signal plug also generates an identification code on four of the digital input lines. Whenever the executive detects a coded plug, it activates the corresponding firmware application module.

The most striking feature of the command module, and of the Unibox as a whole, is that there are no buttons, or meters of any kind, only sockets for the transducer plugs. With the exception of signal traces, which appear on the video display unit, all communication and interaction with the Unibed makes use of the touch sensitive LED character display ('touch-line'). Since the latter can act as a computer terminal, it is available to the application programs for the presentation of numeric data, text information, alarm messages, action requests, etc. Continuously updated values of the more important parameters are displayed here whenever a signal is monitored. Interaction between system and user is basically initiated and controlled by the computer. Once an application has been activated by plugging in the required signal, the user is guided through procedures by prompts from the application program appearing on the touch-line. Certain actions, such as limit setting can be performed at any time and are initiated whenever the computer senses that a character of a given command module has been touched.

The video display unit is, like the command module, a computer peripheral. It operates entirely under control of the microcomputer. The unit is capable of displaying four signal traces with calibration lines, as well as 32 lines of 32 characters each of textual information. Signal traces are displayed with normalised gain, mnemonic identification and an indication of the exact range.

The microcomputer, is responsible for controlling the entire system, handling the signal display and providing the link to the nurse station if required. The system uses a Digital Equipment LSI-11 microcomputer, chosen for its flexible architecture, range of support software, and the availability of a large number of compatible PDP-11 computer systems already in use at the development site. Both monitor and application programs are 'firmware' programmable read-only memory (EPROM) with random-access memory (RAM) as working area. New applications are debugged using a development system with MOS read/write memory and down-line loading from a 'host' PDP-11/10. Once debugged, adding a new application is a matter of programming the EPROM, plugging it into the LSI-11 and adding a suitably coded transducer plug with appropriate signal conditioning.

The Unibed firmware consists of a system executive and a set of application programs for handling the various physiological monitoring functions. Some applications (ECG, pressures, temperatures, fluid output) are primarily intended for continuous monitoring while others are by nature relatively infrequent measurements (thermodilution cardiac output). Some 'continuous' measurements may only be performed, intermittently (certain pressures), depending on the protocol to be followed by the nurse. The following example of an application (cardiac output measured by thermodilution) gives a good impression of the way in which the system interacts with the user. The module is activated whenever the executive detects the connection of a properly coded plug. The command module responds by displaying the cardiac output signal designator and a key for changing preset measurement parameters.

✳✳✳

C.O   PAR

Touching the designator 'key' starts the measurement and the command module then directs the procedure.

C.O   INJECT   10 mL AT   0 °C   PAR

When the application program detects an acceptable thermodilution curve it will integrate the signal and compute the cardiac output using the Stewart-Hamilton formula.

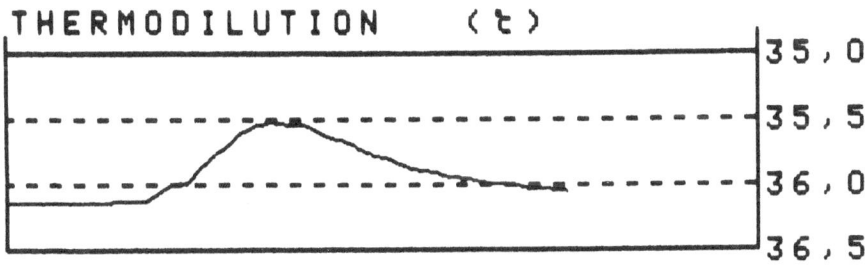

THERMODILUTION   (°C)
35,0
35,5
36,0
36,5

C.O   4.8   PAR

Communication between application modules is possible. The thermodilution module checks the ECG module to see if the heart rate is available and, if so, calculates the stroke volume.

ECG 74   LIM

C.O 4.8 SV 65   PAR

The values for the patient's body surface area, the temperature and
volume of the injectade and the catheter number can be modified by
touching the PAR key. The module will respond by displaying the
default numbers; touching the individual digits will increment their
values.

C.O BS 0.0 0   TI 0 0   VI 1 0   7F

C.O BS 1.0 0   TI 0 0   VI 1 0   7F

C.O BS 2.0 0   TI 0 0   VI 1 0   7F

Returning to the cardiac output display, by touching the C.O. key,
will recalculate the values using the newly entered numbers. Now,
using the body surface area, the application module also computes
the cardiac and stroke index.

C.O 4.8 CI 2.4 SV 65 SI 32 PAR

3.6.4. CONCLUSIONS

Over the last two decades, computers have become an integral part of
the concept 'Intensive Care' and few large CCU's or ICU's lack some
type of computer assistance. Third generation, microcomputer based
systems are helping to solve many of the earlier problems. Features
such as touch sensitive keys or screens (eliminating keyboards) and
integrated front-end with automatic gain control, together with
simplified procedures, are greatly increasing user acceptance. The
basic signals monitored, however, are virtually unchanged. The
pattern recognition programs for monitoring which are in general use
today are still susceptible to artifact.
Yet ECG quality, for instance, is still mainly a question of correct
electrode placement, ensuring good contact and keeping the patient
quiet. Pressures, and cardiac output, are monitored with in-dwelling
catheters, with all their attendant risks. The techiques available
for improving signal quality may be unpleasant for the patient and
may not be completely without risk. Non invasive methods for pressu-

re and flow measurement are still in their infancy and the problems of new electrode systems, such as oesophageal leads, are far from solved. Yet now that sufficient computer power can be available at every bed it is surely time to start concentrating on new techniques and new applications as well as on improving existing ones. Computer systems should be used to improve patient care in the wider sense of these words. We must await in depth evaluations of third generation systems to see whether or not they fulfil this aim and provide a truly valuable aid for the clinical staff of the CCU.

REFERENCES

1. Shubin H, MH Weil, MA Jr Rockwell: Automated measurement of arterial pressure in patients by use of a digital computer. Med Biol Eng 5: 361, 1967.
2. Osborn JJ, JO Beaumont, MA Raison, et al: Measurement and monitoring of acutely ill patients by digital computer. Surgery 6: 1057, 1968.
3. Neilson JM, CW Vellani: Computer detection and analysis of ventricular ectopic rhythms. In: Quantitation in cardiology (Boerhaave series), ed HA Snellen, HC Hemker, PG Hugenholtz and JH van Bemmel, p 117, Leiden University Press, 1972.
4. Cox JR, FM Nolle, HA Fozzard, et al: AZTEC, a preprocessing program for real-time ECG rhythm analysis. IEEE Trans Biomed Eng BME-15: 128, 1968.
5. Feldman CL, PG Amazeen, MD Klein, et al: Computer detection of ventricular ectopic beats. Comput Biomed Res 3: 666, 1970.
6. Gardner RM, HR Warner, AF Toronto, et al: Automated computer-based bedside monitoring of post-operative cardiac patients. Digest 7th Int'l Conf Med Biol Eng, Stockholm 7: 300, 1967.
7. Sheppard LC, NT Kouchoukos, MA Kurtts, et al: Automated treatment of critically ill patients following operation. Ann Surg 168: 596, 1968.
8. Osborn JJ, JO Beaumont, JCA Raison, et al: Computation for quantitative on line measurements in an Intensive Care Ward. In: Computers in Biomedical Research, Vol. III, RW Stacy and B Waxman Eds, Academic Press, New York, 1969.
9. Miller AC, JAC Russel, PR Harris, et al: A modular approach to an intensive care patient monitoring system. Proceedings DECUS conference, Fall 1969.
10. Sheppard LC, NT Kouchoukos, JF Shotts, et al: Regulation of mean arterial pressure by computer control of vasoactive agents in post-operative patients. Proceedings Computers in Cardiology, IEEE Computer Society no. 75CH1018-1C, p 91, 1975.
11. Drazen E, AE Wechsler: Evaluation of computer-based patient monitoring systems. By Arthur D. Little, Cambridge, Massachu-

124

setts, National Center for Health Services Research and Development No. HSM 110-70-406, 1973.

12. Willems JL, J Peperstraete: Cardiac arrhythmia monitoring based on special purpose analog-and micro-processors within the E.E.C., survey report contract 338-77-7 ECI B, Leuven, Belgium, October 1978.

13. Zeelenberg C, MR Hoare, WAH Engelse, et al: Arrhythmia monitoring at the Thoraxcentrum, Rotterdam. Proceedings Computers in Cardiology, IEEE Computer Society no. 74CH0879-7C, p 203, 1974.

14. Zeelenberg C, LS Deutsch, WAH Engelse, et al: Experiences with implementing ARGUS in a cardiac surveillance unit. Proc Trends in computer-processed ECG's, p 31, Amsterdam, 1976.

15. Zeelenberg C, WAH Engelse, LS Deutsch: A hierarchical patient monitoring computer network. Proc. Computers in Cardiology, IEEE Computer Society no 77CH1245-2C, p 439, 1977.

16. Deutsch LS, AH Engelse, C Zeelenberg, et al: The Unibed patient monitoring system: a new approach for a new technology. Medical Instrumentation, vol 11, no 5, p 274, 1977.

DISCUSSION: CHAPTER 3

Chairman: P.G. Hugenholtz

DISCUSSION CHAPTER 3

Paper 2: Hemodynamic monitoring in AMI for prognosis assessment of survival and incidence of reinfarction.

BENEKEN: From one of your slides that related the cardiac index with wedge pressure, there was a kind of uniform relationship between the two. Did you ever test the prognosis if you use only one of these variables? If this relationship is similar then you may not need both.

RUDOLPH: No, until now we didn't do it but I believe it would be enough to measure the pulmonary capillary wedge pressure in order to get a good information on the hemodynamic status of the patient.

HUGENHOLTZ: I can give a partial answer to Dr. Beneken. We have looked at this problem sóme years ago. Multivaried analysis showed that three factors had independent information, although they were closely related: 1) the pulmonary capillary wedge, 2) the cardiac output and the mixed venus oxygen saturation, 3) the diastolic systemic blood pressure.

I think one of the recommendations again from this Group to the European Community Authorities should be that attention should be given to the patients who have borderline but distinct abnormalities in these three parameters. These seem to require further intensive attention. Our low mortality rates in the coronary care unit may be possibly related to the attention we have paid to that group. We now have experience with over 225 balloon pump cases, many of which now are selected from this in between group. We actually have now a trial where we assign, randomly, patients with a big myocardial infarction, usually anterior, with a moderate elevation of pulmonary capillary wedge and with or without change in mixed venus oxygen saturation, to pump versus non pump. We hope in a year to be able to report whether this has decreased the mortality in that group.

Perhaps later we will all talk about the significance of other indicators in terms of their prognosis, because we should try to make a stratification of the risk of the patient. Again there I think we have a lot of work to do before we can made a definite decision. But the coronary care unit has a role in this research for trying to reduce this 10 % mortality even down to 5 %.

PESOLA: I'd just like to ask Prof. Rudolph how the patients were treated, because I am a little bit surprised that there was no change in wedge pressure with time. And I wonder for instance, if they had afterload reduction as part of their treatment.

RUDOLPH: Our conclusions are mostly based on patients with normal cardiac output and normal wedge pressure. This is our biggest group.

Paper 3: Hemodynamic monitoring in AMI: significance of prognostic indexes.

JULIAN: One hears a great number of papers on prognostic indexes validated on retrospective data and one would always like to see the same prognostic index validated prospectively. And this very seldom happens. Can you tell me whether you have validated your data prospectively? In other words, having elaborated your prognostic index have you then applied it to a new population of patients?
MARCHIONNI: No, this index is not verified a priori, up to this time, it is verified only a posterior. Our program is obviously to verify this index based on this previous 227 patient series to a next series of patients.

Paper 5: Prognostic indexes, trend detection and prediction techniques.

HUGENHOLTZ: Thank you very much, Prof. Beneken, for reminding us of what we should be doing. The problem I always find with this is a bit like weather forecasting. You have these wonderful predictions of what we ought to know, and of what we ought to do, but I always get wet because I don't carry my coat with me when it seems to be raining. Perhaps we could have just one set of data at one given time that at least are in close approximation in time and then the patient wants to sleep, and you have to go away. So it's very difficult to get the data to fit what you need for your model.
BENEKEN: Well, the essential point that I wanted to make is that we should not look into one signal by itself but at a cumulation of different signals. You just supply the data which you have already available and then by doing this kind of analysis you can find out for instance, that a certain signal is not important because it's redundant. And there is no way, by intuitive means, to find this out. This is one example where, in fact, this kind of approach can yield to reduction of the load to the patient. I am applying this approach to all patients in the operative theatre where you measure circulatory and respiratory variables, temperatures, the blood chemistry and so on. We already observe that the whole procedure becomes more stable, that less anesthetic needs to be given to the patient and that the patients wake up in a much better condition than they did before.

Paper 6: Lines of development of instrumentation for hemodynamic monitoring in CCU.

BALCON: Thank you for a beautiful illustration of what can be done. I'd just like to know how you eventually store the information of each patient for subsequent group statistical analysis?

ENGELSE: This is just the beginning and the nurses station, that I described, will eventually be connected to a larger computer system for data reduction, and for transmission of information to a central computer.

BALCON: Our experience with the PDP 9, which gave us 24 hour plots turned out to be used very little. There were few people who analysed some groups of patients for prognostic index in terms of that data, but the majority of the patient records are still nicely stacked somewhere in the corner. So we have put the routine of storing at a very low level of our priorities. There is a 24 hour time plot which comes off the printer and goes into the patient record, and the rest is thrown away.

CAMERINI: My question is a general one thinking to what Maseri said today, if you are thinking of the mean coronary units in the Community. I would like to ask the speakers and our Chairman, which are the indications for hemodynamic monitoring in patients who are in a mean coronary care unit? Have we to catetherize all patients, or just a group? And which type of patients need hemodynamic monitoring? Is it correct to go on with pharmacological intervention, as afterload reducing, or what you like, without hemodynamic monitoring? Are we suggesting that all coronary units, there are about 150 I think in Italy, and I don't know the number in Europe, need a hemodynamic facility, or not? Thank you.

HUGENHOLTZ: I think it is a terribly relevant question and I would take the prerogative of the Chair to try and formulate an answer and then ask for dissident opinions. First of all, there is the matter of size and organization. I believe that if you cannot staff, run and occupy efficiently a four-bed unit as a minimum, you shouldn't begin with hemodynamic monitoring. The four-bed or higher unit should have, I believe, some beds instrumented for monitoring the right side of the heart through a Swan-Ganz and arterial pressures. I think these parameters are useful for the control of the level of infusion of drugs. If you begin with that type of pharmacological intervention, or you do balloon pumping, or you are having a link with the surgical unit, you must have these facilities.

MASERI: I believe that at the present state of knowledge the selection of patients to be monitored invasively depends largely on the current research problems the unit is involved in. We did not have a Cardiac Surgery in Pisa so far, thus we were not under the pressure nor under the attraction of generalized surgical approach nor of balloon pumping. Our research interests were lately concentrated on monitoring preinfarction angina, thus we confined ourselves to monitoring only the really unstable patients who represent about 5 % of our population of patients with acute myocardial infarction. We found that clinical experience gained by dealing with these patients over the years, non invasive measurements and chest X-ray are usually sufficient for a satisfactory medical treatment of the patients. How about you Dr. Julian, what's the percent of patients who you submit to hemodynamic monitoring in your unit?

JULIAN: It is about 5 %.

BERNARD: I think that we agree that if you have a research unit and if you are experimenting new drugs, you need to have hemodynamic control. But is it of value to put a catheter and to measure pressures and cardiac output in all patients of your unit to determine prognostic indexes? In my opinion, it is research work, very interesting research work, very heavy research work, but it should perhaps be said in the records.

HUGENHOLTZ: I think there should be still such a thing as is called the clinical judgement. I think that if the patient looks good and he has had his classic infarct but he is pain free then we quiotly leave him in his little corner, and we don't touch him. But I thought we only were talking about the patient who has troubles, and when he has troubles which is again initially a clinical judgement, then the small unit I don't think should hold that patient. I think that patient should be transferred to a larger unit which has the facilities. And that particular step having been done, then the package available for the monitoring can increase to what we have been talking about earlier.

MASERI: I'd like to have your opinion, and the opinion of the audience on two points. Besides the identification of the patients who would benefit from invasive hemodynamic monitoring. 1) It is important that we realize that it's not only a matter of equipment. It is also a matter of training and basic preparation of the people in charge of the coronary care. So it is not enough that we do have facilities for cardiac catheterization and for putting in a Swan-Ganz. Care in the sense of following very carefully the patient is even more important than this simple fact of having the facilities for putting in catheters. 2) Should we have intermittent measurements from time to time, invasive or not invasive and if so, how often? Do you think that studies should be done to try to evaluate how much we gain by having a continuous computerized monitoring with trend analysis rather than intermittent measurements which are a much simpler thing?

JULIAN: I am very worried about what recommendations we might produce. I known in my own particular area we have 20 coronary care units but only 2 of these are, have the equipment and more importantly the expertise to do detailed hemodynamic studies. And I am sure this is not unique to our experience. Dr. Hugenholtz says, 'Okay, we should identify the high risk patients and transfer them'. But this is really not very practicable when if we take Prof. Rudolph's material, there is quite a substantial percentage of patients who have hemodynamic disturbances in the sense of raised coronary wedge pressures, or low outputs. It's maybe, 20 or 30 %; it is a significant per cent. We can't transfer all those patients to a unit; and I think we have got to accept therefore that what we call district hospitals have to use the simplest non invasive methods of assessing these patients. And the kind of things that Dr. Hejkkilä referred to is something that almost anybody could do. And I think we have got do depend on these things. And we have to define, obviously on research units which must correlate the hemodynamic data with the simple clinical, and non invasive data. And that's what we still have to do satisfactorily, I think. But I don't see any way in which we can expect a universal application of hemodynamic monitoring.

HUGENHOLTZ: So your answer to the organizational question that Dr. Maseri posed is the hierarchy of systems must be built out there where this local or regional situation lends itself for district hospitals versus overhead type of hospitals. That is an individual choice that has to be made by the local circumstances. I would strongly subscrive to that opinion, but it still has to be a two-tier or perhaps three-tier approach in which the quickness of the transport to the communications determines the outcome of the patient. It is not that we don't have the techniques. It is the delay in getting them from the front to the hospital basically which is what it's all about.

The second point that Dr. Maseri raised is the matter of what is the value of continuous monitoring and of the display. I think Chierchia's paper has shown very beautifully that you can see things better if you have, shall we say, a trend recording and trend plot. And I think Beneken would go along as that is a beautiful set of data to work from, if you had to really go and use mathematics thereafter. And we've chosen it as we've shown in the last two slides; we showed to have that option available from the many that we have discussed in the past with our doctors. So I'm a step ahead of you in the sense that I am convinced that any modern device used in an intensive care setting of the top tier must have trend plots of this type available because there is little doubt that they will show you at unpredictable moments highly relevant information.

PRASQUIER: I would like to ask a question on rather a different topic. Cardiac rupture is one of the most significant causes of mortality in our coronary care unit. It has become something which I do not see any preventive measure for. And this has been more than 30 % of our mortality in the last times, so I just wonder what we could do to reduce this kind of mortality?

FERUGLIO: Yes, 27 % of our deaths in the coronary care units are due to rupture.

DISTANTE: On my thesis which was on rupture of the heart, as a complication of myocardial infarction in CCU in Pavia, I found a 25% incidence of rupture as cause of death without the use of cortisone.

HUGENHOLTZ: We have been running in the 15 % range, no more.

MARCHIONNI: We had a 30 % incidence rate of cardiac rupture as causes of death in a series of 500 deaths controlled with autoptic study.

HUGENHOLTZ: I think the very 'first perspective everybody in this room should have relates to the fact that CCU's are only one cork in a total system of care. In other words, what we are talking about in what is necessary in these different levels requires, first of all, decision making of high level, high quality at the beginning, that is, the general practitioners. And the training that Dr. Maseri brought up I think should be an activity of this group, the carrying out of this type of information, how to choose, with what to choose, is one of the jobs of this group. And my final comment is that for those of you who are interested, we have now made an admission sheet for patients with acute myocardial infarction which after 4 years of trying with fellows and trainess is quite acceptable to all staff. These forms are available and if everybody would fill in the same forms reliably, perhaps we could start getting some vital statistics.

CHAPTER 4

CLINICAL ASPECTS AND NEW RESEARCH LINES ON PREINFARCTION
ANGINA

4.1. INTRODUCTION

A. Maseri

This session deals with a rather different aspect of those that have been discussed yesterday and this morning, because it is meant to explore the problems of the coronary care in the research environment for the definition of fields of possible future, concerted research.

The mean field of interest, so far, has been that of detection and prevention of arrhythmias. We have heard this morning and in the second part of yesterday afternoon, that interest is now expanding to the detection of pump dysfunction in acute myocardial infarction either by non invasive techniques, as we heard yesterday, or by invasive techniques as we have been discussing this morning. Something caught my attention as I heard Professor Hugenholtz saying: 'I don't know how, but for many, many years we just didn't look at something which now appears to give good results. We haven't looked at myocardial infarction patients with echocardiography and yet we are discovering that this technique may give us unexpectedly useful information at a relatively low price'. Thus I wish to invite you to try and apply this logic to two examples that came up in discussion this morning and that just serve the purpose of introducing this session.

A. We heard in the presentation of Professor Hugenholtz that about 25 % to 30 % of the patients admitted to their CCU's, were admitted because of risk of infarction, indicated by some premonitory signs. So patients with 'impending infarction' represent a rather high proportion of those admitted to CCU.

B. We heard from Professor Rudolph that a sizable number of patients had reinfarction, during their stay in CCU.

Indeed, just in these patients we could be able to prevent infarction altogether. Therefore, these are two aspects that stimulate my personal interest. Although the general trend, especially in the United States, in the environment of research in coronary care, is entirely oriented towards a reduction of infarct size, I believe that the following areas deserve interest:

1. the investigation of the patients admitted because of threatening myocardial infarction, if we could begin to understand something about the causes of myocardial infarction in these patients, we could treat them specifically and try to prevent the infarction;

2. the possibility of preventing reinfarction, which as we heard, occurs rather frequently;

3. the possibility of identifying the 25 %–30 % of patients who are going to die because of cardiac rupture.

4.2. PREINFARCTION ANGINA: REVIEW OF 67 CONSECUTIVE PATIENTS ADMIT-
TED TO CCU
R. Rocci, F. Mauri, A. Mantero, F. Faletra, F. Rovelli

4.2.1. INTRODUCTION

A clinical syndrome whose cardinal feature is changing pattern of
previous stable angina or new appearance of progressive angina is
frequently reported during the period immediately preceding myocardial infarction. Forthy three per cent of 377 patients admitted to
our Coronary Care Unit for acute myocardial infarction from January
1977 to June 1978 experienced this 'preinfarction' angina.
A study of this population is quite difficult because, unfortunately, patients come to our observation when myocardial infarction has
already taken place. We decided therefore to study people admitted
during the same period with similar symptoms, generally grouped
under the term 'unstable' angina, since their progression to myocardial infarction is frequent (1-4). We limited our observation to
this relatively short period of time in order to collect patients
admitted with uniform criteria and who received substantially the
same treatment.

4.2.2. PATIENTS

Our report refers to 67 patients admitted to Coronary Care Unit of
Centro Cardiologico A. De Gasperis for
1. prolonged or recurrent pain not relieved by usual therapy in
   patients with known chronic angina
2. first appearance of pain consistent with a cardiac origin unrelated to obvious precipitating factors
in whom myocardial infarction could be excluded on admission on the
basis of electrocardiograms and serum enzyme levels.
They represent 7.8 per cent of 849 patients admitted to our Coronary
Care Unit during the same period, and should be considered a selected population because only patients with relevant symptoms have
been sent to intensive care.
These patients have been divided in three groups:
A. Group I : Progressive angina, including 34 subjects suffering
   from chronic angina who experienced a sudden increase of frequency of spontaneous pain or prolonged pain not relieved by usual
   treatment.
B. Group II: Recent angina, including 20 subjects who experienced

Table 1

		I	II	III
AGE	MEAN	53.7	55.6	52.9
	± S.D.	9.5	10.3	9.1
SEX	M	27	16	13
	F	7	4	0

Table 2

	I	II	III
Smoking	25	12	9
Inheritance	13	8	4
Hyperlipidemia	11	6	0
Hypertension	6	5	2
Diabetes	5	0	0

for the first time in the few days before admission prolonged or recurring anginal pain, not related to obvious precipitating factors.

C. Group III: Variant angina, including 13 patients in whom pain at rest was accompanied by transient ST segment elevation.

Average age, 54 years in total population, did not differ in the three groups. Also sex distribution, with prevalence of males, did not significantly differ in the three groups (Table 1). Incidence of main risk factors for coronary disease (inheritance, diabetes, hyperlipidemia, hypertension, smoking) arc summarized in Table 2. Here again no difference has been found between the three groups. Physical examination has been generally non specific. Only in 4 patients of group I we did find signs of left ventricular failure.

Table 3. Control ECG

	I	II	III
Normal	11 (32 %)	8 (40 %)	6 (46 %)
Altered ST-T	23 (68 %)	10 (50 %)	7 (54 %)
Previous M.I.	10 (29 %)	7 (35 %)	4 (30 %)

Table 4. ECG changes during angina

	I	II	III
Unchanged	8	6	0
Altered ST-T	16	6	12
Arrhythmias	3	1	2

4.2.3. RESULTS

Control electrocardiograms are summarized in Table 3. A normal
electrocardiogram has been found in 32 per cent of patients with
progressive angina, in 40 per cent of patients with recent angina
and in 46 per cent of patients with variant angina. Incidence of
signs of previous myocardial infarction was 29 per cent in group I,
35 per cent in group II, 30 per cent in group III respectively,
while altered ST-T segments has been found in 68 per cent of group
I, 50 per cent of group II, 54 per cent of group III. Twelve lead
ECG tracings were recorded in 48 patients (72 %) during episodes of
angina: 34 (70 %) exhibited ST-T changes, 14 (27 %) resulted
unchanged (Table 4). A low incidence in of arrhythmias was observed
in all groups.
Complete hemodynamic study with coronary arteriography and left
ventriculography has been performed in 53 patients; in one patient
ventriculography could not be performed for the appearance of intense pain after coronary arteriography and in another patient examination was stopped after ventriculography without performing coronary
arteriography because of hypotension.
Its generally accepted that multivessel disease is frequently found

Table 5

Vessels involved organic stenosis 50 %	I	II	III
0	1 (3 %)	1 (8 %)	1 (8.5 %)
1	7 (24 %)	7 (54 %)	6 (50 %)
2	8 (28 %)	4 (30 %)	4 (33 %)
3	13 (45 %)	1 (8 %)	1 (8.5 %)

in unstable angina (3, 5, 7). We found high incidence of three vessel disease only in group I (progressive angina). Data suggest that number of vessels involved seems to be mainly related to time course than to clinical syndrome (Table 5). Proximal left anterior descending artery was very often involved (59 %) of cases. Significant stenosis of left main coronary artery was found in 5 subjects, while in one subject transient spasm of the same vessel could be demonstrated. The 8 per cent incidence of left main coronary artery stenosis is the same that we found in a review of 1200 consecutive coronary arteriograms (7). The 24 per cent incidence of 1 vessel disease in group I and 52 per cent in groups II and III considered together, does not differ from what we found in 370 consecutive arteriograms of patients who underwent bypass surgery from 1970 to 1975.
In order to evaluate the functional significance of coronary lesions we divided the left ventricle into six areas according to coronary branches distribution as shown in Fig. 1.
Considering for each patient the number of left ventricular areas supplied by coronary branches showing critical stenoses (75 %), we did not find any difference between the groups (Table 6).
Overall left ventricular function resulted generally preserved in our patients just as reported by others (3, 5). As would be expected from a greater incidence of multivessel disease we found more frequent signs of altered left ventricular function in group I (Table 7).
Forty nine patients (73 %) were treated with isosorbide dinitrate in an average daily dosage of 60 mg. In 30 patients (44 %) this treatment was associated with calcium antagonists (Nifedipine, average daily dose 40 mg or Verapamil, from 240 to 480 mg). We associated betadrenergic blocking agent (Propanolol, average daily dose 160 mg) in 6 patients. Calcium antagonists alone were administered in 10 patients. Different treatments were used in 8 patients (Fig. 2).
Response to medical treatment in the first ten days after admission

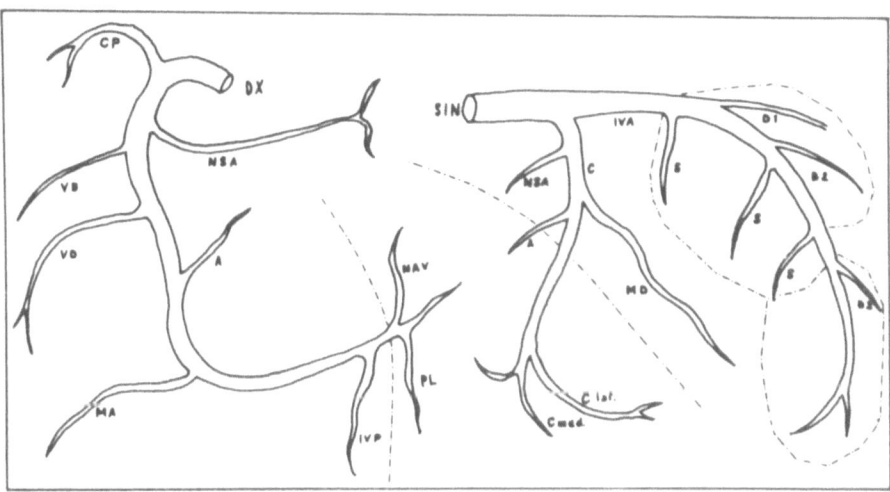

Fig. 1.

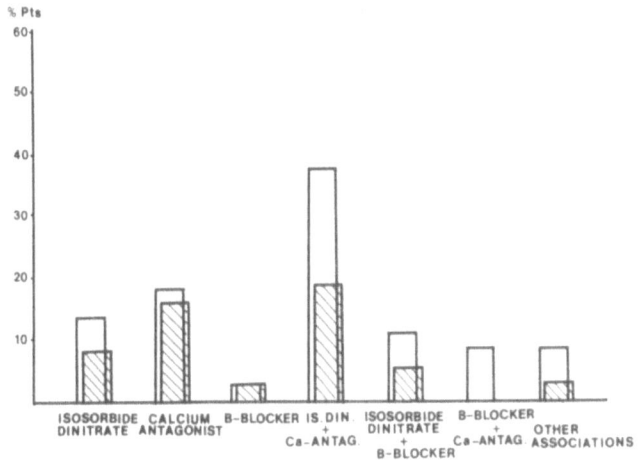

Fig. 2.

is summarized in Table 8. Complete relief from pain was achieved in 33 patients, partial relief in 24. Ten patients developed acute myocardial infarction. Two patients died, one after extensive myocardial infarction, the other of intervening pneumonia ab ingestis due to resuscitatory monoeuvres after an episode of ventricular fibrillation. All patients were treated with anticoagulants.

Patients in whom symptoms did not subside in spite of full medical therapy and complete bed rest and in whom coronary arteriography demonstrated proximal severe obstructive lesions (90 %), underwent aorto-coronary bypass surgery where the anatomical conditions were met.

140

Table 6

		I	II	III
Areas sup- plied by critically stenosed branches	MEAN	3.50	3.30	4.30
	$\pm$ S.D.	1.40	1.60	1.30

Table 7. Left ventriculography

	I	II	III
Normal	7	3	3
Segmental hypokinesia	9	8	6
Diffuse Hypokinesia	2	1	0
Segmental akinesia	8	1	0
Aneurysm	5	2	2
Mitral Regurgitation	2	1	0
LVEDP 25 mmHg	4	2	0

Table 8. Response to medical treatment
(First 10 days from admission)

	I	II	III
Complete relief of pain	15	14	6
Partial relief of pain	15	3	4
Myocardial infarction	4	3	3

These selection criteria make any comparison between operated and non operated impossible. Coronary bypass surgery was performed in 32

Table 9. Surgical treatment: short term outcome

	I	II	III
Deaths	4	2	1
M.I.	2	1	1
Favorable Outcome	11	3	7

patients (48 %), total number of grafts being 61. In one case aneurismectomy and in another case infarctectomy was also performed. Results are reported in Table 9. Seven patients died, four during emergency surgery, three during elective surgery. Four patients developed intraoperative myocardial infarction. A high mortality rate was observed in patients who undergo emergency surgical procedu res (50 % over a total of 8 cases); in patients submitted to elective surgery the mortality rate was 12.5 % over a total of 24 subjects. Twenty one patients were discharged symptom-free.

4.2.4. DISCUSSION

Rate of progression to myocardial infarction has been almost 15 %, which is very high if we consider the very short period of observation, but it does not significantly differ from what we found in previous series (10.4 %) (8) and from those reported by Duncan (9) and by Gazes (2) (respectively 13 and 17 %).
In attempt of defining criteria that could enable us to predict a poor short term outcome in individual patients, we tested the significance of the following parameters using the chi-square test corrected for non continuous data: clinical grouping, total number of risk factors, recurrent pain (three or more times daily despite rest and therapy), unequivocal ST changes during angina, coronary vessel involvement.
A higher rate of myocardial infarction was found in group III (variant angina), but difference does not reach statistical significance (Table 10). Data definitely exclude short term prognostic value of prior chronic angina in our cases. The number of risk factors does not seem to alter short term prognosis. Rate of myocardial infarction is higher in patients suffering recurrent pain while in hospital, altough it does not reach significance. ST changes during symptoms do not significantly define a subgroup with higher incidence of myocardial infarction, while recurrent angina criterion plus ST changes reaches statistical significance. Coronary vessel

Table 10. Myocardial infarction rate in groups

M.I.

I	4 (11.7%)
II	3 (15 %)
III	3 (23 %)

involvement, tested as number of stenosed main branches or number of areas supplied by stenosed coronary vessels, is not a good index of short term evolution to myocardial infarction. Similarly a poor left ventricular function is not related to short term outcome. The value of these abnormalities on long term prognosis should be tested.

4.2.5. CONCLUSIONS

Medical treatment has brought complete relief from pain most patients and a more stable condition in many others. Early surgical treatment leads to high hospital mortality and high incidence of perioperative myocardial infarction.
Early hemodynamic study does not give short term prognostic informations, while it is possible to indentify on clinical basis higher risk patients. The occurrence of acute myocardial infarction in these patients is frequent, thus this population may favour the study of the mechanisms of acute myocardial infarction.

REFERENCES

1. Krauss KR, AM Hutter, RW De Sanctis: Acute coronary insufficiency: course and follow up. Circulation 45 (Suppl. I): 66, 1972.
2. Gazes PC, EM Mobley, RC Duncan, et al: Pre-infarctional (unstable) angina: A prospective study; ten year follow up. Circulation 48: 331, 1973.
3. Bertolasi CA, JE Tronge, CA Carreno, et al: Unstable angina. Prospective and randomized study of its evolution with and without surgery. Am J Cardiol 33: 201, 1974.
4. Conti R, JR Gilbert, M Hodges, et al: Unstable angina pectoris: randomized study of surgical vs. medical therapy. Am J Cardiol 35: 129, 1975.
5. Scanlon PJ, R Nemickas, JF Moran, et al: Accelerated angina pectoris: clinical, hemodynamic, arteriographic and therapeutic

during chest pain (49 with ST segment transient depression; 8 without ST segment abnormalities during monitoring; 8 without ECG recording during pain).

Each group of patients was further divided into the following subgroups (gr.):

A. gr.1: Crescendo angina 'de novo' (4 weeks), in a patient previously free of symptoms – 40 patients in Gr. P. vs 16 patients in Gr. C (p< 0.02).

B. gr.2: Accelerated angina occuring in a patient with previously stable angina and/or old myocardial infarction: 25 patients in Gr. P vs 38 patients in Gr. C (p=0.05). In 20 patients of this subgroup (3 in Gr. P, 17 in Gr. C) the diagnosis of old myocardial infarction was made on the basis of residual Q waves in the ECG

C. gr.3: Unstable angina after recent (4 weeks) myocardial infarction: 11 patients in Gr. P vs 11 patients in Gr. C (n.s.).

D. gr.A: Prolonged pain at rest lasting more than 15 minutes, and/or status anginosus – 27 patients in Gr. P, vs 39 patients in Gr. C (n.s.).

E. gr.B: Frequent episodes of anginal pain lasting less than 15 minutes: 49 patients in Gr. P vs 39 patients in Gr. C (n.s.).

F. gr.To: Patients neither treated with antianginal drugs, nor operated (0 in Gr. P vs 11 in Gr. C).

G. gr.T1: Patients treated with antianginal drugs (betablockers; perhexiline; nifedipine; isosorbide dinitrate) – 24 in Gr. P, vs 17 in Gr. C (n.s.).

H. gr.T2: Patients operated without previous medical treatment: 17 patients in Gr. P, vs 17 in Gr. C (n.s.).

I. gr.T3: Patients operated after treatment with antianginal drugs: 35 patients in Gr. P vs 20 in Gr. C (n.s.).

Sex ratio, mean age, prevalence of risk factors (family history; hypertension; diabetes; serum colesterol 300 mg/100 ml; 20 or more cigarettes/day) were not statistically different in the two groups. Episodes of anginal pain during monitoring in coronary care unit averaged 3 $\pm$ 1.8/day in Gr. P vs 3.9 $\pm$ 2.9/day in Gr. C (n.s.). Syncopes were observed in 32.9 % of the Gr. P patients vs 7.7 % of the Gr. C patients (p<0.01).

The percentage of patients with normal resting ECG was higher in Gr. P (31.6 %) than in Gr. C (10.7 %: p 0.02). However, abnormalities of repolarization were observed in the same percentage of patients in both groups: 64.5 % in Gr. P vs 63.2 % in Gr. C. Residual Q waves, in subgroup 2, were present in 44.7 % of the Gr. C patients vs 12 % of the Gr. P patients (p<0.01).

Atrio-ventricular block was observed during chest pain in 10.5 % of the Gr. P patients vs 4.6 % of the Gr. C patients (n.s.). During anginal attack, ventricular premature beats (>5/minute) and ventricular tachycardia were statistically more frequent in Gr. P patients than in Gr. C patients, respectively.

The subjects with single vessel disease and normal arteries or without significant (70 %) stenosis were more in Gr. P (66.7 %) than in Gr. C (36.9 % : p= 0.05). In 27 patients (26 Gr. P, 1 Gr. C) coronary vasospasm was observed during a spontaneous ischemic episode. The spasm involved one vessel in 20 patients, two vessels in 6 patients, three vessels in 1 patient (right coronary 17; left anterior descending 13; left circumflex 4; left main artery 1). After sublingual nitroglycerin, the spasm was no longer visible, and the arteries appeared completely normal in 9 cases, and involved by atherosclerotic lesions in 26 cases.

According to left ventricular cineangiography, 34.3 % of the Gr. P patients had poor left ventricular function (diffuse hypokinesia and/or aneurysm) vs 56.3 % of the Gr. C patients: this difference was not statistically significant.

Over an average follow-up period of 34.8 months (Gr. P + Gr. C), 35 deaths occurred - 23 in hospital and 12 later on. Average follow-up duration was not significantly different in Gr. P (33.3 months) and Gr. C (37.6 months). Total mortality was higher in Gr. C (39 %) than in Gr. P (13.1 %: p<0.05). In both subgroups 1 (angina de novo) and 3 (angina following recent myocardial infarction), the incidence rate of mortality was not significantly higher in Gr. C than in Gr. P. Only in subgroup 2 (accelerated angina following previous stable angina), was the difference statistically significant: 45.1 % in Gr. C vs 12 % in Gr. P (p<0.05).

In both the P and C groups, ventricular arrhythmias and conduction disturbances during chest pain did not influence later mortality. In Gr. P, mortality was not significantly different in patients with (4/26: 15.4 %) or without (6/49 : 12.2 %) coronary spasm. The difference in the incidence rate of mortality was significant only in medically treated patients (gr. T0 + T1): 60.6 % of these patients died in Gr. C vs 24 % in Gr. P (p<0.05). In the subgroups of surgically treated patients (gr. T2 + T3), mortality was higher in Gr. C (22.2 %, vs 7.7 % in Gr. P), but the difference did not reach the significance level.

Thirtyfive patients developed an acute myocardial infarction:
- 28 in hospital: 10 within the day following coronarography (4 deaths). 3 in the subgroups of medical treatment (3 deaths) and 15 in the subgroups of surgical treatment (4 deaths).
- 7 late: 6 in the subgroups of medical treatment (2 deaths) and 1 in the subgroups of surgical treatment (0 death).

The incidence rate of subsequent myocardial infarction was not significantly different in Gr. P (21.4 %) and C (29.2 %). Lethal infarctions were more frequently observed in Gr. C (11/65) than in Gr. P (2/76: p<0.01).

At the time of the last follow-up examination:
- 44 of the 64 survivors reexamined in Gr. P (68.8 %) were pain free

vs 20 of the 37 survivors reexamined in Gr. C (54 %): the difference was not significant;
- 20 of the 64 survivors in Gr. P (31.2 %) had persistent or recurrent angina (3 cl. I NYHA; 14 cl. II; 3 cl. III-IV), vs 17 (46 %) of the 37 survivors Gr. C (4 cl. I; 8 cl. II; 5 cl. III-IV). The differences were not significant;
- in the medical subgroups T0 + T1, persistent or recurrent angina was observed in 10/19 survivors in Gr. P (52.6 %) vs 7/9 survivors in Gr. C (77.8 %): the difference was not significant;
- in the surgical subgroups T2 + T3, persistent or recurrent angina was observed in 10/45 survivors in Gr. P (22.2 %) vs 10/28 survivors in Gr. C (35.7 %): the difference was not significant; (in each P and C group, the percentage of improved patients was higher in surgical subgroups than in medical subgroups but the difference did not reach the significance level);
- in Gr. P patients, 15/22 (68.2 %) with coronary spasm were pain free, vs 29/42 (69 %) without coronary spasm.

4.3.3. DISCUSSION

A small number of studies has been aimed at comparing unstable angina with and without ST segment elevation. In a recent paper, Plotnick and Conti (13) have attempted to evaluate the significance of the direction of the ST segment shifts during chest pain in patients with unstable angina. The present study is in agreement with the results of their comparison between Gr. P and Gr. C patients with regard to clinical, ECG and angiographic data: the proportion of patients with recent angina and with normal resting ECG is higher in Gr. P; life-threatening arrhythmias are more frequent in this group; normal vessels or single vessel disease are encountered more frequently in Gr. P. Reciprocally, Maseri (12) found that anginal attacks with ST segment depression were encountered only in those patients with double or triple vessel disease.

Spontaneous coronary artery spasm, during angiography, not observed in Plotnick and Conti series (13), and rarely observed by Besse (2) was not uncommon in our patients: 26 of the 75 angiographied patients in Gr. P (34.7 %), 1 of 65 angiographied patients in Gr. C (1.5 %). Maseri (12) reported that, during the anginal attack 'all patients with ST segment elevation had vasospasm localized to one of the major branches, often resulting in complete occlusion'.

It has been asserted that unstable angina with transient ST segment elevation carries a poor prognosis, with great risk of myocardial infarction and death. The severe ischemia observed during anginal attacks, with frequent life-threatening arrhythmias and/or conduction disturbances, appeared to justify the presumption of a poor prognosis. As a matter of fact, ventricular arrhythmias and conduction disturbances did not increase the mortality in our Gr. P and Gr. C patients. Lopes (10) reported a similar experience.

The clinical course of Prinzmetal's angina is not well known, because its 'natural' history is potentially modified by medical or surgical treatment. According to MacAlpin (11), who reported 1 sudden death and 1 non lethal myocardial infarction in 10 patients (7 of them followed up for more than 5 years) 'the prognosis of the patient with variant angina pectoris is probably not as bad as has been suggested by others'. Besse (2) reported 5 deaths and 7 non lethal myocardial infarctions in a study of 29 medically treated patients (average follow-up duration: 19.3 months). In the present study, we observed 6 deaths and 2 non lethal myocardial infarctions in 25 medically treated patients (average follow-up duration: 33.3 months). The medically treated patients, in both C and P groups of this study, are those who were not considered as candidates for surgery: patients with little or no coronary artery disease, or with very severe coronary artery disease and poor ventricular function. Patients with no coronary artery disease were present in Gr. P only. Percentages of patients with double or triple vessel disease, and/or with poor ventricular function were significantly higher in Gr. C. Mortality was also significantly higher in this subgroup (60.6 % in medically treated Gr. C patients, vs 24 % in medically treated Gr. P patients). In surgically treated patients, mortality was also higher in Gr. C (22.2 %, vs 7.7 % in Gr. P) but the difference was not statistically significant (in surgical patients the difference between Gr. P and C is significant with regard to angiographic extent of coronary lesions, but not with regard to alteration of left ventricular function).

These observations are in agreement with the several studies which correlate prognosis of coronary artery disease with angiographic extent of lesions and with alteration of left ventricular function. The lower mortality in preinfarction angina with transient ST segment elevation coincides with a higher percentage of patients with little or no coronary disease in this type of unstable angina, and it is important to emphasize that the presence of coronary spasm in Prinzmetal's angina does not increase the mortality rate.

Ruggeroli (14) and Stenson (15) reported that transient ST segment elevation in post infarction angina implies a poor prognosis. Haiat (8) and Trigano (16) did not confirm this opinion. In the present study, the incidence rate of mortality is high in post infarction angina (gr. 3: 31.9 %) and not significantly different in Gr. P (27.3 %) and C (36.4 %).

The high percentage of patients developing an acute myocardial infarction within three months following the onset of unstable angina is well documented (6, 7, 18). Recent studies (4, 5) stated that the incidence of in hospital myocardial infarction is higher in surgically treated patients than in medically treated patients. In the present report, there is no statistically significant difference between Gr. P and Gr. C with regard to incidence rate of subsequent myocardial infarction - neither in medically nor in surgically treated patients, but the incidence of lethal myocardial infarction is higher in Gr. C.

Persistent or recurrent angina is no uncommon in patients with preinfarction angina. Prospective randomized (1, 3) and retrospective studies (5, 9) stated that the percentage of improved patients is higher in surgical subgroups. The present study is in agreement with these earlier reports: 17/28 (60.7 %) in the medical subgroups are symptomatic, vs 20/73 (27.4 %) in the surgical subgroups. The incidence rate of persistence or recurrence of angina, in medical and surgical subgroups, is lower in Gr. P patients, but the difference is not statistically significant.

In conclusion, it has been written that preinfarction angina with ST segment elevation 'represents only one aspect of a continuous spectrum of acute myocardial ischemia', which, sometimes, may coexist in the same patient with angina at rest with ST segment depression (17). However we believe that, in preinfarction angina, transient ST segment elevation defines a subset of patients characterized by less angiographic extent of the coronary artery disease, higher incidence of coronary spasm, and lower mortality rate even though their risk of subsequent myocardial infarction and/or persistent or recurrent angina appears to be the same as in the absence of ST segment elevation during chest pain.

REFERENCES

1. Bertolasi CA, JE Tronge, MA Riccitelli, et al: Natural history of unstable angina with medical or surgical therapy. Chest 70: 569, 1976.

2. Besse P, P Pribat, M Sicart, et al: Aspects actuels de l'angor de Prinzmetal. Ann Cardiol Angéiol 25: 421, 1976.

3. Conti CR: Current status of randomized prospective study on unstable angina. Adv Cardiol 22: 130, 1978.

4. Conti CR, A Hutter, R Russel, et al: Unstable angina: NHLBI random trial. VIIIth World Congress of Cardiology, Tokyo 1978, Abstr 5-7, p 28.

5. Delahaye JP, P Touboul, J Delaye, et al: Unstable angina: medical or surgical treatment? VIIth European Congress of Cardiology, Amsterdam 1976, Abstr 201.

6. Duncan B, M Fulton, SL Morrison, et al: Prognosis of new and worsening angina pectoris. Brit Med J 1: 981, 1976.

7. Gazes PC, EM Mobley, HM Faris, et al: Pre-infarctional (unstable) angina - A prospective study. Ten year follow-up. Circulation 48: 331, 1973.

8. Haiat R, Ch Halphen, P Chiche: Valeur pronostique des sus-décalages transitoires du segment ST au cours des reprises évolutives de l'infarctus du myocarde à la phase aigué. Coeur Med Int 15: 163, 1976.

9. Hultgren HN, JF Pfeifer, WW Angell, et al: Unstable angina: comparison of medical and surgical management. Am J Cardiol 39: 734, 1977.

10. Lopes MG, AP Spivack, DC Harrison, et al: Prognosis in·coronary care unit noninfarction cases. JAMA 228: 1558, 1974.

11. MacAlpin RN, AA Kattus, AB Alvaro: Angina pectoris at rest with preservation of exercise capacity. Prinzmetal's variant angina. Circulation 47: 946, 1973.

12. Maseri A, A Pesola, M Marzilli, et al: Coronary vasospasm in angina pectoris. Lancet 2: 713, 1977.

13. Plotnick GD, CR Conti: Transient ST-segment elevation in unstable angina. Clinical and hemodynamic significance. Circulation 51: 1015, 1975.

14. Ruggeroli CW, K Cohn, M Langston: Prinzmetal's variant angina: a pathophysiological and clinical kaleidoscope. Circulation 48 (suppl. 4): 211, 1973 (abstr).

15. Stenson RE, MD Flamm, BL Zaret, et al: Transient ST segment elevation with post-myocardial infarction angina: prognostic significance. Am Heart J 89: 449, 1975.

16. Trigano JA, G Chiesa, C Diard, et al: Altérations électrocardiographiques de type angor de Prinzmetal en phase aigué d'infarctus du myocarde. Arch Mal Coeur 70: 901, 1977.

17. Severi S, A Maseri, M De Nes, et al: Clinical, coronarographic and prognostic aspects of variant angina. Study of 138 patients Trans Europ Soc Cardiol 1: 49, 1978.

18. Vakil RJ: Preinfarction syndrome - management and follow-up. Am J Cardiol 14: 55, 1964.

4.4. PROGNOSIS OF ANGINAL PATIENTS IN CORONARY CARE UNITS
S.Severi, P. Marzullo, D. Rovai, A. L'Abbate and A. Maseri

4.4.1. INTRODUCTION

Coronary care units have been mainly devoted to the care of patients
with myocardial infarction, but it is important to recognise the problem of those patients, admitted to a CCU because of recurrent
anginal attacks, who are under a high risk of sustaining a myocardial infarction.
Therefore, we selected for study 138 consecutive patients with
angina at rest and a history of "crescendo" angina, a syndrome known
to evolve frequently into acute myocardial infarction (1-3), during
the four weeks immediately preceding hospital admission.

4.4.2. MATERIAL AND METHODS

The study-group consisted of 127 males and 11 females aged from 35
to 65 years, in whom typical transient S-T segment changes could be
documented during at least one anginal attack. Patients with known
ischemic heart disease, who during anginal attacks did not exhibit
detectable S-T segment changes, did not enter the study. All had
angina at rest and 96 also suffered from exertional angina; 48 had
had a previous myocardial infarction.
Continuous electrocardiographic monitoring was performed and standard 12 lead electrocardiograms were recorded during several episodes of chest pain.

4.4.3. RESULTS

Eightyseven patients showed transient ST segment elevation, during
most of their attacks of angina; 51 showed only transient ST segment
depression. The characteristics of these patients are shown in Table
1.

It can be seen that patients with ST segment depression had a higher
incidence of old myocardial infarction. Usually, they had an abnormal ECG under basal conditions and a positive stress test. The
average number of attacks per day was higher in those patients with
ST segment elevation as compared to those with ST segment depression.
Coronary arteriography was performed in 107 patients. Severe coronary artery disease was more frequent in the patients with ST segment

Table 1

	Old M.I.	Abnormal Resting ECG	Positive Exercise ECG	Average N° of Daily Attacks
Pts with ST ↑ (87)	25	63	67	3
Pts with ST ↓ (51)	22	42	47	1

Table 2

	0 Vessel Disease	1 Vessel Disease	2 Vessel Disease	3 Vessel Disease
Pts with ST ↑ (71)	3	29	20	19
Pts with ST ↓ (36)	1	5	11	19

depression (Table 2).

Coronary arteriography, performed during an ischemic attack, showed coronary vasospasm in 28. Acute myocardial infarction occurred in 18 (20 %) of the patients who had ST segment elevation during angina and in 6 (11 %) of those who had ST segment depression. Coronary arteriography performed in 12 patients before the occurrence of AMI, showed single vessel disease in 1 case, double vessel disease in 4 and triple vessel disease in 7. In all cases, except one, myocardial infarction developed in the heart wall corresponding to the ST segment changes during angina and supplied by a coronary vessel which had significant atherosclerotic stenosis and in which spasm was demonstrated during angina.

None of the patients with ST segment depression during the ischemic episodes died or developed severe arrhythmias, such as ventricular fibrillation or tachycardia or complete atrio-ventricular block. Fifteen of the patients with ST segment elevation developed severe arrhythmias during the resolution phase of some of their attacks; in these patients we were unable to identify any features of predictive value.

Frequent attacks of ST segment elevation was a consistent finding among the four patients who died; all had severe coronary atherosclerotic disease. Two died of massive myocardial infarction and two of intractable ventricular arrhythmias.

4.4.4. CONCLUSIONS

The results clearly illustrate that patients in whom frequent ischemic attacks with ST segment elevation occurr are very likely to develop acute myocardial infarction or to die suddenly from a ventricular dysrhythmia during the admission period. This poor prognosis in patients with ST elevation has also been observed by others (4-6), but has not be related to the frequency of attacks.
It is also clear from our results, that the development of acute myocardial infarction or of fatal dysrhythmias is associated with the presence of severe coronary artery disease. However, severe coronary artery disease is also found in those patients with ST segment depression who have, on admission, a much lower incidence of acute myocardial infarction and no mortality. Therefore, the severity of the coronary artery disease is not the only factor affecting prognosis. Taking into account the above findings and also considering the fact that the subsequent AMI almost always develops in the electrocardiographic leads previously showing ST segment elevation during the ischemic attacks, it would appear that functional changes in the coronary arteries also affect prognosis. The high incidence of MI in this population indicates that they require hospitalization in a CCU and that they may provide the opportunity for the study of the mechanisms responsible for AMI (7,8) and hence the development of interventions for its specific prevention.

REFERENCES

1. Short D.: The management of the patient with angina. Editorial. Am. Heart J., 94: 135, 1977.
2. Gazes P.C., F.M. Mobley, H.M. Faris, et al.: Preinfarctional (unstable) angina. A prospective study. Ten year follow-up. Circulation 48: 331, 1973.
3. Heng M.K., R.M. Norris, B.N. Singh, et al.: Prognosis in unstable angina. Br. Heart J. 38: 921, 1976.
4. Silverman M.E., M.D. Jr. Flamm: Variant angina pectoris. Ann. Intern. Med. 75: 339, 1971
5. Bobba P., C. Vecchio, J. Salerno, et al.: L'angina pectoris con transitorio sopraslivellamento del tratto S-T; Variante di Prinzmetal e forme similari. Giorn. Ital. Cardiol. 2: 1050, 1972.
6. MacAlpin R.N., A.A. Kattus, A.E. Alvaro: Angina pectoris at rest with preservation of exercise capacity: Prinzmetal's variant angina. Circulation 47: 946, 1973.

7. Maseri A., A. L'Abbate, G. Baroldi, et al.: Coronary vasospasm as a possible cause of myocardial infarction. A conclusion derived from the study of preinfarction angina. New Engl. J. Med. 299: 1271, 1978.
8. Braunwald E.: Coronary spasm and acute myocardial infarction. New possibility for treatment and prevention. Editorial. New Engl. J. Med. 299: 1301, 1978.
9. Delahaye J.P., Kraus R., Janin A., Gaspard P., Touboul P.: Preinfarction angina comparison between angina with and without S-T segment elevation.

4.5. HEMODYNAMIC MONITORING AND PHARMACOLOGICAL TESTS IN PATIENTS
WITH PREINFARCTION ANGINA IN CCU.
L. Tavazzi, JA. Salerno, M. Ray, M. Chimienti, A. Medici, M.
Previtali, G. Specchia, P. Bobba

4.5.1. ECG AND HEMODYNAMIC MONITORING DURING ISCHEMIC EPISODES AT
REST.
In this communication we wish to report some aspects of our experience with hemodynamic monitoring and pharmacological tests in patients
with angina at rest studied in CCU.
We performed continuous 6-lead ECG recording for several consecutive
days in 63 patients, and both ECGraphic and hemodynamic monitoring
in 48 patients.
The first remarkable finding emerging from the analysis of the
ECGraphic data in patients with angina at rest was the frequency of
ischemic episodes without a pain. Only 4 of the 31 selected patients
undergoing continuous ECG monitoring for 2 or more days showed no
painless episodes and in the remaining 27 patients 1536 of the
recorded ischemic episodes were painless, while only 332 were accompanied by pain, thus 4.6 painless episodes occurred for each painful
one. Duration was one factor involved in determining the presence of
pain. Fig. 1 shows the correlation between the lenght of the
episodes and pain: episodes lasting more than 5 minutes were usually
painful while shorter ones were generally painfree. This behaviour
was consistent in most patients but the duration critical for pain
was very different from patient to patient. It is also evident that
episodes lasting 3 minutes or less were very frequent. Both painfree
and painful episodes were usually associated with clear ventricular
function impairment. Fig. 2 shows an example of a recording taken
during the night in a sleeping patient. The ECG shows a sequence of
episodes of ST-segment elevation each lasting about 1 minute. Systolic pulmonary artery pressure initially increased and did not change
substantially during the subsequent ischemic episodes; diastolic
pulmonary pressure always increased with each upward shift of the
ST-segment. Systemic diastolic blood pressure remained almost unmodified while systolic pressure decreased, particularly during the
first two ischemic episodes. Heart rate increased only slightly,
simultaneously with the ST-segment elevation. In patients with angina at rest and ST-segment elevation, a repetitive sequence of
ischemic episodes with a similar hemodynamic pattern as reported in
Fig. 2 is very common, and may continue almost unmodified night and
day even for several days. Less frequently seen is an increase in
blood pressure associated with the ST-segment elevation; an example

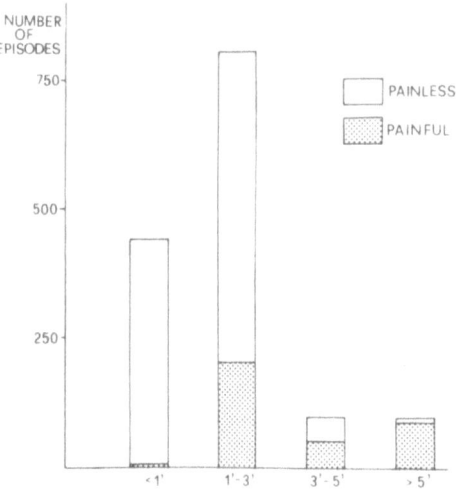

ANGINA AT REST
RELATIONSHIP BETWEEN
DURATION OF ISCHEMIA AND PAIN

Fig. 1. Relationship bet-
ween duration of ischemia
(ECG changes) and presence
of chest pain in patients
with angina at rest.

of this, recorded in 1 of 6 patients presenting such an increase, is
shown in Fig. 3. Several patients alternated episodes of ST-segment
elevation, ST-segment depression and simple T-wave voltage or polarity changes. All these findings indicate that myocardial ischemia is
an extremely dynamic and changeable phenomenon. In our experience
patients showing only ST-segment depression during ischemic attacks
generally have fewer ischemic episodes than those showing ST-segment
elevation.

Hemodynamic monitoring allows quantitative determination of the degree of cardiocirculatory impairment caused by myocardial ischemia.
Examples of the hemodynamic patterns observed during ischemic episodes with ST-segment elevation are reported in Figs. 2 and 3 and
during those with marked ST-segment depression in Figs. 4 and 5. In
one patient (Fig. 4) ST-segment depression gradually increased;
simultaneously pulmonary artery pressure, which was normal in basal
conditions, progressively increased; blood pressure rose after the
first ECG changes and cardiac output did not change markedly. After
nitroglycerin all parameters returned to baseline. In another
patient (Fig. 5) more severe hemodynamic impairment was evident.
Moderate ST-segment depression, present in basal conditions, rapidly
increased followed soon after by a decrease in blood pressure;
pulmonary artery pressure increased and heart rate also rose and a
pattern of severe subclinical left ventricular failure was observed.
It must be noted that systolic pulmonary pressure increased much
more than the diastolic, probably reflecting an increased right

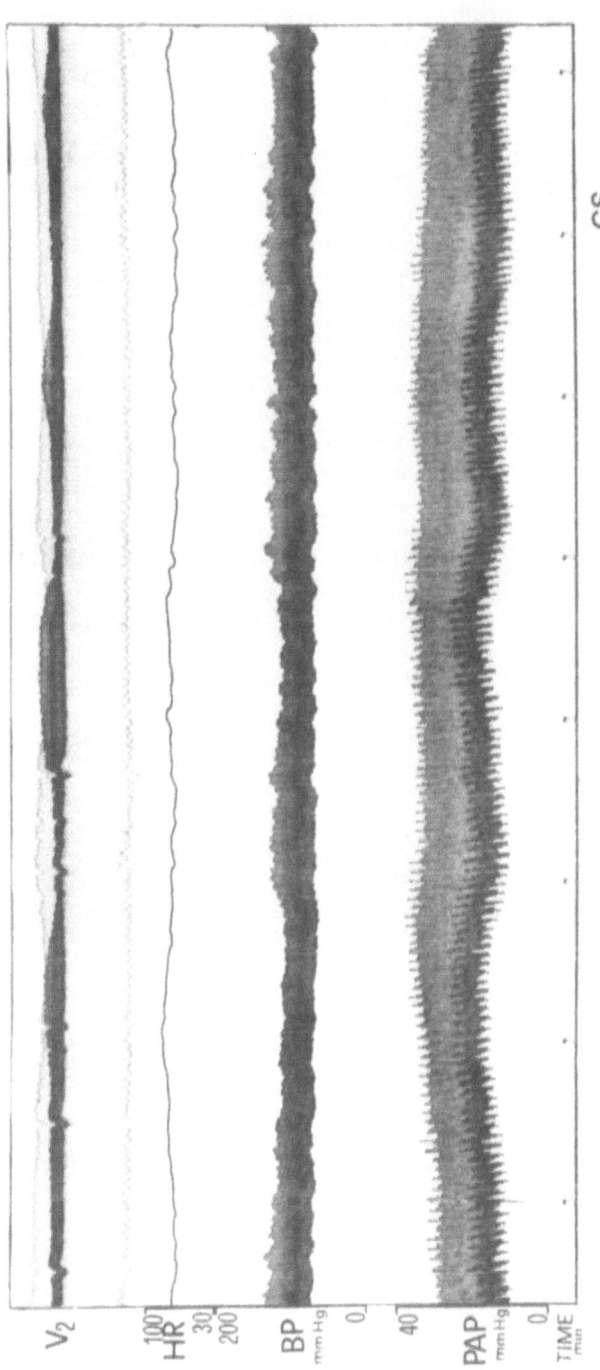

Fig. 2. Repeated painless ischemic episodes, characterized by ST-segment elevation in lead V2 recorded in a sleeping patient. HR: heart rate; BP: systemic blood pressure; PAP: pulmonary arterial pressure. See text for further explanation.

158

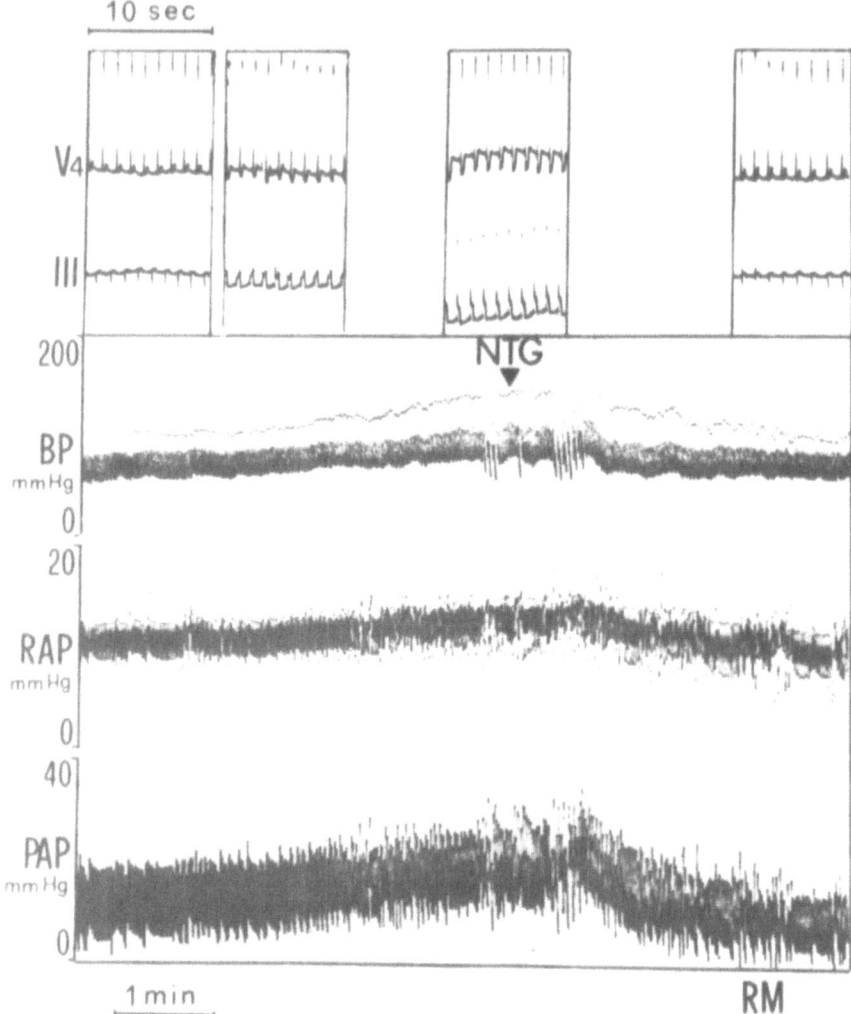

Fig. 3. Ischemic episode at rest. The hemodynamic tracings and ECG
were recorded simultaneously on different recorders at different
paper speeds. The ECG strips are presented here in approximate
chronological correspondence with the hemodynamic events. No hemodynamic changes are seen before the onset of ST-segment elevation in
lead III and specular ST-segment depression in lead V4; subsequently, systemic blood pressure (BP), right atrial pressure (RAP) and
pulmonary artery pressure (PAP) increase simultaneously, while in
lead III the R-wave becomes higher and ST-segment elevation increases. After sublingual 0.3 mg nitroglycerine (NTG) both ECG and
hemodynamic parameters return to baseline. During the ischemic episode some extrasystoles appear.

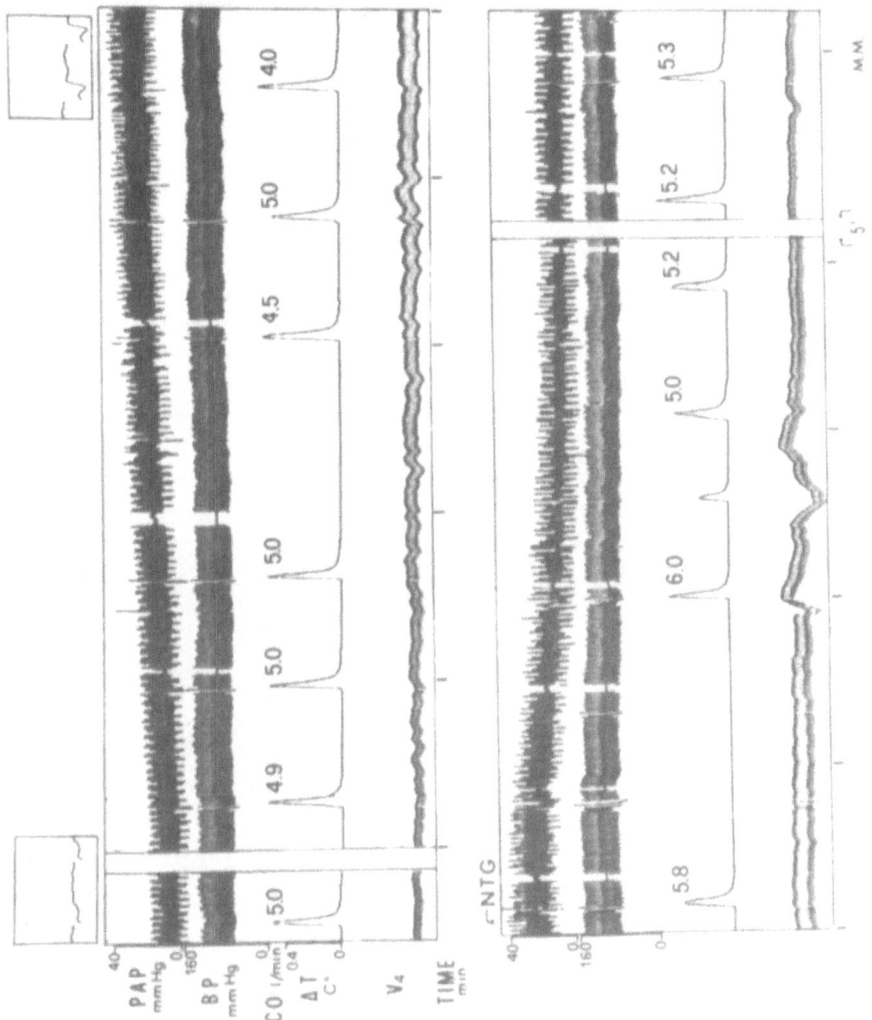

Fig. 4. Ischemic episode at rest. Top panel: in basal conditions slight ST-segment depression is present, which then increases markedly (as far as 5 mm) over 4 minutes (lead V4). Pulmonary artery pressure (PAP) increases simultaneously, and soon after systemic blood pressure (BP) also rises, while cardiac output (CO) decreases slightly. Heart rate (HR) increases from 78 to 82 per minute during the ischemic episode. Bottom panel: after sublingual 0.3 mg nitroglycerine (NTG) PAP and BP rapidly decrease, CO increases above the basal value and ST-segment depression gradually decreases. Return to baseline values is reached 9 minutes after NTG administration.

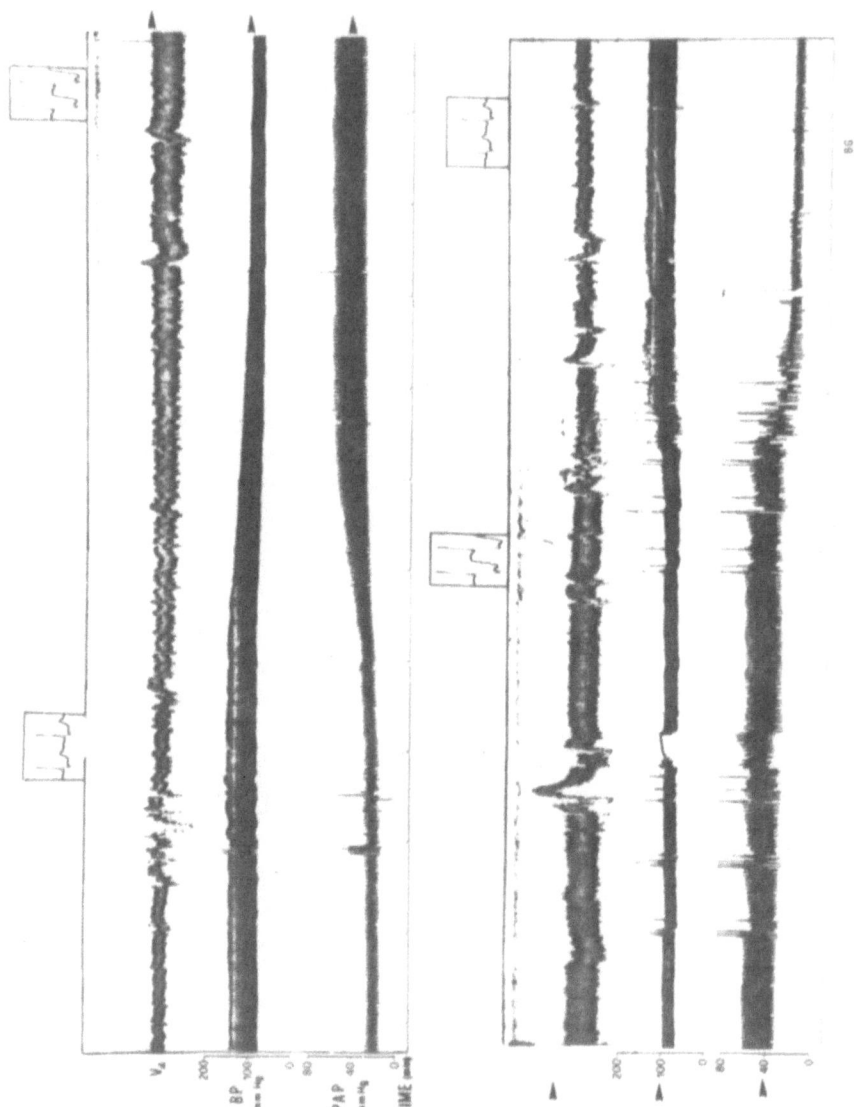

Fig. 5. Ischemic episode at rest. Under basal conditions moderate ST-segment depression is present. Hemodynamic parameters remain unchanged when ST-segment depression (darker zone in lead V4) and R-wave voltage begin to increase. Soon after, both systolic and diastolic blood pressure (BP) decrease rapidly and simultaneously, and pulmonary artery pressure (PAP) increases. As shown in the short ECG strips recorded at higher paper speed (25 mm/sec) heart rate also increases (from 104 to 136 per minute). After sublingual nitroglycerin (0.6 mg) ST-segment depression diminishes, BP and PAP rapidly return to baseline. The strips are continuous. See text for further explanation.

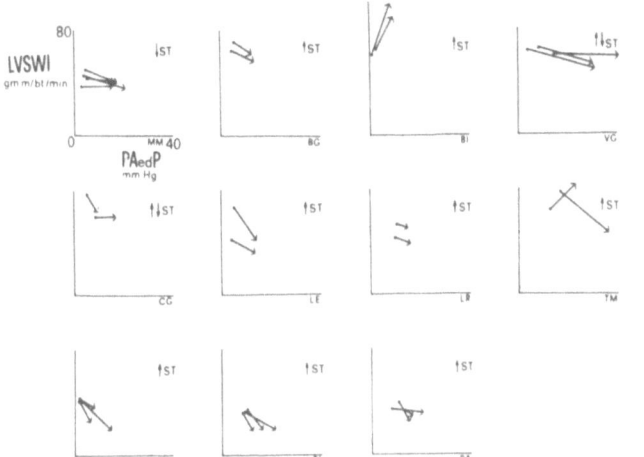

Fig. 6. Changes in left ventricular function during two or more ischemic episodes in 11 patients with angina at rest. The baseline values and maximal changes in left ventricular stroke work index (LVSWI) and pulmonary artery end-diastolic pressure (PAedP) are plotted. The final values for x and y are the same in all graphs. See text for further explanation.

ventricular contractility due to autonomic reflexes. The hemodynamic situation quickly returned to baseline after NTG-induced reduction of ST-segment depression. In Fig. 6 changes in left ventricular function observed during two or more ischemic episodes in some patients are reported. Left ventricular function was usually compromised during transient myocardial ischemia; the degree of hemodynamic impairment may very greatly from patient to patient, but usually it is roughly similar in any one patient during different ischemic episodes.

In agreement with previous observations (1-3), the most important finding from a pathophysiological point of view was the systematic absence of significant increases in heart rate and blood pressure prior to the occurrence of ischemic episodes at rest.

4.5.2. PHARMACOLOGICAL TESTS.

As for the pharmacological tests, we evaluated the effects of dipyridamol and ergonovine maleate in patients with angina pectoris and in control subjects. Since dipyridamol has been observed to induce myocardial ischemia in a very high percentage of patients with angina, it has been proposed as diagnostic test (4). It has also been documented that ergonovine maleate induces coronary spasm

and myocardial ischemia especially in patients with ST-segment elevation during ischemic episodes (3, 5-16). Our main findings are
summarized below.

Dipyridamol (0.75 mg/Kg i.v. in 10 minutes) was administered to 69
patients with angina pectoris and to 22 control subjects during
continuous ECG recording: 22 patients had angina at rest, 7 angina on
effort and 40 angina both at rest and on effort. ECG signs of
myocardial ischemia appeared - that is, the test was positive - in
all patients with angina on effort and in 48 % of the patients with
angina both at rest and on effort; no ECG changes were observed in
the 22 patients with angina exclusively at rest, nor in control
subjects. We therefore conclude that the dipyridamol test lacks
sufficient sensitivity as a diagnostic test of angina but seems
specific; moreover some relationship seems to exist between the type
of angina and the test response. There also seems to be a relationship between coronary lesions and dipyridamol effects; the test was
positive in 31 %, 66 % and 45 % of the cases with critical stenoses
involving 1, 2 and 3 coronary vessels respectively, while it was
negative in all patients with normal coronary arteries or subcriti-
cal coronary lesions. Therefore a positive test suggests the presence of critical coronary stenosis. Dipyridamol seems to provoke
myocardial ischemia by stealing the blood flow from regions supplied
by vessels with critical lesions in favour of better perfused
myocardial areas (17). The positivity of the dipyridamol test in
angina on effort and the negativity in angina at rest might be
interpreted, in the former, as indicating that the pressure-flow
equilibrium in the coronary districts is favourable for the steal
occurrence and could contribute to inducing myocardial ischemia
during effort.

The ergonovine test provides different information. The test was
performed in CCU in 113 patients with angina pectoris and in 46
control subjects during continuous ECG recording. Ergonovine induced
the appearance of ECG signs of myocardial ischemia in 80 % of 40
patients with angina at rest, in 84 % of 62 patients with angina
both at rest and on effort, and in only 18 % of 11 patients with
angina exclusively on effort. It was negative in all control subjects. We therefore conclude that the ergonovine test is specific,
shows good though not absolute sensitivity in angina at rest, and
that the test response is correlated with the type of angina. In our
patients no correlation was found between test response and coronarographic findings in control conditions, while in several patients
undergoing coronary angiography during an ergonovine-induced ischemic attack coronary spasm was observed and a close relationship was
found between the constricted vessel and the localization of the ECG
signs of ischemia (3, 5, 7, 8). Furthermore coronary angiography,
performed in 5 patients during both spontaneous and ergonovine-
induced ischemic episodes, showed spasm in the same site of the same

coronary artery (15, 16). Similar findings have been reported by other Authors (7, 14).

In agreement with these findings suggesting that ergonovine provokes myocardial ischemia by inducing a primary reduction in blood supply, in 70 % of 33 patients with angina at rest in whom the ergonovine test was performed in CCU during hemodynamic monitoring, careful analysis of the initial ECG and hemodynamic events showed no changes in those parameters, implying an increase in myocardial demand before the ischemic changes. In the remaining 30 %, blood pressure increased moderately before the ECG changes (systolic increment ranging from 5 to 28 mmHg, mean $\pm$ S.E. 12.2 $\pm$ 2 mmHg). In 14 patients both spontaneous and ergonovine-induced ischemic episodes were recorded and in 10 the ECG and hemodynamic changes observed were in the same direction. In addition in 90 % of 51 patients in whom only 12-lead ECG recordings were evaluated during both spontaneous and ergonovine-induced ischemic attacks, the alterations were similar.

In conclusion, the appearance of ECG signs of myocardial ischemia after ergonovine represents a specific sign for diagnosis of ischemic heart disease. The similarity of the electrocardiographic, hemodynamic and coronarographic findings during spontaneous and ergonovine-induced ischemic episodes may suggest a common pathophysiological mechanism, namely coronary spasm.

Finally, we compared the effectiveness of some antianginal drugs in preventing both spontaneous and ergonovine-induced ischemic episodes (Fig. 7). The protocol for prophylaxis of the spontaneous episodes included a sequence of two 48-hour periods of placebo and drug followed by two other 24-hour periods of placebo and drug. Six-lead ECG's were continuously recorded.

Eight patients were treated with 15 mg NTG ointment every 6 hours: the ischemic episodes disappeared in 5 patients and markedly decreased in 3. The average daily number of episodes was 10.7 during placebo administration and 0.6 during NTG (p<0.001). In 7 of these patients ergonovine administration after placebo induced an ischemic attack which was relieved by sublingual NTG. When the test was repeated 1 hour after NTG ointment (15 mg), another ischemic attack occurred in 6 patients. Thus, NTG ointment in the doses used was effective in preventing the spontaneous ischemic episodes in the majority of patients with angina at rest but was ineffective in preventing the ergonovine-induced episodes in the same patients. Moreover when the ergonovine-induced anginal attacks arose after application of NTG ointment they were less easily interrupted than those arising after placebo. The average doses of NTG necessary for relieving the ischemic episodes were 1.04 $\pm$ 0.3 (S.E.) mg in the former and 0.67 $\pm$ 0.1 (S.E.) mg in the latter (ns). Similar results were obtained when nifedipine was used according to the previous protocol. In 11 of 14 patients with angina at rest the ischemic

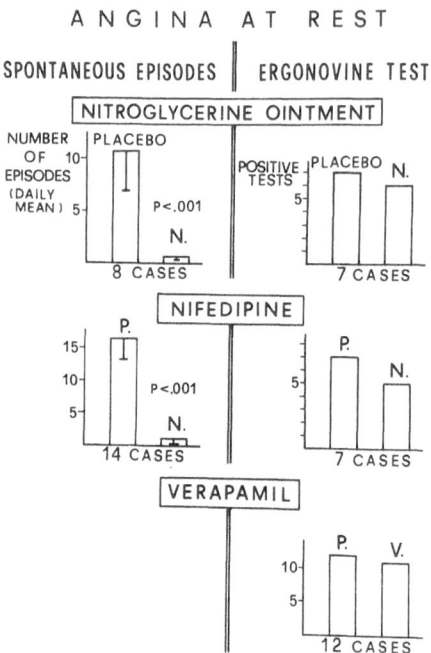

Fig. 7. Effectiveness of nitroglycerin ointment and nifedipine in preventing spontaneous ischemic episodes at rest and lack of effectiveness of the same drugs and verapamil in preventing ergonovine-induced ischemic attacks. See text for further explanation.

episodes were completely abolished after nifedipine, in 2 they were markedly reduced, and in the other no effect was observed. The average daily number of episodes decreased from 16.5 during placebo to 1.1 during nifedipine treatment (p<0.001). The doses used ranged from 60 to 120 mg daily. In 7 of these patients the ergonovine test was performed; it was positive in all of these after placebo; 30 minutes after 20 mg nifedipine sublingually it was again positive in 5 patients and negative in only 2. The doses of nitroglycerine necessary for interrupting the ischemic episodes after placebo and nifedipine were similar: 0.58 ± 0.1 (S.E.) mg and 0.45 ± 0.2 (S.E.) mg respectively (ns).

Verapamil (10 mg i.v.) was also ineffective in preventing the ischemic episodes induced by ergonovine in 11 out of 12 patients in whom it was tested.

Why the drugs used were unable to prevent ergonovine-induced myocardial ischemia is not clear. It may be that the ischemic stimulus provoked by egonovine is simply much stronger than the spontaneous one (s) or it may be qualitatively different or perhaps ergonovine acts beyond the site of action of these antianginal agents during the sequence of events leading to myocardial ischemia. At any rate, the ergonovine test seems of no use in testing the potential effectiveness of antianginal drugs.

In conclusion ECG, and hemodynamic monitoring in patients with angina at rest in CCU provides information about the frequency of ischemic episodes, presence or absence of pain, site and extension of myocadial ischemia, hemodynamic impairment consequent to ischemia and possible pathophysiological mechanism. This information is essential in establishing the severity of the disease, potential risk, and therapeutical approach.

Since acute myocardial infarction is frequent in these patients, understanding of the mechanism responsible for the transient ischemic attacks may also shed light on possible pathogenetic mechanisms of myocardial infarction.

REFERENCES

1. Guazzi M, A Polese, C Fiorentini, et al: Left and right heart hemodynamics during spontaneous angina pectoris. Comparison between angina with ST-segment depression and angina with ST-segment elevation. Br Heart J 37: 401, 1975.

2. Chierchia S, C Marchesi, A Maseri: Evidence of angina not caused by increased myocardial metabolic demand and patterns of electrocardiographic and hemodynamic alterations during 'primary' angina. In Primary and secondary angina pectoris. Ed by Maseri A, Klassen GA, Lesch M Grune and Stratton, New York, 1978, p 145.

3. Tavazzi L, JA Salerno, M Ray, et al: Acute myocardial ischemia induced by ergonovine maleate in patients with primary angina. In Primary and secondary angina pectoris. Ed by Maseri A, Klassen GA, Lesch M Grune and Stratton, New York, 1978, p 247.

4. Tauchert M, DW Behreubeck, J Hotzel, et al: Ein neuer pharmakologischer Test zur Diagnose der Koronarinsuffizienz. Dtsch Med Wshr 101: 35, 1976.

5. Specchia G, L Angoli, E Bramucci, et al: Ergonovine maleate in coronary arteriography. Cardiology (in press).

6. Higgins CB, C Wexler, JF Silverman, et al: Spontaneously and pharmacologically provoked coronary arterial spasm in Prinzmetal variant angina. Radiology 119: 521, 1976.

7. Specchia G, E Bramucci, A Mussini, et al: Il test all'ergonovina maleato in coronarografia. Atti Società Italiana di Cardiologia (in press).

8. Maseri A, A Pesola, M Marzilli, et al: Coronary vasospasm in angina pectoris. Lancet 1: 713, 1977.

9. Bertrand ME, C Laisné, JM Lefebvre, et al: Le spasme des arteries coronaire. Arch Mal Coeur 70: 1233, 1977.

10. Shroeder JS, JC Bolck, RA Quint, et al: Provocation of coronary spasm by ergonovine maleate. New test with results in 57 patients undergoing coronary arteriography. Am J Cardiol 40: 487, 1977.

11. Curry RC, CY Pepine, MB Sabom, et al: Effect of ergonovine in patients with and without coronary artery disease. Circulation 56: 803, 1977.

12. McLaughlin PR, PW Doberty, RP Martin, et al: Myocardial imaging in a patient with reproducible variant angina. Am J Cardiol 39: 126, 1977.

13. Nelson C, B Nowan, H Childs, et al: Provocative testing for coronary arterial spasm: rational risk and clinical illustration. Am J Cardiol 40: 624, 1977.

14. Heupler FA, WL Proudfit, M Razavi, et al: Ergonovine maleate provocative test for coronary arterial spasm. Am J Cardiol 41: 631, 1978.

15. Specchia G, E Bramucci, L Angoli et al: Spontaneous and provoked coronary artery spasm: are they the same? Europ J Cardiol 6: 581, 1978.

16. Bramucci E, G Specchia, S De Servi, et al: Riproducibilità del quadro clinico elettrocardiografico e coronarografico dello spasmo coronarico spontaneo mediante ergonovina maleato. Giorn Ital Cardiol 8: 489, 1978.

17. Becker LC: Conditions for vasodilator-induced coronary steal in experimental myocardial ischemia. Circulation 57: 1103, 1978.

4.6. THE IMPORTANCE OF EVALUATING CORONARY RESERVE IN ANGINAL PA-
TIENTS IN CCU

A. Biagini, M.G. Mazzei, C. Carpeggiani, D. Rovai, A. Maseri

4.6.1. INTRODUCTION

Following a recent series of observations in our own institution as
well as in several other centers (1-6), it appears of relevant
practical importance to establish the different mechanisms of angina
pectoris in patients admitted to CCU for frequent anginal attacks.
Angina at rest may occur because of the exaustion of coronary
reserve due to an excessive increase in cardiac work in the presence
of severe atherosclerotic stenoses, or because of a sudden reduction
in blood supply.
The correct management of patients admitted in CCU for frequent
anginal attack requires the identification of the pathogenetic mechanisms that cause the anginal attacks. Therefore in order to establish whether the episodes of angina at rest occurring in patients
admitted to our CCU were caused by an increase in the hemodynamic
factors conditioning the myocardial oxygen demand (beyond the limits
of their coronary reserve set by the presence of coronary stenosis
(7)), we decided:

1. to obtain measurements of the heart rate (HR) and blood pressure
   (BP) at the onset of transient ST-T changes observed on the CCU
   monitor, before the onset of the chest pain (when possible);
2. to compare the values of the double product (HR x systolic BP)
   reached at the onset of pacing-induced angina with that determined at the beginning ST-T changes occurring at rest.

4.6.2. MATERIALS AND METHODS

We studied fifteen consecutive patients (aged from 36 to 68 years)
admitted to our CCU for frequent attacks of angina at rest. All the
patients gave their informed consent to the study. None of the
patients showed serum enzyme elevation or permanent electrocardiographic changes suggestive of acute myocardial infarction during the
period of study. All had severe angina at rest, 12 had also angina
on effort, 7 has suffered a myocardial infarction (4 anterior and 3
inferior). Symptoms had begun between 1 and 198 months prior to
admission. After the admission in the CCU the ECG was continuously
monitored and for each patient several episodes of angina at rest
were recorded. The blood pressure was measured by a nurse at the

early onset of the anginal attack and a 12 lead electrocardiogram
was obtained as soon as possible. The atrial pacing test was usually
performed on the day after an episode of angina at rest at the same
hour.
A Cordis bipolar French 4 catheter was inserted percutaneously into
right antecubital vein and positioned in the right atrium in a low
threshold area. The pacing was started at 100 beat/min and the
pacing rate was increased in increments of 10 beats/min after 1
minute at each level. The blood pressure was measured with a
cuffmanometer at the beginnig of each step and every 30 seconds.
The pacing was discontinued at the onset of clear ischemic alteration on the ECG or at the beginning of pain or on the appearance of
A-V block not responsive to atropine 1 mg iv.
Twelve patients also underwent a triangular bycicle ergometer stress
test some days after the pacing test.
Coronary arteriography and left ventricular angiography were performed by the Judkins technique (8) in 13 patients.

4.6.3. RESULTS

No complications were observed during the study; 12 patients showed
typical ischemic ECG alterations. Only 4 patients developed angina.
No ECG changes or pain were observed in the remaining 3 up to a
value of HR of 160/min for 3 minutes. Eight patients had spontaneous
episodes characterized by ST depression, 3 patients by ST elevation
and 4 patients alternated in different episodes ST depression with
pseudo normalization of negative T wave during the pacing test on
the same leads.

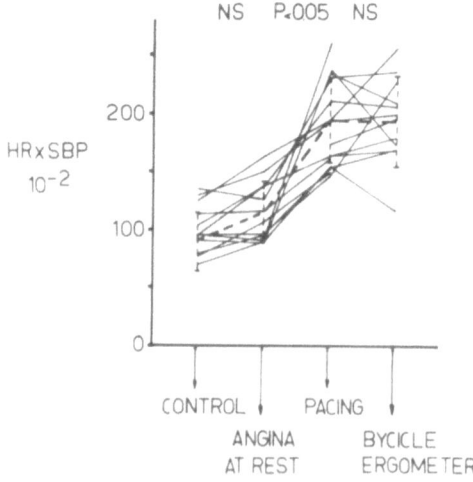

Fig. 1.

Table 1. Angiographic findings

Normal	1
1 Vessel disease	2
2 Vessel disease	4
3 Vessel disease	6

The average double product was 96.7 $\pm$ 21.4 mmHg/min in resting condition, 116.6 $\pm$ 25.9 during the spontaneous episode of angina, 196 $\pm$ 39.2 during the pacing test and 195.3 $\pm$ 36.9 during the bicycle ergometer stress test (Fig. 1).
All the episodes of angina at rest are not preceded by increase in heart rate but by a small increase in blood pressure probably related to the delay from the onset of the ischemic attack to the measurements of blood pressure. Indeed, the values of blood pressure recorded in the late phase of the ischemic attack are always higher than the values at the onset of ST segment changes or at the onset of pain.
The angiographic findings observed in our patients are summarized in Table 1. Considering significative a reduction of the lumen greater than 75 %, 6 patients had triple vessel disease, 4 patients had double vessel disease, 2 patients had single vessel disease and 1 patient had normal coronary vessels.

4.6.4. DISCUSSION

In our patients the level of double product at which the ischemic alterations occurred was significantly lower in the spontaneous episodes than during the pacing and the stress tests. Moreover, the ECG changes observed during the spontaneous episodes appear to be more severe than those recorded during the pacing test, thus indicating a different degree of ischemia in the two situations.
Our data, in agreement with a recent report (9), demonstrate that even in patients complaining of severe limitation of exercise tolerance, the comparison of the double product level at the onset of a spontaneous anginal attack with that reached during a positive pacing test is a simple procedure for evaluating whether or not angina at rest is caused by an exaustion of coronary reserve or by a functional factors such as coronary vasospasm.
This conclusion is supported by the finding that the degree of coronary obstructions in patients with 'stable' angina and in those with 'unstable' angina are markedly similar. We believe that vasospastic angina is quite a sizeable portion of the patients with

unstable angina.

Considering that the vasospasm has been defined a proved hypothesis for variant angina (10), that its importance has been also demonstrated in the pathogenesis of angina at rest with ST-segment depression (2, 11), and finally that it is indicated as a possible cause of myocardial infarction (12), we think that, for a rational therapeutical approach, the presence of a coronary vasospasm has to be investigated in patients admitted to a CCU for frequent anginal attacks at rest.

These conclusions do have important therapeutical implications because interventions aimed at reducing myocardial O_2 demand do not find any rationale in those patients, but favourable results have been reported with nitrates (13), with calcium antagonist (14) and with perhexiline (15).

We would like to point out that the treatment of vasospastic angina remains empirical and symptomatic until the causes of vasospasm and the possible feed back mechanisms controlling its reversibility or irreversibility are elucidated.

REFERENCES

1. Maseri A, R Mimmo, S Chierchia, et al: Coronary spasm as a cause of acute myocardial ischemia in man. Chest 68: 625, 1975.

2. Maseri A, A L'Abbate, A Pesola, et al: Coronary vasospasm in angina pectoris. Lancet 1: 713, 1977.

3. Maseri A, O Parodi, S Severi, et al: Transient transmural reduction of myocardial blood flow, demonstrated by thallium-201 scintigraphy as a cause of variant angina. Circulation 54: 280, 1976.

4. Wiener L, H Kasparian, PR Duca, et al: Spectrum of coronary arterial spasm. Clinical, angiographic and myocardial metabolic experience in 29 cases. Am J Cardiol 38: 945, 1976.

5. MacAlpin RN, AA Kattus, AB Alvaro: Angina pectoris at rest with preservation of exercise capacity: Prinzmetal's variant angina. Circulation 47: 946, 1973.

6. Scherf D, J Cohen: Variant angina pectoris. Circulation 49: 787, 1974.

7. Braunwald E: Control of myocardial oxygen consumption, physiologic and clinical consideration. Am J Cardiol 27: 416, 1971.

8. Judkins MP: Percutaneous transfemoral selective coronary arteriography. Radiol Clin North Am 6: 467, 1968.

9. Berndt TB, J Fitzgerald, DC Harrison: Hemodynamic changes at the onset of spontaneous versus pacing-induced angina. Am J Cardiol 37: 938, 1976.

10. Meller J, A Pichard, S Dack: Coronary arterial spasm in Prinzmetal's angina, a proved hypothesis. Am J Cardiol 37: 938, 1976.

11. Maseri A, S Severi, M De Nes, et al: Variant angina: one aspect of a continuous spectrum of vasospastic myocardial ischemia. Am J Cardiol 42: 1019, 1978.

12. Maseri A, A L'Abbate, G Baroldi, et al: Coronary vasospasm as a possible cause of myocardial infarction. A conclusion derived from the study of preinfarction angina. N Engl J Med 299: 1271, 1978.

13. Parodi O, A Maseri, I Simonetti: Management of unstable angina at rest by verapamil. A double blind cross over study in CCU. Br Heart J (in press).

14. Afzal Mir M, EM Kafetzakis: Assessment of perhexiline maleate in angiographically proven intractable angina: a double-blind trial. Am Heart J 96: 350, 1978.

DISCUSSION: CHAPTER 4

Chairman: A. Maseri

DISCUSSION CHAPTER 4

Paper 1: Preinfarction angina. Review of 67 consecutive patients admitted to CCU.

Paper 2: Clinical coronarographic and prognostic aspects of preinfarction angina.

Paper 3: Prognosis of anginal patients in CCU.

MASERI: These three papers have something in common. They show that patients with angina admitted to a coronary care often go on to develop myocardial infarction in spite of our therapy, and, at least according to our experience, the infarction develops, in the same area where they showed signes of ischemia during angina.

BALCON: We treated 70 patients with recurrent attacks of pain at rest for 48 hours with beta-blockers and nitrates. In 42 of the patients the pain went away in 48 hours. In 28 it continued and in 27 of them who had coronary stenoses we went on immediately to surgery one of them died, and 2 suffered myocardial infarctions; so our surgical mortality was very much lower in the acute situation. Of the 42 patients in whom pain was relieved in 48 hours, 25 had coronary stenoses, 19 of those were treated surgically, 7 of them because they came back again with a second episode of pain. One of those died and 2 had myocardial infarction. None of the medically treated patients had myocardial infarction or died. Overall surgical mortality for patients with rest angina (44 of them) was 4.6 % and the myocardial infarction rate 9.2 %. So that isn't a lot different from the overall surgical mortality for any other group of patients.

HUGENHOLTZ: We have studied 122 patients with angina at rest, but not containing any true Prinzmetal. Our therapy, has been massive beta-blockade for a period of at least 8 hours, usually it went for 24 hours, and this gave complete relief in all but 22. These 22 then were pumped. And the striking thing of these pump cases was that all became symptom free without further analgesics within an hour. These 22 were pumped for varying periods of time, all succesfully weaned, one sustained an infarction, all 22 subsequently were submitted to coronary arteriography and most of them operated at a much later date when they were cooled off. So we would concur with Dr. Balcon that the infarction rate can be low, the death rate can be low. The only thing where we differ is we don't have surgery immediately available. Our surgeons feel that, if you put an acute case in, it really pushes two routine cases out of the way. So this is why we have gone to the pump and we report really excellent results with it.

MASERI: I think that the experience of Dr. Balcon and Dr. Hugenholtz is very encouraging and we must admit that after all we are dealing with something of which we do not understand exactly the mechanism, or if we understand the mechanism, we don't understand the causes of the mechanism. Since it's very difficult to have the appropriate therapy, empirically I would stay with the therapy which produces the best results. I think however, that it's difficult to rationalize exactly the 'why' these interventions are effective, I think that it would be interesting to try and find a better medical therapy if possible, rather than rely on surgery, which can be performed with good results only in a few centers.

DISTANTE: I would like for Dr. Maseri to tell his thought about what, in perspective, we should consider as a maximum, optimal medical therapy. Because I think, what strikes me looking at data from different centers is that, both from American centers and European, there is quite a striking difference in type of medical management that these centers use. So the way of judging optimal medical therapy before surgery may be arbitrary.

MASERI: Well, I can only say that you're right, the medical therapy in different places is different. And therefore the results of so called 'optimal medical therapy' are different. For example, somebody is happy with the 'massive' doses of beta-blockers, somebody is not; we are not, personally. In the United States, if the patient does not respond to four to six tablets of propanolol, that's a non-responder, so he goes to surgery.

I would like to get away from this to get on the lines of the perspectives of research in coronary care. Just to cast a stone on the pool, we believe it's remarkable that you get infarction always in the same area where you before had transient ischemic changes: this could be a clue.

HUGENHOLTZ: With these 122 patients we think we are on the right track when we say first medical therapy. The only point where I agree with you is that it is not inevitable your beta-blockers work, and I took the 22 out, who went to the pump. We are now going to perspectively study randomly assigned beta-blocker versus calcium antagonist to see whether there's a difference there. But we're not going to do anything different. If they don't respond within 24 hours, and I think we'll bring that period even back to less, then they go on the pump, or if I have the same surgeon standing by as Dr. Balcon has, I would send them on the surgery.

Paper 4: Hemodynamic monitoring and pharmacological tests in patients with preinfarction angina in CCU.

Paper 5: Evaluation of coronary reserve in anginal patients in CCU.

MASERI: We can open the discussion on these two papers that have something in common, because they try to find out the cause of angina before treating the patient. Perhaps if we can begin to understand why the patient gets angina, maybe we can develop more rational forms of therapy.

PRASQUIER: Dr. Biagini, one of the factors that you don't take into account when you study the double product, at rest and during pacing, is that these patients, might be in left heart failure and actually the heart's size tends to increase when they rest. The second question is, I would like to ask Dr. Maseri and the audience, what is the present experience with the isotopic studies during the rest angina, and do the perfusion studies add something to our understanding of the mechanism of the pain?

BIAGINI: When we performed our tests we recorded at the same time the echocardiogram in order to detect the dimensions of the left ventricle. We tried also to augment the volume of the ventricle, by putting up the legs of the patient. The results show that the size of the heart has little influence on the pressure-rate product at which the patient has the alteration of the electrocardiogram or pain.

MASERI: As to the second question, the isotope studies that have been performed as well as coronary sinus thermodilution studies, presented as case reports in different laboratories, showed that there is a large reduction in perfusion during these attacks of angina regardless of whether the ST segment is elevated or depressed, but they don't tell us anything about the cause of this reduction in perfusion, whether it is caused by platelet aggregation or by a spasm or the combination of the two.

BALCON: It really relates to what Dr. Tavazzi's saying, and I'm sure you would be interested. We've now had two patients with attacks of spontaneous angina at rest, to whom we have given ergometrine and reproduced angina without coronary spasm, but with very large changes in preload and afterload, particularly preload, end-diastolic pressure going up to 50 in the left ventricle. And I just wonder what that's all about. Perhaps you can help me.

TAVAZZI: In our experience an increase in heart work is not important in determining the ischemic attack.

MASERI: If I may add to that, I would just say that the interesting aspect of this problem is not so much that there is or not a coronary spasm, but rather that angina comes about from a mechanism different from that traditionally assumed of an excessive increase in myocardial demand exceeding the possibility of supply.

Should we say that within the perspectives of a clinical investigation in coronary care, the problem of investigating the cause of angina at rest in CCU is something which is worth proposing?

TAVAZZI: I should like to make some comment about the use of beta-blockers, as the drugs, the sole drugs for defining if the patient is respondent or not respondent to medical therapy. I disagree about this point. I think that many patients, or some of the patients can be well controlled by calcium antagonists or isosorbide dinitrate and cannot be satisfactorily controlled by beta-blockers.

HUGENHOLTZ: We simply have taken beta-blockers because we wanted to make our treatment uniform, and we've reported what we've seen. But I have a question for you. You seem to direct the discussion toward what are the mechanisms, because it can't just be, let's say, the standard, there must be something more behind it. Now we feel the same way, and we've been trying to figure out a way in which we could determine whether or not platelet aggregation was such a causative moment. And so we started to look at the literature, and it turns out that nobody, apparently, has sampled, in the coronary sinus, the breakdown products of platelet aggregations in the form of serotonin.

ROSSI: When I was in the United States I studied serotonin effects on dogs. And I produced a diffused small myocardial infarctions by very slight and very low doses of endoaortic infusion of serotonin in the dogs.

MASERI: Well, that is very interesting information. Coming back to beta-blockers, Guazzi pointed out that his patients were responding only to very high doses, much higher than those which would gave complete beta-block. At that level, they may be active in some other place rather than just reducing myocardial consumption. I would like to ask Dr. Julian's opinion if he thinks that the patient with angina at rest before being treated aggressively should be investigated also aggressively. I don't know how aggressive we can consider the procedure of putting in a catheter to see whether there is an increase in heart rate and blood pressure causing the anginal attack or of performing a pacing or an exercise stress test, compared to putting in an aortic balloon or having a by-pass operation.

JULIAN: First can I just say one thing, I don't think anybody has mentioned the provocation of angina by beta-blockers, because I think this sometimes occurs. And I must say we seem to have a much lower incidence of medical failure than, for example, Dr. Balcon has, and also we have a much lower incidence of ST segment elevation. I think this obviously represents different populations that we are looking at. And we have something like a 90% or more resolution of pain within, say, 24 hours or so, or virtual resolution, or diminution of pain. With beta-blockers and in some cases with niphedipine and nitrates. We always use nitrates, and some cases respond very quickly to nitrates alone. But we would normally use beta-blockers. But if they were not responding quickly, we'd use niphedipine. We have found, with that kind of regime, there are only 3 or 4 patients per year in our unit who we feel worried about, and whom we would then put on the balloon pump with a view to coronary angiography. We tend to put them on the balloon pump before we do coronary angiography and then take them directly to surgery, if that's what they seem to need.

MASERI: Yes, but what I am asking is, why prior to balloon pumping you don't perform hemodynamic monitoring and stress testing to try and find out the cause of the attacks?

JULIAN: I'm not quite sure what one gets out of that.

MASERI: Well, if you see that the attack comes out of the blue, without any change in heart rate, without any change in blood pressure, at much lower work loads of those tolerated during a stress test, then these stenoses are not the limiting factor responsible for his attacks at rest.

HUGENHOLTZ: What would we learn? I mean, our experience is as has been said, we see these 4 or 5 years in this area, I've talked about this over several years, and those are the ones whom you've done everything for medically. The balloon goes in and it has this dramatic effect on the pain, so decompression and the law of Laplace, whatever, after the reduction, it seems to be the mechanism. When they go to coronary arteriography after that, they always have a lesion, and then they go on to surgery if they are operable. So I wouldn't find that a fruitful population to look for the mechanisms such as you want to elucidate. There is a committment from the service who have worked for that patient 24 hours. They are not really eager to rock the boat. It seems to be just getting back under control, and I would not find that population to be a just population to find out mechanisms.

MASERI: Although, from the empirical point of view I might agree with you, the problem is this: do you think that you are following a rational approach for that patient by having the balloon and the operation? His coronary stenosis may be the bystander rather than the culprit. By finding out the cause of his attacks you might perhaps get to a new form of medical treatment and achieve the same result without having balloon or without having by-pass.

HUGENHOLTZ: The best way of finding out whether you're alive is to stay alive. I mean, I find this not the right population to ask these fundamental questions on. They are usually under stress. The whole situation is under stress, and we do find that we have no deaths, and we have few infarctions. So I won't rock the boat. And I don't care about the mechanism, thank you. I'm trying to relieve the patient's pain; I'm trying to avoid myocardial infarction and I'm trying to keep him alive. These are the three goals that Beneken asked us for. I think we shouldn't delude him that we are confused about our aims. Hell; no. Pain should go away, infarction should be prevented, and death should be avoided. And I'm perfectly willing to investigate, but I would do that in a cath. lab. for example, if you have that patient who has an angina and you don't find the obstruction, and we all have them, and then to pace these and then to look at these mechanisms, this is what we are doing now, and there we are putting coronary sinus catheter in and try to sample for serotonin and for other things. And this is where I'm perfectly willing to go along with the protocol with you, but not in a CCU.

MASERI: CCU and cath. lab. are the same thing because it's the patient problem. I have to solve the patient problem, because, between the balloon pumping and the operation, you have to go to cath.lab. anyway, so the investigation can be done one way or another.

Furthermore, I think, how many places are so equipped that to relieve the patient's symptoms and to keep the patient alive, it is possible to do counterpulsation and by-pass surgery? As you've seen in Italy, we have heard of the experience of Milan, which is not encouraging although they are the number one cardiac surgery center in Italy, I think that it is not economic, it is not atraumatic because you have to put the balloon, you have to operate the patient which can be successful only in few experienced centers as it is yours. If we understand more, perhaps we would achieve exactly the same result as you are in a cheaper way.

BALCON: Can I say that you're absolutely right. It's a question of attitude. We're a very surgically orientated center, and I'm quite sure we could achieve medical results better than those we do if we tried very hard. But we don't try very hard, because in any event, if those patients just became ordinary stable anginas, they would have gone through the mill and been operated on. So it's really a question of expediency for us. That's what would happen anyhow.

MASERI: This brings about another problem, which is, whether the patients may be candidates for by-pass surgery to improve prognosis, rather than to treat the cause of their anginal attacks at rest. That is different concept and in that respect we can open a interminable discussion.

HUGENHOLTZ: The first argument you began with, is we must study the mechanisms of angina pectoris better. I agree. All I said is I don't want to study them in that subset of the population whom I've had in the CCU for 24 hours on maximum drug therapy and who still have pain and for whom I must do something. And I've found the pump to work. And then it goes down the line as we all do. So all I'm arguing is it's not that particular patient I'm willing to put into the pot to be studied. I'm saying, that patient who comes in primarily for the first time, he has stable angina and he is being studied and doing the study in the cath. lab., we pace him and then we get pain out of him or whatever, there is a preparation which I'm willing, as a doctor, to take on my back to do some further study to look at the mechanisms. That was argument number one. Argument number two, where you start saying, or it's really three, surgery may not be the answer because after all we've had the other panaceas before, etc., that can counter by simply looking at what the long-term results of coronary artery by-pass surgery are. And I'm getting very impressed, not only from our survival curves, which is the ultimate argument, but more so about the fact that most of them have a perfect restoration of cardiac function if you do the right operation at the right time. So I would take that part out of the equation, you see, and I would go back to that I'm willing to study the mechanisms but then, under what I consider control circumstances and not something where the whole situation has become so unstable that I find the situation as thin as an egg.

MASERI: Unfortunately, if you want a rational rather than an empyrical treatment for these patients, it is them who you must study.

ROCCI: I just wanted to ask Dr. Hugenholtz, how long does the preparation of the balloon pumping take and how many people are involved in this operation? How many people in the team?

HUGENHOLTZ: Well, I'll give you a little round about answer, because I know what you're after. What you're after is the discussion of how much really does this take out of a unit in terms of manpower, etc. I could give you a figure, and the figure is that it takes us now three-quarters of an hour to do the balloon pumping. But that's only a figure; and that was achieved after a lot of disasters. We began at the beginning by being extremely negativistic about the balloon pump as a concept. Then we shifted the site, where the balloon was inserted, to the operating room. We made deals with the operating room nurses that there wouldn't be any delay in terms of cleanliness of corridors when the patient passed, etc., I won't belabour the point. At this particular point, the whole thing takes three-quarters of an hour; it's a surgical procedure, it's a medical decision. Consulting is kept down to a minimum and the nurses themselves take care of the machine and there is no extra nurse involved. And the whole thing has become decompressed to a routine affair from being one major achievement, so to speak, and to simple, routine procedure, no more, no less. But it takes time, and it takes steps and preparation.

CHAPTER 5

PRECORONARY CARE

5.1. INTRODUCTION
R. Balcon

We heard yesterday about the birth of coronary care units and about the enermous information that we gathered by continuous monitoring of patients and how this led to the understanding that life-threatening arrythmias occurred early in the course of the disease and that there was aq fairly rapid exponential decay in their incidence as the hours went by. The study in our area of London looking at whole community as opposed to any hospital group of patients with myocardial infarction, showed that approximately two-thirds of all deaths from myocardial infarction occur outside hospital. One of the first people to appreciate this and do something about it is sitting before us and will be talking in a moment, but Frank Pantridge started his first mobile coronary unit in 1966, and although, in Europe, I don't think his ideas have been followed very extensively, for practical reasons in the Unietd States they certainly have. In some centers such as Seattle they have taken the coronary care right into the community, into factories, you can lift up a telephone and say: I have a pain in my chest, please come.

In this session we will discuss the problems of pratical feasibility and of benefits of a mobile care system and of staffing of ambulances of their dedication to coronary patients only. We will also discuss, at the light of our personal experience, the possibility of an integrated graded system of care with transfer of critically ill patients from peripheral units to centralized specialized centers where they can benefit of sophisticated expertise and of technology too expensive to be distributed to all units.

5.2. A MOBILE SERVICE FOR INTRA-AORTIC BALLOON ASSISTANCE IN CARDIO-
GENIC SHOCK AND REFRACTORY ANGINA.
K. Jennings, N. Brooks, M. Cattell, C. Warnes, R. Balcon

Intra-aortic balloon assistance (IABA) reduces myocardial oxygen
consumption by decreasing aortic impedance and increases myocardial
oxygen supply by increasing aorto-coronary pressure gradient and
thus coronary flow. It has therefore been used to treat acute
manifestations of coronary artery disease, in particular, cardioge
nic shock and recurrent angina at rest. We are reporting a pilot
study for the use of IABA in this way. The only new feature of
management was the despatch of an emergency team consisting of
cardiologist, surgeon and cardiac technician to the referring hospital in the hope that IABA could be achieved early.

5.2.1. CARDIOGENIC SHOCK

This condition has a high mortality whatever form of treatment in
used (1-2). Patients survive the initial event and then there is
progressive deterioration presumably due to increasing left ventricular damage until death ensues. The earlier treatment can be applied
therefore, the more chance of success. In 18 months 33 patients were
considered for treatment with IABA. It was established in 31. The
balloon could not be inserted in 2 patients with peripheral vascular
disease, both of these subsequently died. IABA was established
before transfer in 12 patients after an average of 15 hours cardiogenic shock, after transfer in 16, after 17 hours. Two patients died
during transfer. Three patients admitted directly were treated after
an average of 4 hours cardiogenic shock, so that despite immediate
response to emergency calls IABA was still delayed if the patient
was being treated in another hospital. The mean systolic blood
pressure for all patients was 78 mmHg. (range 50 - 90 mmHg).
Hemodynamic improvement occurred in 27 patients, the mean systolic
blood pressure (with the device on standby) rising to 116 (range 90
- 140) mmHg in 24 hours. Ten of these 27 patients who improved
underwent angiography. Eight were found to have major stenoses of 3
vessels and 2 of 2 vessels. All had poor left ventricular function
as assessed by left ventricular angiogram. The mean ejection fraction was 33. The mean left ventricular end diastolic pressure was
23 (range 8 - 40) mmHg. Eight of the 10 investigated patients
proceeded to aortocoronary bypass grafting. Three of these patients
survived and reinvestigation in 2 - 6 months revealed that 5 of the

6 grafts were patent but the left ventricular angiogram was unchanged. Six of the patients who were not investigated or treated surgically survived to leave hospital. The overall survival rate for all patients with cardiogenic shock was 28 % and was not affected by where IABA was instituted.

This survival rate is similar to other reported results (3).

The chief factor which affected survival was the duration of cardiogenic shock before IABA was started. The average time was 9 hours (range 5 - 12 hours) for the 9 survivors and 21 hours (range 8 - 72 hours) for those who died. No patient who survived had cardiogenic shock for more than 12 hours before IABA. This difference is statistically significant (P < 0.01). There was no difference between the duration of IABA between those who survived and those who did not. (5 and 5.75 days respectively), nor between the patients treated surgically and the remainder of the group. All of the survivors maintained or increased their urine output whilst those who died had a falling output. The difference between urine flow in these 2 groups is significant (P<0.05) at 48 hours. This analysis has shown that early treatment with IABA is essential to obtain optimal results. It interrupts the cycle of deterioration that presumably leads to death in patients with cardiogenic shock. Our pilot scheme has demonstrated the feasibility of taking IABA to the patients but success depends on early recognition in the referring hospital and prompt treatment. There are relatively few complications of IABA and the treatment is well tolerated by the patients. There is no doubt that patients who would survive without IABA will be treated if an aggressive policy is pursued, but we believe this is acceptable.

5.2.2. REST ANGINA

Rest or unstable angina can be successfully treated by IABA (4). Eleven patients with continuing cardiac pain at rest who had been treated for at least 24 hours with beta-adrenergic blocking agents and regular sublingual Isordil were treated with IABA. Other similar patients were treated without IABA. Pain was relieved quickly by this treatment in all, although one patient died suddenly before investigation. The remaining 10 underwent angiography and 7 were found to have major stenoses of 3 vessels and 3 of 2 vessels. Left ventricular angiography was normal in 4 and there were regional wall contraction abnormalities in 6. The mean left ventricular end diastolic pressure was 25 mmHg (range 7-50 mmHg). The 10 investigated patients all underwent aortocoronary bypass grafting, one dying in the early post-operative period of ventricular failure. The others have been followed for 2-24 months and 7 are free of pain and the other 2 have grade 1 angina. In the year that the last 3 of these patients were admitted a total group of 70 patients were treated for rest angina, 28 of whom didn't settle on treatment with beta-blocking agents and regular Isordil. All were investigated (3 on IABA) and 25 of these underwent surgery with 1 death. The overall operative mortality for patients with continuing rest pain was therefore 5.5 %. The risks of surgery are therefore higher in this group than in our patients with stable angina (< 3.0 %) but the relief of symptoms was similar.

5.2.3. COMPLICATIONS OF INTRA-AORTIC BALLOON PUMPING

In 2 patients the balloon could not be inserted because of peripheral vascular disease. Three patients had evidence of acute ischaemia and the limb required urgent embolectomy. Two further patients had late intermittent claudication and are awaiting corrective surgery.

1. In conclusion, IABA was effective in cardiogenic shock if started early enough but the provision of an emergency team alone was not sufficient to ensure this.
2. In our experience, continuing rest angina is almost always associated with severe 2 or 3 vessel disease and requires surgery. The intermediate phase can be managed successfully with IABA but we do not believe it is essential.

REFERENCES

1. Lown B, C Vassaux, WB Hood, et al: Unresolved problems in coronary care. Am J Cardiol 20: 494, 1967.
2. Dietzman RH, RA Ersek, CW Lillihei, et al: Low output syndrome: recognition and treatment. J Thorac Cardiovasc Surg 57: 138, 1969.
3. Scheidt S, G Wilner, H Mueller, et al: Intra-aortic balloon counterpulsation in cardiogenic shock. Report of a co-operative clinical trial. N Engl J Med 288: 979, 1973.
4. Gold HK, RC Leinbach, MJ Buckley, et al: Refractory angina pectoris: Follow-up after intra-aortic balloon pumping and surgery. Circulation 54 (supp III): 3, 1976.

186

5.3. PREHOSPITAL CORONARY CARE
J.F. Pantridge

The community mortality from the coronary attack is of the order of
40%. More than two-thirds of the deaths from the coronary attack
occur outside hospital. It is claimed that the Coronary Care Unit
will reduce the hospital deaths by one-third. However even if every
patient with a coronary attack were admitted to an efficient Coronary Care Unit the effect on the community mortality would not be
greater than 4.5 %.
Deaths from the coronary attack among the younger age groups occur
soon after the onset of symptoms. Thus Bainton and Peterson (2)
showed that among males aged 50 and less, 63 % of deaths occurred
within one hour. The Framingham study (3) showed that 61 % of
coronary deaths among patients of both sexes under the age of 65
occurred within one hour. It is thus clear that the major problem of
coronary deaths is outside hospital.
More than 90 % of sudden deaths, that is deaths within one hour of
the onset of symptoms, result from ventricular fibrillation (4). In
1966 it was shown that the correction of ventricular fibrillation
outside hospital was a practical proposition (5, 6). The first
prehospital coronary care scheme in Belfast was incorporated into
the existing emergency system. This was possible since the ambulance
depot for the whole city, population 450,000, is in the grounds of
the main teaching hospital, the Royal Victoria Hospital. One of the
fifty ambulances in the depot was reserved for coronary patients.
When a call was received from the General Practitioner or member of
the lay public the ambulance proceeded to the patient. This ambulance was staffed by a junior doctor and coronary care trained nurse.
One-third of the population of Belfast is remote from the Royal
Victoria Hospital and located on the other side of the river. To
provide coronary care for this area a mobile unit operates from a
district hospital. Since the district hospital has no ambulance
depot a mini-vehicle is used to transport the doctor, nurse and
required equipment to the patient. Either the doctor or the nurse
will accompany the patient to hospital in the ambulance when this
eventually arrives. The other individual will drive the mini-vehicle
back to base.
There has been a proliferation of mobile coronary care units in the
U.S.A. Most of these are staffed by emergency medical technicians.
Some achieve remarkable success. In the year 1977 Cobb's unit in
Seattle had 110 longterm survivors among patients who had ventricular fibrillation outside hospital (7). The majority of these had

ventricular fibrillation before the mobile team arrived. The population of Seattle is approximately half a million. Cobb's data therefore show that more than 200 lives per million population may be saved each year from the correction of ventricular fibrillation outside hospital. However, in Seattle, only 25 % of patients in whom resuscitation is attempted outside hospital are longterm survivors. This undoubtedly relates to the limitations of cardiopulmonary resuscitation. Kouwenhoven's data (8) show that during chest compression the arterial pressure is of the order of 80 mmHg and between compressions around 20 mmHg. Thus the mean arterial pressure during cardiopulmonary resuscitation is less than 70 mmHg. An arterial pressure of less than 70 mmHg will not be adequate for the perfusion of ischemic areas in the myocardium. Thus progressive myocardial damage is likely to occur. This may explain the inverse relationship between the duration of cardiopulmonary resuscitation and the chance of longterm survival.

When hospital Coronary Care Units were initiated the emphasis was no immediate cardiopulmonary resuscitation followed by defibrillation. The emphasis in most hospital Coronary Care Units now is on immediate correction of ventricular fibrillation. Improvement in the salvage of patients with ventricular fibrillation outside hospital will occur when the emphasis is on the correction of ventricular fibrillation at the earliest possible moment. This implies the widespread availability of small portable inexpensive defibrillators. Unfortunately this objective has been hindered by the proposition of the Purdue workers, Tacker and Geddes, that one-third of patients over 70 kilo will not be defibrillated by conventional defibrillators which store 400 Watt seconds. Tacker and Geddes have suggested that defibrillators storing as much as 1000 Watt seconds should be available.

The contention that defibrillators storing more than 400 Watt seconds are necessary is not supported by the Belfast experience. Indeed a prospective study of 233 episodes of ventricular fibrillation indicated that successful correction was possible in 95 % with a delivered energy not greater than 165 Watt seconds. Among the few patients who failed to convert with low energy there was not a single example of failure to convert ventricular fibrillation with 400 Watt seconds stored that is a delivered energy of 320 Watt seconds.

In addition to the correction or prevention of ventricular fibrillation outside hospital, prehospital coronary care will influence mortality by its effect on infarct size. A salutary effect on the ultimate size of the infarct should result from immediate correction of the autonomic disturbance at the onset of acute myocardial infarction. Among patients seen within 30 minutes of the onset of the infarct one-third will show evidence of sympathetic overactivity and half will show evidence of parasympathetic overactivity. A normal blood pressure and normal heart rate will be evident in only 17 %. Twenty-two percent of patients seen within 30 minutes of the onset of infarction will have a systolic blood pressure not greater than 80. In almost all of these patients the hypotension is associated with bradycardia. Correction of bradycardia by atropine will result in most cases in an almost immediate rise in blood pressure. Early acute AV block usually associated with profound hypotension will respond to atropine although the dose required will be greater than that needed for the correction of sinus bradycardia. The correction of vagal overactivity frequently unmasks sympathetic overactivity. Evidence of sympathetic overactivity when first seen or when unmasked by atropine is readily corrected by a beta blocking agent given carefully in aliquots with the object of obtaining a heart rate in the region of 90. Data from the operation of the Belfast mobile coronary care unit in 1969 showed that in patients seen within 3 hours the incidence of cardiogenic shock was 4 % and hospital deaths 10 %. Among patients seen after 3 hours the incidence of cardiogenic shock was 13 % and hospital deaths 19 %.

REFERENCES

1. Pantridge JF, AAJ Adgey, JS Geddes, et al: The acute coronary attack, Pitman medical, Tunbridge Wells, 1975.
2. Bainton CR, DR Peterson: Deaths from coronary heart disease in persons fifty years of age and younger. A community-wide study. New Engl J Med 268: 569, 1963.
3. Gordon T, WB Kannel: Premature mortality from coronary heart disease. The Framingham study. Am J Med Ass 215: 1617, 1971.
4. Adgey AAJ, PG Nelson, ME Scott, et al: Management of ventricular fibrillation outside hospital. Lancet 1: 1169, 1969.
5. Pantridge JF, JS Geddes: Cardiac arrest after myocardial infarction. Lancet 1: 807, 1966.
6. Pantridge JF, JS Geddes: A mobile intensive care unit in the management of myocardial infarction. Lancet 2: 271, 1967.
7. Cobb LA: Personal Communication, 1978.
8. Kouwenhoven WB, JR Jude, GG Knickerbocker: Closed-chest cardiac massage. Am J Med Assoc 173: 1064, 1960.
9. Tacker WA Jr, FM Jr Galioto, E Giuliani, et al: Energy dosage for human trans-chest electrical ventricular defibrillation. New Engl J Med 290: 214, 1974.

5.4. A PROSPECTIVE RANDOMIZED STUDY ON THE EFFECTIVENESS OF A MOBILE CORONARY CARE UNIT (MCCU) IN GOTHENBURG
S. Holmberg and B. Wennerblom

5.4.1. INTRODUCTION

It has been demonstrated that mobile coronary care units reduce mortality in the early, pre-hospital phase of acute myocardial infarction. Results from previous studies have also suggested that hospital mortality could be reduced if the patients are brought under care earlier by the help of a MCCU.
The reported good results have raised the question whether the same results could be obtained in Sweden. It is, however, difficult to predict the efficiency of mobile coronary care units in Sweden from information collected from other countries, because there are many differences among countries concerning emergency medical care. In Sweden for example, general practitioners are rare and patients usually seek medical advice directly at hospitals. They are since a long time authorized and encouraged to order an ambulance in all emergency situations for transport to the hospital without previous contact with a doctor.
Before accepting this new type of medical management we decided in 1972 to perform a prospective randomized trial on the effectiveness of a mobile coronary care unit in Gothenburg.
Gothenburg is a city with 450,000 inhabitants. During the time of the study Sahlgrenska Hospital was the only hospital in the city and equipped with a six bed coronary care unit. The ambulance organization in the city is centralized and all ambulance transport controlled from an Ambulance Center (AC). Any person may contact this centre directly by phone and order an ambulance. The paramedical staff in the Ambulance Center are trained in making preliminary judgements as regards the severity of an illness. This experience and the centralized ambulance organization made it possible to organize a randomized procedure in the AC.

5.4.2. PILOT STUDY

To find out the efficiency of the AC staff in detecting acute myocardial infarction (AMI) a pilot study was performed in 1973 during a twelve week period. The AC staff were given criteria for suspecting acute myocardial infarction as shown in Table 1.
During this study the staff only noted the patients they suspected

Table 1. Criteria for suspecting AMI.

---

1. Chest pain, starting or significantly worsening within 48 hours

2. Sudden dyspnoea without known pulmonary disease or previous similar attacks

3. Sudden unconsciousness without known epilepsy

---

to have an AMI and no extra medical attention was given to these
patients outside or within the hospital.
During the same twelve week period all patients arriving at the
hospital alive with the definite diagnosis of AMI were identified
and the hospital mortality was retrospectively analyzed.

5.4.3. RESULTS

During the twelve week period there were 2,100 acute ambulance calls
(Fig. 1). The AC staff suspected an AMI in 311 patients, 215 of
which were less than 75 years of age. The hospital records of these
215 patients were retrospectively reviewed concerning the final
diagnosis and mortality (Table 2).
Sixteen patients had suffered a sudden cardiac death outside hospital. Forty eight patients had an AMI which means that the AC staff
made a correct diagnosis in 21 percent of the 215 patients. Besides

PILOT STUDY 12 WEEKS 1973

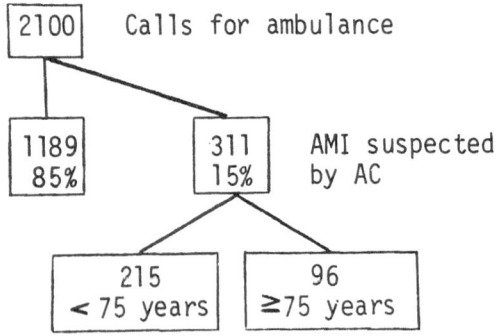

Fig. 1.

Table 2.　　PILOT STUDY 12 WEEKS 1973

DIAGNOSIS IN 215 PATIENTS (< 75 YEARS)
SUSPECTED BY AMBULANCE CENTRE (AC) TO
HAVE AMI

Sudden coronary death outside hospital	16	
AMI	48	21%
Probable AMI	2	
Angina pectoris	27	
Chest pain	4	
	97	45%
Other cardiac disease	28	13%
Non cardiac disease	37	17%
Leaving hospital the same day	53	25%

these, 13 percent had other cardiac diseases and 17 percent had variety of non-cardiac diseases. In the latter group surprisingly few patients, with epilepsy (one patient) or alcoholic problems (4 patients), were included in the study. Twenty-five percent of the patients could leave the hospital on the same day. Thus 75 percent were admitted to hospital for further examination.

During the same period 165 patients below the age of 75 years with definite diagnosis of AMI were admitted to the hospital alive (Fig. 2). Eighty eight (53 percent) of them had been brought to hospital by ambulance and this need for ambulance transport was made

PILOT STUDY 12 WEEKS 1973

All patients (< 75 years) with AMI arriving
in hospital alive

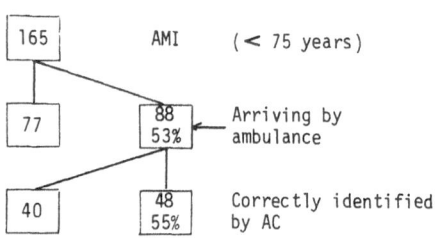

48/165 = 29% of patients with AMI arriving
in hospital alive could be identified by AC   Fig. 2.

by the AC staff. Forty eight of these patients (55 percent) were
correctly identified by the staff as suspected AMI. The pilot study
thus demonstrates that only half of the patients send for an
ambulance when they get symptoms of AMI. It also demonstrates that
only 29 percent of all patients with AMI admitted alive into the
hospital could be identified by the AC staff, a lower figure than we
had hoped for. However, the hospital mortality in the ambulance
transported group was 32 percent compared to only 12 percent mortality in the other group (Fig. 3). Those who died in the ambulance
group also had a median survival time that was much shorter than
that of the non-ambulance group.
Even though the group of AMI identified by the AC staff was small it
seemed to be a group with a remarkably high hospital mortality. This
encouraged us to perform the originally planned study.
    The aim of the prospective randomized study on the effectiveness
of a mobile coronary care unit was to elucidate the following:
1. the effect of a MCCU on mortality in the early, pre-hospital
   phase of AMI,
2. the effect of a MCCU on hospital mortality,
3. to test the function of a MCCU operated by ambulance drivers and
   CCU nurses without the participation of a doctor.

5.4.4. ORGANIZATION AND EQUIPMENT

The MCCU was stationed within the hospital and staffed with two
ambulance drivers temporarily working in the CCU and two CCU nurses.
It was equipped with a battery operated defibrillator with an
oscilloscop and a tape recorder for continuous recording of ECG. All
drugs usually given in the CCU in the initial phase of AMI were

PILOT STUDY 12 WEEKS 1973

ALL PATIENTS (< 75 YEARS) WITH AMI
ARRIVING IN HOSPITAL ALIVE

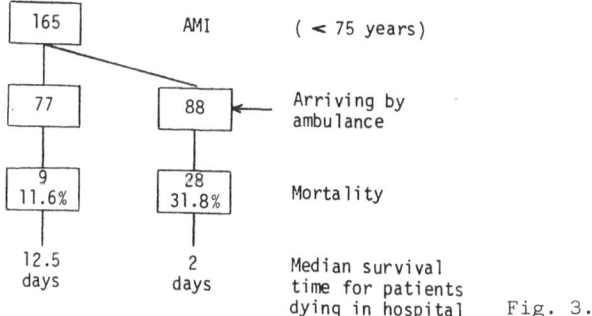

Fig. 3.

available in a specially prepared container with loaded syringes and ready for immediate administration. The nurses followed strictly the standard protocols and were allowed to administer the drugs for the same indications as in the CCU. Equipment for radio communication was available in the ambulance providing nurses the possibility of consulting a cardiologist during transport, but this was never used. The randomization procedure was carried out by the staff in the AC by help of sealed envelopes containing information whether a MCCU or standard ambulance should be used. Precautions were taken to prevent the staff from detecting the information inside the envelopes and it was also checked that the envelopes were taken in consecutive order and that the AC staff acted according to the information. When a patient with suspected AMI was identified an envelope was opened. If the standard ambulance was to be used routine procedures were started by alerting a standard ambulance. If the patient was allotted to the MCCU group this was immediately reported to the CCU over a direct telephone line. The ambulance staff started from the hospital on the average of one minute following the telephone call. The transport to the patient was made at the highest possible speed using sirenes.

After reaching the patient an ECG recording was started as soon as possible and the patient treated till otpimal conditions were achieved for transport back to hospital. As far as possible the patient was kept calm, free of pain and if dyspnoic always given furosemide and oxygen before commencing transport. The transport back to hospital was performed at a lower speed to avoid stress and anxiety. From the moment the patient arrived in hospital the treatment was the same for both groups. The standard ambulance patients were met at the entrance of the hospital by the MCCU team and both groups were immediately transported to the CCU and treated there according to the standard protocols for this unit. The study was run during the day time Monday through Friday and thus covered approximately a 1/4 of the hours of a week. The study started in October, 1973, and has been running intermittently till April, 1978. It was stopped approximately three months each summer and some weeks each winter. The total number of hours during which the study was run amounts to approximately one year round the clock.

The randomization procedure was easy to carry out in the ambulance center and the procedure only caused delays in action of a few seconds. It should be pointed out that for statistical reasons 60 percent were planned to be randomized into the MCCU group and 40 percent to the standard ambulance group (ST.AMB.).

5.4.5. RESULTS

Nine hundred fifty four patients were included in the study (Fig. 4). Eighty eight percent were randomized to the MCCU. A number of patients over 75 years of age were initially included because of lack of information of their age at the time of randomization. These patients and some additional patients that refused to go back with

ALL PATIENTS IN RANDOMIZED STUDY

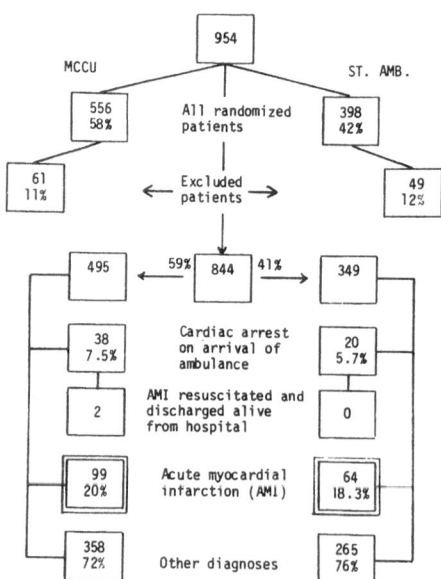

Fig. 4.

Table 3.

AMI PATIENTS IN RANDOMIZED STUDY

	MCCU	ST. AMB.
No. of patients	99	64
Mean age	63.8 years	63.1 years
Previous AMI		
0	55 %	66 %
≥1	45 %	36 %
Previous LHF	30 %	30 %
angina pectoris	55 %	56 %
hypertension	31 %	40 %
diabetes	11 %	16 %

the ambulance, mainly alcoholics, and a few patients with known epilepsy that had had an attack were excluded from further analysis. Eight hundred forty four patients were included in the final analysis. Fifty one patients were found to be in cardiac arrest on arrival of the ambulance. Of these, two-belonging to the MCCU group - were resuscitated and discharged alive from hospital. No patients in the standard ambulance were successfully resuscitated. Among those being alive on the arrival of the ambulance 163 patients got the final diagnosis of acute myocardial infarction (AMI). Ninety nine patients (61 percent) belonged to the MCCU group. The same distribution between the two groups was thus seen in the patients with AMI as in the total patient material.

A comparison between the patients with AMI in the two groups concerning pre-hospital characteristics demonstrate that the groups are similar (Table 3). There is a tendency for the MCCU group to have had more previous AMI, 45 compared to 34 percent. The proportions of the patients having previous left heart failure, angina pectoris, hypertension and diabetes are essentially the same in both the groups. From these data it appears that the two groups of patients are comparable.

Table 4.

AMI PATIENTS IN RANDOMIZED STUDY

DELAY FROM ONSET OF SYMPTOMS TO AMBULANCE CALL

	MCCU	ST. AMB.
Unknown	0	5
< 30 min	18/99 = 18%	9/59 = 14%
< 1 hour	35/99 = 35%	17/59 = 29%
< 2 hours	53/99 = 53%	30/59 = 51%
Median delay	92 min	117 min (59 pat.)

The delay from the onset of symptoms to the ambulance call shows a wide variation in both the groups from less than one minute to several days (Table 4). There is a tendency in the MCCU group to have more patients with a delay less than one hour and the median delay time also appears to be slightly shorter. This is, however, difficult to evaluate as information was lacking in five ST. AMB. patients. The median delay time for that group could vary from 94 to 130 minutes depending on whether these five patients had a very short or a very long delay time.

5.4.6. MORTALITY

In this study, mortality in the pre-hospital phase of AMI was slightly influenced by the MCCU. Two out of 38 patients having cardiac arrest on the arrival of the MCCU could be resuscitated and discharged alive from hospital. Two additional patients in the MCCU group had suffered ventricular fibrillation during transport to hospital and were successfully resuscitated and discharged alive from hospital. Correspondingly 2 patients in the standard ambulance group had a cardiac arrest during transport but could not be resuscitated.

Table 5.

AMI PATIENTS IN RANDOMIZED STUDY

	M o r t a l i t y	
	MCCU	ST.AMB.
No. of patients	99	64
Dead		
outside hospital	1	2
in hospital		
0-24 hours	6 = 6%	12 = 18%
> 24 hours	10	7
In hospital	16 = 16%	19 = 31%
Total	17 = 17%	21 = 33%

The hospital mortality was, however, significantly influenced by the MCCU (Table 5). There was a 16 percent mortality in the MCCU group compared to a 31 percent hospital mortality in the ST.AMB. group, a significant difference ($p < 0.05$). The difference was most marked during the first 24 hours where six patients (6 percent) died in the MCCU group compared to twelve patients (18 percent) in the ST.AMB group ($p < 0.01$). The three patients dying of AMI during transport, one in the MCCU group and two in the ST.AM.B. group should be included with all the patients with AMI that were alive on the arrival of the ambulance bringing the total mortality for the groups to 17 and 33 percent respectively. The hospital mortality in the ST.AMB. group of 31 percent is almost identical to what was found during the pilot study of AMI patients transported to hospital by ambulance (32 percent). The difference in mortality could possibly be artificial and explained by different criteria for the diagnosis of AMI in the MCCU and ST.AMB. groups. A higher mortality in the non-AMI group transported with the MCCU would cancel the favourable results reported here. An additional analysis of the mortality for all patients arriving alive at the hospital and not diagnosed as AMI was done (Table 6).

Of 360 patients in the MCCU group not developing AMI there were four

Table 6. Mortality in patients arriving alive in hospital not developing AMI.

	MCCU	ST.AMB.
No. of patients	360	265
Hospital deaths	4 (1.1%)	8 (3.0%)
– thereof in cardiac disease	1	4

hospital deaths (1.1 percent) and of these one was caused by cardiac disease. In the 265 standard ambulance cases not developing AMI there were eight deaths (3.0 percent) and of those four were caused by cardiac disease. Thus, even in patients not developing AMI there is a tendency to lower hospital mortality in the group transported by a MCCU.

DISCUSSION: CHAPTER 5

Chairman: R. Balcon

DISCUSSION CHAPTER 5

Paper 2: A mobile service for intraaortic baloon assistance in cardiogenic shock and refractory angina.

HUGENHOLTZ: We have reported the results of our series of patients with cardiogenic shock in the American Journal of Cardiology and our series has since increased to 60 patients treated with balloon pumping and with more than 55 % survival, long-term. We have found that it is the patient started on the pump with more than six hour delay who is at greatest risk of not surviving; and the second thing is the age.
MASERI: Could you comment on the complications you have had with balloon pumping?
HUGENHOLTZ: Several centers have quite a variable degree of complications. Maybe we have been lucky. Our main complications have been local vascular problems. We've had a number of people that we just couldn't get in, and I consider that not quite a complication, but the pump couldn't be used. The striking thing, in our experience, has been the marked thrombocytopenia. The membrane is supposed to be non allergenic or traumatic to the thrombocytes, but they are going down, and I'm wondering, is this therapeutic platelet aggregation that we are causing.
TAVAZZI: Dr. Balcon, please explain your indication to the application of the balloon in patients with angina at rest, because I have seen that some patients had normal left ventricular end-diastolic pressure.
BALCON: Well I believe that balloon pumping is one way of relieving continuing chest pain. And as I said this morning, the other way is with simple medication. And there was a time, there was a period, when we were planning a triumph of both forms of treatment. And these eleven patients were in the pilot study. We actually don't use it any more for rest angina, unless we are planning a surgical approach. So we don't really have indications. They were the same as for any other group of patients with continuing angina. It was just that form of treatment, which as you know was being advised by the Mass General and various other places. And we abandoned the trial after a while because it didn't seem right to go on.
JULIAN: I think we need to define which patients, if any, are benefited. I'm not convinced absolutely. I know everybody agrees that the patients look wonderful on the pump. They look nice and pink, and then they die, all of them do. So I think what we really need to know is which patients do benefit. Now you won't find that out simply by treating a lot of patients. You'll find it out by

preparing different groups of patients, some of whom are treated and some of whom are not.

HUGENHOLTZ: I don't feel today, sorry to say this perhaps, from me, as a scientist, that I can deny a person who's in shock and who comes into my hands within six hours and who is young, the pump. And I know this is bad science but we are not alternating or randomly assigning these people to medical versus surgical therapy. I think medical treatment, including dopamine, to my view, is murder.

JULIAN: Dr. Balcon was talking about a group of patients we would all agree as being shocks, I think. And we know that the mortality in such a group is of the order of about 80 %. If you lower the age group and modify things, you will get that natural mortality below 80 %. I don't known what the natural mortality in your patients would be.

HUGENHOLTZ: I'm simply saying that when we look at our data we found two discriminating factors: it was those who where below 60 and who came in within six hours who did the best.

JULIAN: From the point of view of the purpose of this meeting, we need to be able to tell people in what we call district hospitals which patients, if any, should be directed to yours or Dr. Balcon's organization. And we need to have a very clear definition of the criteria. And we will only do this if we have controlled experiments to define these populations.

HUGENHOLTZ: Yes and no. I think I can give some criteria by which we can tell the physicians around us these are the patients we want you to send us. I'll accept the chest film and the physical examination and the low peripheral blood pressure and the lack of urine produc- tion, if they do come in with a balloon catheter in their urinary tract; but I concur with him that I cannot force these people to do a catheterization or some other hemodynamic investigation because then it takes so long and they don't have the facilities. But when we perform hemodynamic monitoring and they are in the class 3 to 4 MIRU and they have the shock syndrome, then they get the pump. My only issue with you is that today I wouldn't personally want to do this thing, although I know it's against the grain of me as a scientist. I could have done this 33 years ago when we started. And it's sad, that once you are in the thing, you move or you have a certain committment to this, and then it's very difficult to set up a control study that is really control.

BALCON: Well I think that we could go on and argue that particular point for a long time, which we shouldn't. Dr. Julian is obviously right.

HUGENHOLTZ: As a scientist, but not necessarily as a doctor.

BALCON: But I was only going to add that you'll have a lot of trouble getting that study done, because this is, you know, the rushing around emergency work area where you see immediate results. And I don't think the protocol would be followed. They'd say, oh well, I know we should have not ballooned that one, but his grandfather was a friend of my uncle; that kind of thing: so we ballooned him. I honestly believe you would have great difficulty in not doing it, because the effect is so immediate and so obvious. And even the nurses would say, well, why aren't you ballooning him?

Paper 3: Mobile CCU's: techniques and management.

Paper 4: A randomized study on effectiveness of mobile CCU's.

BALCON: Can I open the whole subject of mobile coronary care to the audience.
FERUGLIO: We started a regular coronary care unit in 1968 and after about 7 or 8 years we were discouraged with the fact that many of our patients used to come into a coronary care after 7 hours, at the average. So in 1977, starting from June the first, we started with a mobile coronary care unit. According to previous experience, we delimitated a certain area that could be reached by the ambulance in about 20 minutes at the most. The area covered about 280,000 people and the ambulance was run with a doctor on it at disposal 24 hours a day all around the clock and all around the year. At the beginning we tried to reach our people through the doctors, in order to make the doctors aware that this means was at their disposal. But we were also disappointed, because after 6 months we had very poor results. Only about 8 % of the people reaching our coronary care in the hospital used the mobile unit; then we reviewed our policy, and we tried to reach the people through the press, through local television, etc. So the things changed quite a bit. And now, after one year and a half, we have come up, first to 10 % and then to 31 % of the patients admitted to our coronary care now coming through the ambulance and they reach the coronary care within one hour. And I have not reviewed the results, but I think that this was one of the main targets and we are very happy with this. I would say another thing, and this is that the false calls by the people are only 50 %, in our experience. Things have changed completely when we didn't leave on the central ambulance staff the decision to go out with the coronary care unit ambulance or with the standard ambulance. Now they have a specific telephone number, which comes out also on the newspapers among all the other emergency phone numbers, so they call that number and without any specific explanation the coronary care unit goes out with the doctor. We of course advertise this means, especially with patients of high risk, patients discharged from the coronary care, relatives, and people who come to our regular clinics. But I think this is one of the first experiments in Italy, done as a study of course, and we hope to come up with definite results in 5 years, but the first main target after one year of working is that today, 30 % of all our 600 patients admitted to the

coronary care unit come through this means.

HOLMBERG: We send out an intern from hospital and a nurse.

HUGENHOLTZ: All three major cities, including Rotterdam (Rotterdam is the only one that has equipped every ambulance with the minimum package - defibrillator, intervention set, etc. and a single-channel writer) have trained the two people on the ambulance, one is the driver, in all resuscitation techniques. And that system we have run for the last three years, resulting in 88 correct cardiac massages successfully arriving in hospital with 35 % long- term survivors. We are very happy with that. And my question to you is: do you think we are correct in just using only a nurse (they incidentally are allowed to give atropin as well as morphin when necessary), trained in resuscitation techniques? We did not believe we needed a doctor. I couldn't afford them, but we've had no mistakes that I can really detect.

PANTRIDGE: If Dr. Hugenholtz got manpower to put in these balloon pumps, he should have no problems in sending out a doctor in the ambulance. If always seemed to me that if you have a coronary care unit and 90 % of the people in that coronary care unit are either convalescent or moribund, you are employing all of this manpower, looking after patients who are in the hospital, who 90 % of them are either convalescent or moribund. Maybe what you are doing is absolutely right. Maybe your paramedical personnel can be very efficient in your possible CCU's, but I don't think that those people are as good as a well trained nurse, taking with her a young house physician. He incidentally is by law authorized to give intravenous injections. The nurse is not of course.

BALCON: Does anybody have any comment to make about Dr. Holmberg's paper, the randomized trial?

PANTRIDGE: I can't quite understand why randomized trial was necessary. You have a situation here where we know that the deaths outside hospital are due to ventricular fibrillation; that's point number one. Point number two is that we know that ventricular fibrillation can be corrected. So I think it's a matter of arranging how it should be done. I think everybody will agree and in fact I believe even Dr. Hugenholtz will agree that infarct size can be limited.

BALCON: If nobody comments otherwise, I am going to go away with the opinion that mobile coronary care is thought to be desiderable in some form or another. Although, it is probably not necessary to have medical manpower.

JULIAN: I mean the striking thing is that many of us agree exactly with what is being said by Dr. Pantridge and by many others. In fact, as he has pointed out, there are very few mobile coronary care units around, and this applies particularly in Britain; and I think most of us - we had, as you pointed out, a unit in Edinburgh and we had one in Newcastle, and in both cases these were doctor manned and they have now been abandoned because we cannot get the doctors to man them. Now we would like to have them run by paramedical personnel. But for financial reasons and from the need of persuading the paramedical people to get involved in this, this turns out not to be feasable. This may not be a problem in other countries, but in our country this is a very big problem. I don't know whether you have the same problem in London and I don't know whether it occurs in other countries, but we have a very big problem of persuading that either the whole lot should be trained, or one group doesn't like another group to be trained and to be paid more. So there are big political problems which are much more important than the medical problems. This may not apply outside Britain, but it certainly applies in Britain.

PANTRIDGE: There are political and administrative reasons why things are not happening. And I think the reason is our masters, political and administrative, really don't understand what the situation is. You can get all the money you want for balloon pumps and heart-lung machines. No difficulty getting money for those things or getting the money to pay the personnel to run them. But, if you look at the number of lives that can be saved from cardiogenic shock, they are small. By the nature of things, cardiogenic shock means a massive infarct, they cannot be very good lives after that, but we have people dying outside hospital from ventricular fibrillation who've got a very good likelihood of duration of life. There is evidence that the long-term outlook for these people is extremely good. Yet nothing is being done for them for these silly administrative and political reasons. So I think in fact, if you are going to summarize the situation, I would suggest that here is a situation where there are these enormous numbers of lives, numbers of thousands that could possibly be saved and yet nothing is being done about it. And you may or may not say you need medical personnel, but you certainly need personnel of some caliber who can do the various things that can be done.

CHAPTER 6

EXPANDING ROLE OF CORONARY CARE UNIT IN THE COMMUNITY
(Telephone transmission and ambulatory monitoring of ecg)

6.1. INTRODUCTION
L. Donato

The purpose of the final session is to explore the possibility of interfacing better and further the CCU's with the community. We will discuss two subjects, one is telemonitoring and the other one is 24-hour ECG analysis.

Telemonitoring has two kinds of interests: 1) to make possible regular ECG checks in patients that have to receive periodical controls, like pace-maker carrying patients, without having theme move to the center; 2) to record and transmit ECG's to a specialist center from areas like factories, schools, stadiums, when a physician might not be readily available.

The 24 hour ECG analysis it is also interesting from two points of view: 1) that of patients with suspect symptoms that cannot be documented when they come to the hospital but they could be clarified by 24 hour monitoring; 2) that of controlling patients at risk after discharge from hospital and of evaluating individual treatments.

6.2. AVAILABLE TECHNIQUES FOR TRANSMISSION OF BIOSIGNALS FROM
PATIENTS OR FROM PERIPHERALS TO A CENTRAL STATION
P. Mancini

6.2.1. INTRODUCTION

The growing tendency towards the centralization of expertise and the
even improving techniques for the transmission of biosignals represent the rational for exploring the actual possibilities of the
transmission of biosignals, in particular those derived from electrocardiograms to coronary care units.
Better interfacing with the community might improve the cost/benefit
ratio of the Coronary Care Units (CCU). By necessity a CCU must be
equipped with particularly trained personnel, and the possibility of
patients being able to use this expertise for consultation from
their homes appears a possibility worthy of consideration, in view
of the rapid advances in technology. The possibility of the use of
conventional telephone lines for transmitting biosignals has already
been successfully explored and is, at present, a subject of careful
attention.
    The most immediate potential conditions where this technology may
find application is in the transmission of electrocardiographic
tracings for analysis and the transmission of signals from patients
carrying particular apparatus requiring regular or occasional checks
to evaluate the adequacy of their function.

6.2.2. TRANSMISSION OF BIOSIGNALS AND POSSIBLE FIELD OF APPLICATION

Obviously, the telephonic transmission of signals presents some
limitation due to technical reasons. One must remember that telephone lines have been designed for a precise purpose, namely the
transmission of the human voice at a quality level sufficient for
human understanding.
This end can be seen in terms of communication channel bandwidth,
which results in practice and for most public networks to be around
3.000 Hz with an average signal-to-noise ratio of 40 dB. These are
target figures seldom respected due to particular electrical conditions of the line or the switching station which degrade the
communication quality. A better situation is encountered with leased
lines, but they permit only a particular use of telephone transmission. In fact they are not switchable, cannot be shared and are only
suitable for fixed installations.
    With this characteristics of the telephone channel it is necessa-

ry to use suitable interfaces, modem (modulator-demodulator), in order to have the best utilization of the line and to obtain a reliable transmission of the signal. The modem is necessary for adapting the flux of information coming with the signal to be transmitted to the available channel; the information is encoded and decoded by means of one or more modulated carriers.

The modem is also employed to prevent interference, which may be achieved by strictly following suitable standards of transmission with respect to carrier frequency and power.

The problem of a standard suitable for biomedical signal transmission has been considered by several international authorities, in particular by the European Community and by the International Telegraph and Telephone Consultative Committee (CCITT).

The Biomedical Research Committee of the European Community has sponsored various simposia either devoted or related to the topic (Cortona, Stuttgard, Mainz) (1, 2, 3) and the CCITT has established the recommendation v. 16 (1976) (4) dedicated to medical data modems. Various transmission systems are considered on the recommendation, those with either galvanic or acoustic coupling, those with or without simultaneous voice and digital data transmission, and those with one, two or three contemporary signals. However, the attention is pointed towards a specific type of biological signal, the type with a frequency content between 5 and 10 Hz. This is the case for the ECG.

At present, the most frequent application of biomedical data transmission is made in cardiology and we can classify the various systems in four complexity levels.

At a first level we can considere these personal devices capable of transmitting one ECG lead. They are characterized by being very low in cost, are pocket-sized and battery operated and they have acoustic coupling to the microtelephone. This type of device can be useful for emergency use and drug monitoring, due to the possibility of performing rhythm analysis from a selected lead. The principle of operation is very simple; a voltage controlled oscillator is driven by the ECG signal and outputs, into a loudspeaker, a sound with variable pitch. The sound is transmitted through the telephone and received by a demodulator which drives a standard ECGraph. With this type of device it is sometimes possible to check pacemaker carrying patients as well, in order to determine the pacemaker life expectancy by precise measurement of the stimulating frequency.

Devices at a second level of complexity are more adequate for pacemaker checking. In these cases, with a modest increase un cost and dimension it is possible to obtain information on the shape and the parameters of the pacemaker stimulation pulse as well. This facility enables the specialist to evaluate the general electrical condition of the prosthesis and its electrode. The principle of operation in this case is complicated .by the presence of a pulse stretcher which expands the time course of the pacemaker artifact in order to permit its telephone transmission as if it were ECG complex.

A third level of systems is represented by the terminals for the transmission of the ECG to computer aided interpretation units. In this case, more than one signal is transmitted simultaneously, in order to meet with the needs of the various computer programs which often require three contemporary leads for a complete diagnosis. Here the operation of the transmitter is based on multiple carriers indipendently modulated by the signals from the various leads. In this case, it is often difficult to compress correctly all the information to be transmitted into the limited bandwidth of the telephone channel, and when the signal-to-noise ratio of the line is poor a distorted signal is received after demodulation.

Telephone lines permit bidirectional exchange of information and this capability leads to the fourth level of systems. In this class we have a patient terminal capable of transmitting and receiving information. The transmitted information is related to the various biological signals of interest while the received information is the medium through which we obtain the terminal operation controlled by the receiving station. This facility enables the physician to select various functions (change leads, amplification factor, calibrations, etc.) at the patient terminal and permits an optimal utilization of the channel for biosignal transmission. This type of system is particularly useful for remote patient monitoring and will permit, in the future, the delivering of an essential part of hospital cardiac care to the patient's home.

6.2.3. OUR EXPERIENCE

In the past few years we have had the opportunity of developing various types of systems for biomedical data transmission. We started with a simple system for remote pacemaker pulse analysis (5, 6) and we have now reached a new system of ECG telemonitoring with remote controlled terminals (7).

Our aim is to aid all those patients who need periodic and well defined instrumental check-up. This objective requires two contemporary conditions: a reliable care-free patient terminal and a well established medical centre servicing for telephone consultation. At present we are concerned with the first of the above mentioned conditions, which, in our opinion is prioritary. The second condition is not completely manageable by staffs and involves organizational and political problems with the hospital. However, we can say that a well suited technical mean can greatly help, whereas the presence of even a minor technical imperfection could be determinant in the failure of the entire centre's organization.

6.2.4. CONCLUSION

In conclusion, we can say that from a technical point of view the
telephone transmission of biosignals is a well established and well
defined new medical instrument. In many countries there are working
examples of telephone ECG transmission from centre to centre, mainly
where automatic ECG diagnosis is performed. Even pacemaker carrying
patients can profit from simple devices for periodic transtelepho-
nic check-ups.

But, in practice, we think that much work has yet to be done in
the liason between organization and instrumentation before a substantial part of medical assistence might profit from the new telephone
technique in the field of electrocardiology.

REFERENCES

1. Intramural versus extramural care. The reach of technology. International Conference supported by the European Community. Cortona,
   Italy September 22-24, 1975. Published by Commission of the
   European Communities EUR 56 22c, 1976.
2. Medical data transmission by public telephone systems. Proceedings of a workshop organized in Stuttgart, 26-28 November 1975.
   Published by a Commission of the European Communities EUR 5704c,
   1977.
3. Medical data transmission by public telephone systems. 2nd International Symposium - Mainz, June 3-4 1977. Supported by the
   European Community. Published by URBAN - SCHWARZEMBERG - Munchen
   1978.
4. International telegraph and telephone consultative Committee -
   CCITT - Sixth Plenary Assembly - Geneva, 27 September - 8 October
   1976. Orange Book - Volume VIII. 1 - Data Transmission over the
   telephone network. Published by: International telecommunication
   Union - Geneva 1977.
5. Mancini P, R Bedini: A new method for utilizing a standard
   ECGraph for in vivo clinical pacemaker analysis. IEEE-BME 281-
   286, 1975.
6. Mancini P, R Bedini, G Palagi, C Contini, F Pauletti, G Bini: Un
   nuovo dispositivo per il controllo telefonico del paziente porta-
   tore di pacemaker permanente. Bollettino della Società Italiana
   di Cardiologia, vol XX, 1027-1030, 1975.
7. Mancini P, R Bedini, G Palagi, C Contini: A new method for in
   vivo pacemaker electrical analysis for ambulatory and telepho-
   ne-home check. Proc San Diego Biomedical Symposium, vol 15,
   17-21, 1976.

6.3. AUTOMATED SYSTEM FOR INTERPRETATION OF 24-HOUR ECG TAPE RECOR-
DINGS
P.W. Macfarlane, I. Hutton, A. Irving, M.P. Watts, T.P.M. Taylor,
T.D.V. Lawrie

6.3.1. INTRODUCTION

The concept of long-term tape recording of the ECG was first proposed many years ago by Holter (1). However it is only in recent years
that the full benefit of this technique has been realised and there
has been a considerable expansion of facilities for recording and
interpreting 24-hour tape recordings. In some countries bureau services have been established and considerable sums of money are involved in the provision of interpretative services.

On one 24-hour ECG tape there may be of the order of up to
200,000 cardiac cycles to be analysed and this creates a vast amount
of data which requires careful handling if it is not to be wasted in
any way. Conventional methods of interpretation require a physiological measurement technician to review the 24-hour recording normally
replayed at least at 60 times the recording speed. This is a strain
on technicians and indeed is of limited value in that instances of
obviously abnormal rhythm can be easily detected by the technician
but subtle changes in heart rate throughout the 24 hours cannot be
observed. Likewise analysis of fluctuating atrial activity may be
missed and the diagnosis of complete AV block for example may not be
made unless there has been a marked change in heart rate which
causes an alert technician to have a closer look at particular
pieces of recording.

In order to circumvent some of these limitations, there recently has
been a move towards using a digital computer in conjunction with
24-hour analysers to provide a more detailed record of the tracing.
Some limited systems are commercially available and a few more are
likely to be announced in the near future where a micro-processor is
incorporated for simple data logging tasks such as providing a
histogram of RR intervals. Again however this is a limited approach
and in our own laboratory we have developed a more comprehensive
approach for the detailed interpretation of a 24-hour ECG recording.

6.3.2. METHODS

ECGs are tape recorded using Oxford Medical Instruments 24-hour
recorders. The appropriate Oxford compatible tape replay unit is
used and linked to a high speed ECG analyser (Pathfinder) of

Reynolds Medical Electronics. In the normal operation of this analyser, a technician teaches the analyser the morphology of the normal beat and analysis thereafter is completely automatic once the various triggering levels have been set. In our case, for replay to the computer, none of the "hold" switches is set since the tape must not stopped at any stage during the 24 minute replay, even altough arrhythmic events can be detected and automatically printed by the Pathfinder.

The analyser is linked to a PDP8A computer via an interface built in our own laboratory. The output from the analyser consists of the logic pulses, normal and abnormal, together with QRS triggering pulse and the ECG itself. The purpose of the interface is to remove high frequency interface from the ECG signal and to widen the logic pulses so as to allow the computer time to check the logic level. The interface also contains a clock which pulses at a rate of 7.500 Hz. This in turn is used to control the rate of sampling the ECG on the computer AD converter (ADC).

Three signals are input to the computer ADC. As well as the ECG, the two logic pulses are input via this route. There are also three inputs to the computer clock and in particular to the Schmitt triggers which form part of this system. These three inputs include the QRS triggering pulse, the inhibit signal from the analyser (this indicates an excessive amount of artefact) while the third input is from the external clock. This completes the link between the analyser and the digital computer.

From the computing point of view, one or two questions must be answered by the operator before data acquisition commences, e.g. is there a full 24-hour tape to be analysed or is there only a portion? In addition if an estimate of ST trend is required, the operator is asked to adjust the reference point before the onset of the QRS complex and the point at which the ST segment is to be measured. This is accomplished by making use of the fact that the QRS triggering signal occurs after the QRS complex on the ECG is input to the computer. Therefore the reference points for QRS onset and ST measurement are referred to this triggering point, i.e. the respective number of samples prior to the occurrence of the trigger is defined. The computer initially assumes the onset to be 28 samples before the trigger and the ST reference to be 8 samples before the trigger and all three reference points are marked on the ECG which is output via a digital to analogue converter. The operator then adjusts the reference points if necessary by inserting the appropriate numbers into the computer.

The computer will also store a finite number of strips of abnormalities and prior to the onset of data acquisition, the operator can indicate to the programme how many samples of VES for example it is required to store. Likewise the numebr of examples of runs of VES is also indicated to the programme. At the present time up to 30 examples of each type of arrhythmia can be stored with a maximum combined total of 60. These arrhythmias include single VES, couplets, marked arrhythmia (e.g. AF), runs of VT and asystole. The programme is then ready for acceptance of the ECG data, the tape is started and data acquisition commences.

Subsequently, the computer will store for each QRS complex an indication of whether it is normal or abnormal and its relationship to the preceding QRS complex, i.e. the RR interval. In addition the time since the start of the recording is also stored. As previously discussed, an estimate of ST deviation is also stored in 6 bits of the computer word. Finally if the inhibit output of the analyser is switched on, a record of this is also kept. This means that there is too much artefact on the recording for analysis to be undertaken by the Pathfinder. Thus for each QRS complex, three computer words are stored containing all the necessary information.

The sequence of events is as follows. When the QRS triggering signal is obtained, the computer programme is interrupted and measurements are made on the outputs from the logic signals of the analyser. At the same time, the clock counter is transferred to core since this indicates the RR interval, and is then reset to zero. The estimate of the time of day is calculated and stored. If and only if the inhibit pulse is set, the programme is interrupted to prevent analysis at that time.

In addition to the routine acquisition of this QRS data, the ECG is sampled continuously at a rate of 7.500 samples per second, i.e. 125 samples per second in real time. The data is stored in a cyclic buffer and a separate logical analysis determines whether it needs to be transferred to disc for permanent storage at any particular instant. For example if runs of ventricular tachycardia are noted, then the computer will store the data in the buffer at that time. In this way a set of abnormal rhythms can be stored automatically without the need for a technician to observe their presence.

At the end of 24 minutes or less, a complete description of the ECG is then available on disc for further analysis by a separate computer programme.

The analysis begins with a few routine matters such as inserting the patient's name, age and so on for output purposes. The starting time of the 24-hour tape is also input and the critical periods for early or late VES are set up. Normally a late VES is reported if the coupling interval is longer than 0.40 secs. An early VES is reported if the coupling interval is less than 0.40 secs. Prior to analysis the operator can adjust this parameter if it is so desired. Output from the system can be written both to a VDU and also to magnetic tape which is later taken to a similar system where a line printer is available for hard copy of the report.

The basic summary consists of a break-down of the 24-hour recording into 15 minutes periods for which the average heart rate, incidence of VES, early VES, late VES, supra VT and VT is output. In addition, an indication of the percentage artefact in the 15 minute period is also provided since this is a good indication of the reliability of the VES count. For each of these outputs, it is possible to obtain an alternative display in graphical form indicating the variation in heart rate for example over 24 hours. Likewise a graph of the number of VES over 24 hours is obtained. In addition an ST trend graph can also be plotted. This does not give an absolute measurement of ST deviation but provides a trend of the ST amplitude throughout the 24 hours.

Another option which is available is to plot a histogram of coupling intervals over a 15-minute period. This is useful in deciding whether VES are unifocal or multifocal, as in the case of the former a histogram of coupling intervals produces a normal distribution. In the case of the latter there is a scatter or biomodal distribution depending on the complexity of the arrhythmia.

One other very important option is available. This concerns the arrhythmia analysis of the 8 sec. portions of ECGs which have automatically been selected and stored by the digital computer programme. Based on earlier work in our laboratory for routine interpretation of cardiac rhythm in 3-lead ECGs (2, 3) methods were available for analysis of 8 sec. strips of rhythm. These have been incorporated into the programme and therefore up to 40 different rhythm statements can be made from an analysis of the 8 sec. strips.

In parallel with this it is possible to output the various strips of rhythm via the digital to analogue converter. Thus the system automatically capture arrhythmic events, produces an interpretation and outputs the ECG.

6.3.3. DISCUSSION

There is still considerable scope for further development of the analysis programme. For example, the next step might be to obtain a sample of ECG every 15 minutes to provide an analysis of rhythm on a regular basis rather than simply on a random basis depending on the occurrence of any arrhythmic activities. In this way a trend of PR intervals, for example, could be obtained so that more subtle changes in rhythm over the 24 hour period could be detected.

The ultimate aim would be to produce a fully automated report which can make some English language comment on the appearances throughout the 24 hours. Typically the report would indicate whether the rhythm was basically stable or unstable, whether the tracing was technically satisfactory or not and would be able to give an account of the abnormal rhythms if any were detected.

To date the system has proved effective in the trial of a new anti-arrhythmic drug. Without this system, it would have been an enormous task to study the effect of the drug and in particular to determine whether a patient met one of the criteria for exclusion for further study, viz: more than six ectopic beats in one minute. This type of criterion cannot be estimated by any other technique than that described above because commercially available analyser simply count the number of ectopic beats and it would be an impossible task for a technician to stop and start a tape recording at every minute of 24 hours in order to count the number of VES in that time interval. Thus the value of the system has already been demonstrated.

It is worth considering the economics of the approach. The computer hardware cost approximately £ 20,000 although currently available equipment would not cost as much with the possibility of offering an improved performance in respect of disc storage space. The analysing equipment and interface with a few tape recorders has cost the order of £ 10,000. At the present time our throughput is of the order of 25 tapes per week. The current commercial rate for analysis of one tape is £ 50 so that the system virtually pays for itself within six months of installation. Of course, the time taken for a technician to set up the equipment, etc., has to be taken into account, together with incidental costs such as ECG paper and tapes but clearly with the system having an expected life of up to 10 years the cost of installation represents a small sum compared to the cost of having the tapes analysed by a bureau. Indeed the figures above being based on 5 tracings per day clearly underestimate the situation. If the technician were paid solely to do this work, she would be available $7\frac{1}{2}$ hours per day and the number of tracings analysed would increase to the order of 8 giving a proportionate increase in the benefits of utilizing the computer system. It could also be argued that the cost of the computer analysis would be virtually static over the 10 year life of the computer whereas the cost of the bureau service is likely to increase with time.

There is currently a trend to introduce micro-computer assisted analysis of the 24 hour recordings. This is acceptable for producing a histogram of RR intervals over the 24 hours but beyond that there is little that the system can do unless greater storage facilities such as a disc are made available. Whenever the addition of medium scale data storage facilities to a micro-computer is considered, the differentiation between a micro-computer and a mini-computer system becomes somewhat less clear. Likewise the cost of the two systems begins to become similar and the mini-computer system described would seem to offer the best solution to the problem. When the ECG is sampled at 7.500 Hz there is very little time indeed for processing of the signals. Therefore considerations of on-line digital analysis of the high speed replayed ECG must be limited to the technique described above unless special purpose circuitry, e.g. parallel processors, is to be used. It would seem to us that there will be little advantage in changing from the type of system described above to any other approaches incorporating digital processing.

Computer analysis of 24 hour ECG tape recordings has been proved feasible and worthwhile both from the practical and economic points of view. It would seem to us that this is the optimal approach to analysing such tracings and indeed perhaps the only way to cope with the increasing volume of tape recordings accruing from the recognised value of the technique of 24-hour monitoring.

REFERENCES

1. Holter NJ: New method for heart studies, Science, 134: 1214, 1961.
2. Macfarlane PW, TDV Lawrie: An introduction to automated electrocardiogram analysis. Butterworths, London, 1974.
3. Taylor TPM: PhD Thesis. Computer analysis of cardiac arrhythmias. University of Glasgow, 1974.

6.4. A SOFTWARE APPROACH TO RHYTHM AND ST-T ANALYSIS OF 24 HOUR ECG
C. Marchesi, M. Biella, C. Contini, G.F. Mazzocca

6.4.1 INTRODUCTION

The practical limitations encountered in the use of commercially available systems for ECG ambulatory monitoring, led us to the development of the ASTRI (Analisi ST RItmo) computer program, for the analysis of rhythm and ST segment changes.

The major limitations of commercially available systems are the following:
A. required presence of a physician or of a very well trained operator during the analysis;
B. inadequate accuracy of the QRS detection and of the classification of abnormal beats;
C. unreliability of the analysis of the ST-T changes;
D. high cost.

The ASTRI program includes some original features, such as unsupervised analysis and one-pass processing (1-4).

The evaluation of ASTRI is in progress. It is performed on a random basis over the 24 hour recordings and all the rhythm classes recognized by ASTRI are separately evaluated. The present values obtained for specificity and sensitivity of different classes are always more than 90 percent.

6.4.2 MATERIAL AND METHODS

A. Hardware: the present evaluation version of ASTRI runs, in time sharing, on a Hewlett-Packard HP-1000 system composed of:
1. A/D and D/A converters HP 2313.
2. mag tape HP 7970
3. disc unit HP 7905
4. line printer HP 2767
5. 21MX processor HP 2112.

The graphic units used are:
1. Tektronix: 611 storage CRT for threshold control
2. Versatec 1100 for hard copy of histograms and plots
3. ECG recorder for patient record documentation.

The 24 hour ECG was recorded on an Oxford MEDILOG recorder or on an Avionics ELECTROCARDIOCORDER.

B. Software: ASTRI is composed of 5 programs:
SCAR 1 performes the sampling of the ECG signal and its recording on

mag tape at 60 times real-time reduction. The samples are grouped in records of 30 seconds each.

SCAR 2 is an interactive program for selection of thresholds both for the QRS detection algorithm and for beat classification. The ECG signal is presented on the CRT together with markers which point to Q, R, S waves, with a column of three numbers close to each QRS representing the measure of RR interval, QRS duration and a shape factor (Fig. 1). This factor is computed by comparison with a normal beat selected by the operator.

SCAR 3 is the program for automatic analysis. The processing is performed record by record, according to the following operation sequence.

QRS detection: obtained by an algorithm based on the analysis of slopes (5). Every QRS is identified by the three instants of occurance of the Q, R, S waves.

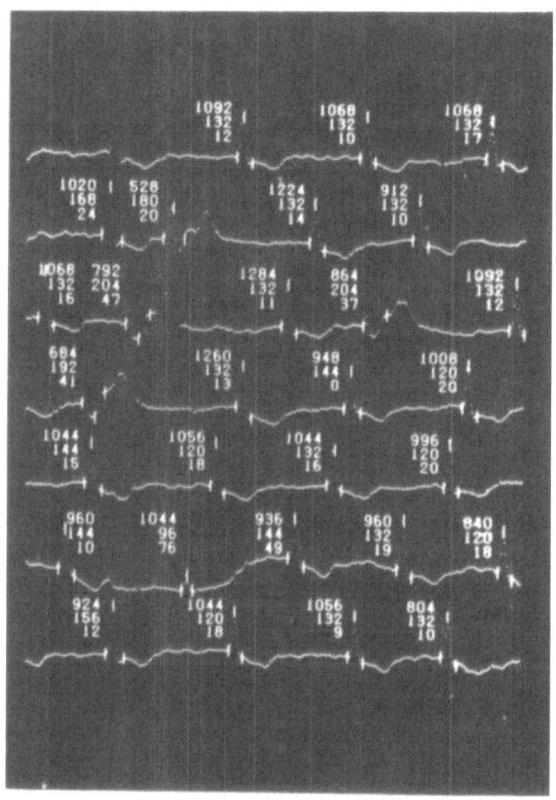

Fig. 1. Display of an ECG record during the set-up procedure.

Cardiac cycle parameters: RR interval, QRS duration, and an integral QRS shape factor are measured on each detected cycle. The shape factor (SF) is obtained by (6):

$$SF = \sum_{i=t_Q}^{t_S} \left| QRS_t - QRS \right|_i$$

where QRS_t is the typical QRS and i points to the samples in the interval Q-S ($t_Q - t_S$).

Classification: based on the cycle parameters using a decision logical scheme; 11 classes are recognized, 6 classes refer to single beats and 5 to sequences of beats. Let I_i (i = 1,6) be binary input functions defining, when set, the following beat features:
I_i = premature, I_2 = wide, I_3 = abnormal shape, I_4 = delayed, I_5 = premature compared to mean value, I_6 = delayed compared to mean value.

The simple beat classes are defined by the following logical equations:

normal $= \bar{I}_1 \cap \bar{I}_3 \cap \bar{I}_4$

premature $= I_1 \cap \bar{I}_2 \cap \bar{I}_3$

premature and abnormal $= I_1 \cap (I_2 \cup I_3)$

delayed $= I_4$

abnormal shape $= \bar{I}_1 \cap \bar{I}_2 \cap I_3 \cap \bar{I}_4$

abnormal shape and wide $= \bar{I}_1 \cap I_2 \cap I_3 \cap \bar{I}_4$.

The definition of the sequence classes are based on the combination of consecutive beats, whose level of abnormality is less restrictive than in the single beat classes:

normal $= \bar{I}_1 \cap \bar{I}_5$

premature $= (\bar{I}_2 \cap \bar{I}_3) \cap (I_1 \cup I_5)$

premature and abnormal $= I_2 \cap (I_1 \cup I_5)$

premature for bigeminisms $= I_1 \cup I_5$

delayed $= \bar{I}_3 \cap (I_4 \cup I_6)$

delayed and abnormal $= I_3 \cap (I_4 \cup I_6)$

Bradycardia of normal beats is defined as a sequence of a consecutive number of delayed beats; bradycardia of abnormal beats is a sequence of delayed and abnormal beats; in a similar way tachycardia are defined by premature or premature and abnormal beats and bigeminy by normal and premature for geminy beats. Table 1 shows all the classes recognized.

Table 1. Classes recognized by ASTRI program.

C_1 : normal beats

C_2 : premature beats with normal QS interval

C_3 : wide or abnormally shaped premature beats

C_4 : delayed beats

C_5 : abnormally shaped beats

C_6 : abnormally shaped and wide beats

B_1 : bradycardia

B_2 : bradycardia of abnormal beats

T_1 : tachycardia

T_2 : tachycardia of wide beats

GE : geminy.

ST-T changes: each ST-T interval is searched for a positive and a negative wave. The sign of the waves is referred to the baseline defined as a straight-line crossing the P-Q intervals of two consecutive beats (5). The areas of the waves, if recognized, are considered ST-T parameters.

Moreover, the reference value of the RR is beat-to-beat self adjusted to follow the slow trends in heart rate. Trends are detected by the Trigg's method (7).

At the end of the processing of a record, the histograms of the distribution of RR, QRS duration, ST positive and negative area and shape factor, are updated.

Finally, a quality control of data is performed record by record, based on the histogram of the shape difference between the typical beat and the dominant beat in each record.

The classes, the histograms, the time plot and, optionally, all the measurements are saved on disc.

SCAR 4 it takes care of the printing of the classification, ST-T measurements, histograms and plots (Figs. 2, 3). It also produces a patient record that summarizes the computer findings.

SCAR 5. This program drives an ECG-strip recorder to obtain a D/A converted version of selected 30 second ECG records from mag tape.

This version of ASTRI is coded in FORTRAN; only the I/O routines are coded in ASSEMBLER. It runs at 20 times real-time reduction.

6.4.3 EVALUATION

The evaluation has been performed following a simple random sampling technique. The samples, which correspond to the records, have been

221

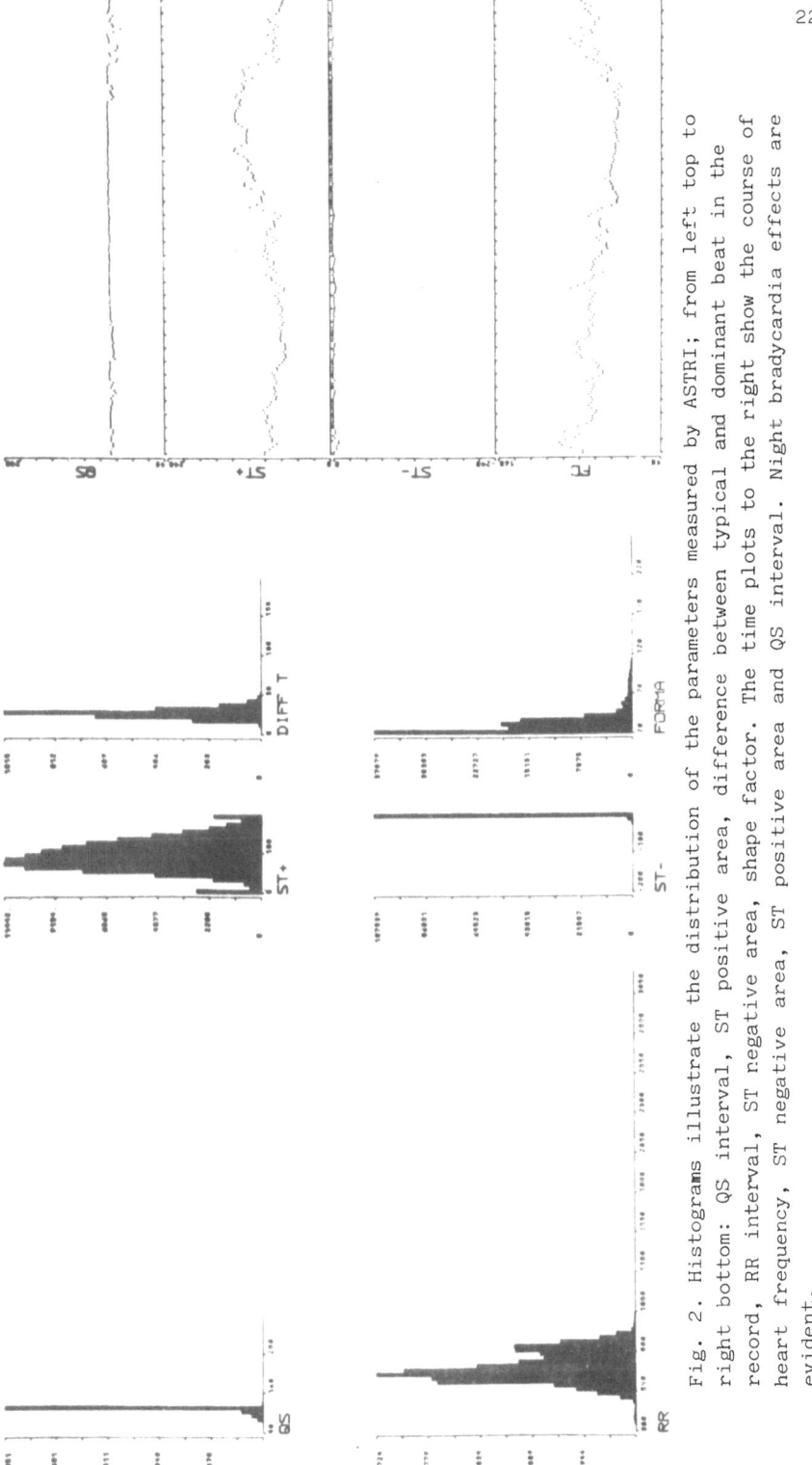

Fig. 2. Histograms illustrate the distribution of the parameters measured by ASTRI; from left top to right bottom: QS interval, ST positive area, difference between typical and dominant beat in the record, RR interval, ST negative area, shape factor. The time plots to the right show the course of heart frequency, ST positive area and QS interval. Night bradycardia effects are evident.

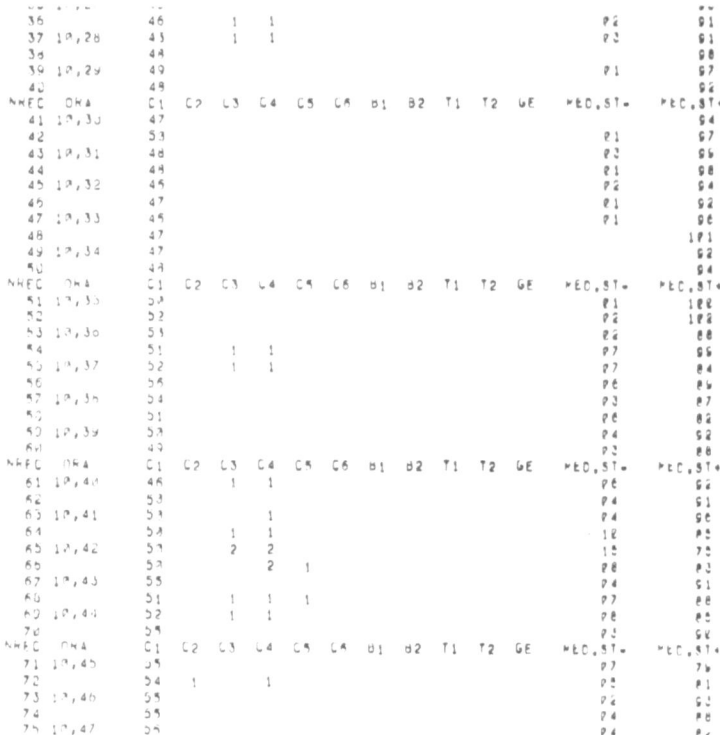

Fig. 3. Computer print-out of the record by record classification.

manually verified by a trained cardiologist. The evaluation procedure is based on the following steps:

A. ECG data are recorded on digital tape and are therefore precisely identified.

B. manual evaluation has been performed by a trained cardiologist not involved in program design.

C. ECG tapes were selected for evaluation if one abnormality class was dominand with an $F \geqslant 0.01$ proportion.

D. abnormal class distribution has been assumed to be random and the binomial model of the proportion between normal and abnormal events has been applied.

In this hypothesis the evaluation of a class C by a sampling of n digital records out of about 3000 (= N) in a 24 hour recording, is performed by a random drawing of a sample of size n from the population of size N in order to verify the condition:

$$P_r (F - f \geqslant d) = p \qquad (1)$$

where f is the proportion of C in the sample, d (>0) is the error accepted a priori with risk p and P_r means "Probability that". The problem is now a one tail test; if a normal distribution is assumed for f, the value of n will be given by (8):

$$n = n_o/(1 + n_o/N); \qquad\qquad n_o = t^2 fq/d^2$$

where $q = 1 - f$ and t is the Student variable for one tail test. These relations hold if n represents isolated events; in our case a cluster sampling has to be performed because the abnormal beats are included in a 30 second record (Fig. 4). The correction factor f_c is then computed (8):

$$f_c = \sum_{i=1}^{N} M_i^2 \, (f_i - F)^2 / N\bar{M}fQ$$

where M_i = size of the i-th sample, $\bar{M}$ = average of M_i.

As balance among various factor we selected:
n = 100
d = 0.3
p = 0.005 (one side t)

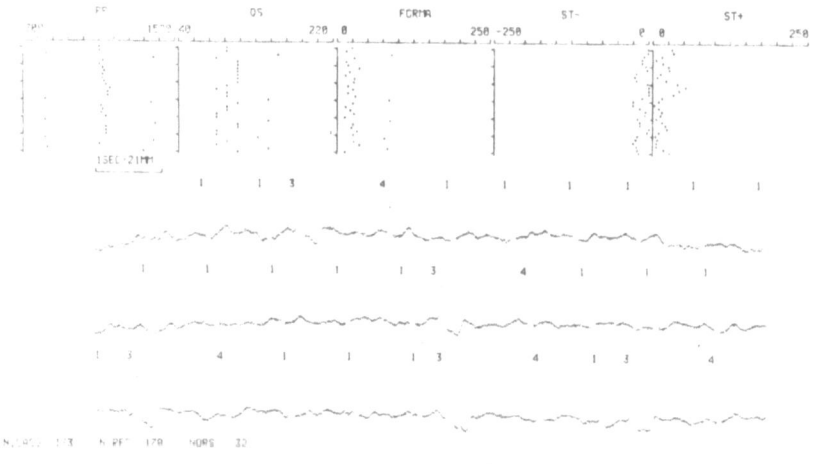

Fig. 4. Typical record format used for evaluation. The time plots have a beat to beat resolution. The number close to R wave is the class number (see Table 1).

Table 2 shows the results obtained so far by the application of this method, where TB are the total beats evaluated, NP is the number of patients so far selected for the evaluation, SENS is the sensitivity of the classification of the class, SPEC is the specificity.

The value of the sensitivity of C4 has been held low to obtain a higher specificity; actually, we have considered non relevant the detection of beats with low delay, while beats with greater delay have to be detected because they may have clinical relevance.

Table 2. ASTRI evaluation preliminary results.

	TB	NP	SENS	SPEC
QRS detection	22933	7	99.89	99.95
C1 (normal)	2118	1	98.91	91.97
C2 (SVE)	10267	3	96.21	98.20
C3 (PVC)	10548	3	95.54	99.97
C4 (delayed)	8316	2	75.68	99.69

6.4.4 DISCUSSION

The evaluation of monitoring systems suffers from the lack of accepted standards; the final answers to this old problem will only come from the access to a classified data base (9-11). At present, the only practical alternative is a man/machine comparison of random sampled data.

Assuming that the data from the literature (12, 13) are comparable with those obtained by our approach, the preliminary statistical results of our evaluation range among the best values of sensitivity and specificity of PVC classification. Moreover, ASTRI appears to be the only system evaluated even when compared with the other classes of abnormality.

Furthermore, in order to evaluate the performance of ASTRI in routine use, we have analyzed some of our ECG records on three commercial systems. The results show that in every case ASTRI allowed the cardiologist to get faster and more reliable information useful to the diagnosis (14).

The results of the statistical evaluation of the cases analyzed so far indicate that the automatic analysis performed by our program is comparable to that achieved by a trained cardiologist. Thus the traditional concept that the "operator interaction is required to monitor classification during the processing" (2) does no longer seem to apply. The higher cost of minicomputer hardware relative to special purpose electronics of commercial systems is compensated for by the greater versatility and by the possibility of updating, transfer of programs and concurrent uses for other jobs.

REFERENCES

1. Marchesi C, C Contini, GF Mazzocca: Minicomputer based cardiac rhythm and ST-T interval automatic analysis in ambulatory monitoring. Abstracts of communications of VIII World Congress of Cardiology, 17-23 September 1978, p 553.
2. Hansmann DR, JJ Sheppard: High speed computer ECG rhythm analysis. Abstracts of communications of VIII World Congress of Cardiology, 17-23 September 1978, p 554.
3. Ripley KL, RM Arthur: Evaluation and comparison of automatic arrhythmia detectors. IEEE Proceedings on Computers in Cardiology, Rotterdam, October 2-4, 1975.
4. Clark KW, RE Hitchens, JA Ritter et al: ARGUS/2H a dual channel Holter-tape analysis system. IEEE Proceedings on Computers in Cardiology, Rotterdam, September 29-1 October, 1977.
5. Marchesi C, S Chierchia, A Maseri: Left and right ventricular pressure monitoring in the CCU. Methods and significance. IEEE Proceedings on Computers in Cardiology, Rotterdam September 29-1 october, 1977.
6. Neilson JM: High speed analysis of ventricular arrhythmias from 24 hour recordings. IEEE Proceedings on Computers in Cardiology, Bethesda, October 2-4, 1974.
7. Trigg DW: Monitoring a forecasting system. Operat Res Quart Pergamon Press, 15: 271, 1964.
8. Cochran WG: Sampling techniques. John Wiley & Sons, Inc, 2nd Edition 1963.
9. Feldman CL: Evaluation of arrhythmia detectors. IEEE Proceedings on Computers in Cardiology, Bethesda, October 24, 1974.
10. Hagan A, et al: Development of a data base for electrocardiographic use. Proceedings of the tenth Bethesda conference on optimal electrocardiography. Am J Cardiol, p 35, 1977.
11. Ripley KL, G Oliver: Development of an ECG database for arrhythmia detector evaluation. IEEE Proceedings on Computers in Cardiology, September 29-1 October, 1977.
12. Hansmann DR, JJ Sheppard, A Yeshaya: Evaluation of the Dyna-Gram Holter ECG analysis system. IEEE Proceedings on Computers in Cardiology, St Louis, October 7-9, 1976.
13. Klein MD et al: A validation technique for computerized Holter tape processing sytems used in drug efficacy testing. IEEE Proceedings on Computers in Cardiology, Rotterdam, Septembe 29-1 October 1977.

14. Contini C, GF Mazzocca, C Marchesi, M Biella: Evaluation and clinical results of ASTRI program for ambulatory monitoring (this book).

6.5. EVALUATION AND CLINICAL RESULTS OF ASTRI PROGRAM FOR AMBULATO-
RY MONITORING
C. Contini, G.F. Mazzocca, C. Marchesi, M. Biella

6.5.1. INTRODUCTION

The ASTRI program (1) has been conceived for the automatic analysis
of rhythm disturbances and ST-T changes, in order to offer an
alternative to commercially available systems, which are unreliable
mainly in the detection of ECG alterations compatible with ischemic
diseases (positive and negative ST changes, negative T wave, etc.).

Its clinical application has been applied to more than 200
patients so far and has followed two distinct phases.
A. The first phase was orientated to the testing and updating of the
program performances. The patients were selected according to the
documented pathological conditions in their ST-T and/or rhythm
disturbances, to stress the program algorithms.
B. In the second phase patients were admitted to 24-hour monitoring
when typical indications existed, like claiming of unstable
symptoms that were undetermined by usual rest and stress ECG
tests.

6.5.2. MATERIAL

A consecutive series of 55 patients was admitted to the study, and
was divided into two groups. The first group consisted of 30
patients who reported symptoms of atypical or typical chest pain and
other forms of dizziness but with no previous positive diagnosis of
ischemic heart disease, based on rest and exercise ECG, and myocardial infarction documented by ECG and serum enzymes.

6.5.3. RESULTS

Table 1 shows the results of the study.
In 13 patients of the first group, no ECG changes were observed, in
17 positive or negative ST-T changes were measured, but only 2
reported episodes of chest pain during the recording. Among the
patients in the second group, 10 failed to show ECG changes; 15
showed positive or negative ST-T changes and only 5 reported episodes of pain during the recording.

We wish to point out that 6 out of 7 patients who reported chest

Table 1. Clinical results of ST-T segment analysis in ambulatory monitoring

	N°	ST→	ST↑	ST↓	ST↑↓	Tot.	Clin.ECG$^+$	Clin.ECG$^-$
Group 1	25	10	4	10	1	15	5	10
Group 2	30	13	1	15	1	17	2	15
Total	55	23	5	25	2	32	7*	25

* Also asymptomatic episodes are present in 6 patients

pain, also had asymptomatic episodes of ST-T changes during ambulatory monitoring.

6.5.4. DISCUSSION

The ASTRI program showed evident advantages when compared with commercial systems; the most significant are listed in the following points:
A. Flexibility (particularly important is the possibility of fitting the QRS detection thresholds to every patient).
B. Reliability of the QRS detection.
C. Very short man-machine interaction time (5-15 minutes, depending on the tracing complexity).
D. Proper quantitative determination of arrhythmias (because of the combination of the shape factor and other time interval parameters).
E. Beat classification is suitable for quantitative diagnostic aid.
F. Comprehensive presentation of all available information allowing the evaluation of antiarrhythmic treatment efficacy.

In our opinion, the most relevant features of ASTRI are the overall flexibility and the moderate interaction required. In the commercially available systems this time may easily exceed 120 minutes in complex tracings, with high incidence of pathological events.

Greater effort was dedicated to the evaluation of the ST-T changes analysis, because the method used is entirely new in ambulatory monitoring and comes from previous experiences in CCU monitoring (2, 3, 4). Commercially available systems are very unreliable, especially in ST-T segment depression diagnosis.

From a clinical point of view, the number of patients in our series is too low to allow definite conclusions about the significance of asymptomatic episodes of ST segment changes, although our findings are in close agreement with those previously reported (5, 6, 7, 8). It is our opinion that presence or absence of chest pain can no longer be considered a significant symptom for evaluating the clinical course and efficacy of therapeutic intervention in patients with previous positive diagnosis.

Some uncertainty about significance of ST-T changes arises when they are present in patients without other evidence of ischemic heart disease. However, recent observations (3, 4) during continuous hemodynamic monitoring in CCU showed that these episodes are relevant, because they are associated with the presence of severe alterations of ventricular function.

It is our belief, however, that the diagnostic possibilities of ambulatory monitoring of ECG are greatly increased by a reliable method of ST-T change analysis, even if this opinion seems to be, as yet, far from being freely accepted by cardiologists who adopt the current commercially available systems.

REFERENCES

1. Marchesi C, M Biella, C Contini, GF Mazzocca: A software approach to rhythm and ST-T analysis of 24 hour ECG (this book).
2. Marchesi C, S Chierchia, A Maseri: Left and right ventricular pressure monitoring in the CCU. Methods and significance. IEEE Proceedings on Computers in Cardiology, Rotterdam September 29 October 1, 1977, pagg. 579-583.
3. Maseri A, R Mimmo, S Chierchia, C Marchesi, A Pesola, A L'Abbate: Coronary artery spasm as a cause of acute myocardial ischemia in man. Chest 68: 625-633, 1975.
4. Chierchia S, C Marchesi, A Maseri: Evidence of angina not caused by increased myocardial metabolic demands and patterns of ECG and hemodynamic alterations during 'primary' angina. In: Pathogenetic mechanism of angina pectoris. Ed A Maseri, J Klassen, M Lesch, New York: Grune and Stratton 1978.
5. Schang SJ Jr, CJ Pepine: Transient asymptomatic ST segment depression during daily activity. Am J Cardiol 39: 396, 1977.
6. Stern S, D Tzivoni: Early detection of silent ischemic heart disease by 24 hour ECG monitoring of active subjects. Br Heart J 36: 481, 1974.
7. Allen R, C Pholan: Silent S-T depression in patients with angina pectoris. Circulation (suppl III) 50: III 122, 1974.
8. Golding R, F Wolfe, D Tzivoni, S Stern: Transient S-T elevation detected by 24 hour ecg monitoring during normal daily activity. Am Heart J 86: 501, 1973.

DISCUSSION: CHAPTER 6

Chairman: L. Donato

DISCUSSION CHAPTER 6

Paper 2: Present techniques for biosignals ambulatory telemonitoring.

HUGENHOLTZ: I have been involved with the use of radio-telephone to see whether cardiac rhythm could be transmitted and analysed during transport phase or in the home, but the experiment turned out to be a failure. Whether it was due to technical problems or the cost of the whole thing or the infrequent use of it, I don't know.

DONATO: Thank you, Paul. Professor Julian.

JULIAN: Dr. Graham Sleyman did organize and train people who had gone out of the coronary care unit to transmit their ECG's over the telephone. The point of this is to identify people who are reinfarcting or having arrhythmias. Technically, it worked extremely well and he got excellent recordings but it was very disappointing in the actual yield. He did pick up a few arrhythmias which they would otherwise have not picked up, but I don't think he felt that it was actually worth the effort.

DONATO: And would that correspond to your opinion?

JULIAN: I think so, because I think it's very difficult for, leaving a side pacemaker checks, the coronary care type patient to know when he's having something. And this has been the problem with self-administration of drugs, etc. We can't identify the patient when the patient can't identify himself.

DONATO: What about using this system to link different levels of hospital, district hospital to main referral centers?

JULIAN: Yes, this has been used of course in a number of parts of the world, with some success.

BENEKEN: I will just briefly comment on the pacemaker application. First of all, a question. I have always understood that the benefits of any telephone communication would not be enough for a proper transmission of the pacemaker pulse itself, so for any shape analysis, it's no good. And then I think with the present extended lifespan and reliability of the pacemakers, I just wonder whether it is not cheaper to let a patient come back to hospital once in a while.

DONATO: Dr. Pantridge, please.

PANTRIDGE: The radio transmission has been used quite extensively in the States. And some people take the view that the paramedicals who go out to do things can be controlled in that they're asked to transmit the ECG's and somebody in the coronary care unit then looks at the ECG and then instructions are given over the radio-telephone, so paramedicals can be more effective. However most people have given it up for the very reason that perhaps 19 times out of 20 it works, and on the very occasion when you really want it, there's some snag in the system.

MANCINI: I want to answer really to the question arising from the pacemaker: before transmitting the signal we stretch the time, in order to obtain bandwidths compatible with telephonic transmission. And what we receive is exactly what you could see in the oscilloscope near the patient. This is accomplished by means of an integrated circuit which accomplishes this operation of stretching and which has a very low cost.

JULIAN: We have used a similar system, a cardio-beeper which trans-mits a sound signal and if there is a risk, it has a decoder. We've used this for people with symptomatic arrhythmias, to transmit their arrhythmia. In fact, it's just to see what we have in fact trained patients to do, is to play the noise from the beeper into their own tape-recorder and bring the tape-recorder in, rather tahn transmit it over the telephone.

I would like to support the approach that Dr. Hutton described, which is similar to our own, we feel that we haven't been able to abandon technician interaction with the system. I'm sure this is still going to be essential, but it's much lower level, much easier, much less tiring if you can run a 24-hour tape literally in 24 minutes and not in the 2 or 3 hours as it may take using another system. So I believe in the use that Dr. Hutton makes of a preprocesser in association with a computer, and I think that's the way things will go. I think the 24-hour tape is now an absolutely vital tool of ordinary clinical practice, as well as a research tool.

HUTTON: I really just want to support Prof. Julian about the same things, that it still takes nearly one hour for the girl to set the machine up, to put it to the computer. So although the actual analysis is done in 24 minutes, it still takes about an hour, so although we are somewhere along the road, we clearly still have some considerable way to get yet.

MARCHESI: We didn't use a Pathfinder, but I don't agree with Dr. Julian's approach, because I think that, with the exception of Pathfinder that I don't know very well, a preprocessing performed conventionally by commercially available machines is not as adequate as required. Thus, the computer comes into operation too late, because data preprocessing is not accurate enough.

HUTTON: Well as a matter of fact I'm quite sure I didn't bring this out in my presentation. The point I was trying to make was that our data was being analysed in two ways: one by the actual QRS morpholo-gists through the Pathfinder; but also rhythm analysis, separately, using a separate program. So in fact we have two forms of analysis of the actual ECG itself.

HUGENHOLTZ: When we met at the working group on Computers in Cardio-logy, in September, we agreed that there would be a cooperative effort to make at least a data base from a series of tapes, through which these various commercial systems could be tested on their reliability, accuracy, sensitivity and specificity. The idea of having some preprocessing appeals to me as a total system, but that's for the rhythm disturbances, and let's just skip these. I'm more interested in what you think about the ST segment. I always led to believe that, even with good instrumentation the assessment of ST segments just still is not reliable enough that you can hang a diagnosis on it. Therefore I would like to ask you, do you have reasons to believe that you are that accurate? And for example, have you tested this series against a standard exercise test on a bicycle ergometer with leads analysed over a shorter period of time? And what degree of advantage did the 24-hour record give above the provocation over short-term exercise?

MARCHESI: I have just some considerations about our method of ST measurements. And my consideration is this one: of course it is new in ambulatory monitoring environment, but the method comes from a long experience in coronary care unit monitoring, there the method is quite well consolidated. But anyway, which is the main difference in our system? When you just take one point, somewhere in the ST interval, as commercial systems do, we have an unstable measurement. If you take areas, you have a more stable measurement, as our records document even in episodes of short duration. This may be crucial because it is in the episodes of small duration that you are losing information, because it is confused with the background noise. We have tested this type of analysis in CCU with independent indicators of ischemia (left ventricular function changes).

DONATO: With the cassette recorder, artifacts may arise at the time of recording. This is something that needs to be checked on. And then finally, which is the significance of ST changes that are recorded sometimes in these patients in the absence of typical chest pain?

HUGENHOLTZ: We don't look at one point of the ST segment under stress either, we take several points, you know we have a computer program for it, and we have increased specificity and sensitivity to quite acceptable levels. And we've debated it, should we go one step further and take the tapes, but current standard quality may not be good enough.

MANCINI: Anybody who has evaluated the performance of this kind of a cassette recorder in order to check the stability of the speed of the motor, the stability of the reproduction of the shape or the other parameters which are related with the further kind of analysis, can find that a very good new unit will give you a stable record if you have fresh batteries. As soon as one uses for the second time a cassette, or you use a not absolutely fresh battery, I suspect that the data loses quality rapidly.

HUGENHOLTZ: And that's why I don't think cassettes today are to be used for that purpose yet.

MASERI: I would like to know what's the problem with the ST segment evaluation? What sort of transient ST change would you accept as a real ST segment change? Say, 3 mm? 4mm? 5 mm? Or what else?

MANCINI: In other words you are moving now from the ability of the system to measure the change to its significance.

HUGENHOLTZ: The closest I can come to an answer is saying that from the exercise ECG literature, 2 millivolts depression are - all right - set against coronary angiography.

MASERI: The problem of 'specificity' and 'sensitivity' in terms of detecting a coronary anathomic stenosis must be reconsidered. For me, it should be compared with some very difficult 'gold standard'; under optimal conditions electrocardiogram detects ischemia: equating a functional change, such as ischemia, with an anatomic alteration cannot be accepted any longer. Electrocardiographic changes should be evaluated versus a 'gold standard' indicative of the presence or absence of ischemia (as indicated by myocardial perfusion changes or lactate production). Accordingly it does not appear correct to compare the results of Holter monitoring with stress testing, they may provide different, complementary information. Myocardial ischemia may result from functional impairment of coronary blood supply not necessarily related to coronary stenoses or to exercise. My point is: if you see a change which is, say, a ST change of 3 millimeters, you would accept it as a real change?

HUGENHOLTZ: For the same reasons that you do not accept that the presence or absence of a stenosis is proof of coronary artery disease, I concur that it's the best I have. That's all I was trying to tell you. I am therefore not willing to accept 3 or any number of millivolts as being the proof of something, because I don't know what the substrate is.

MASERI: If you want to know what sort of relation between the standard coronary care transient changes and some index of ischemia, we do have. In the studies that we have been doing with Drs. Chierchia and Marchesi in the past years, we obtained about 700 hours of recording together with hemodynamic changes. There we can check that the ST changes go hand in hand with simultaneous changes in dP/dt and end-diastolic pressure of the left ventricle. Dr. Marchesi showed an example of ST segment elevation taken with a commercial cassette. Would you buy that as a true ST segment elevation, or could that be an artifact?

HUGENHOLTZ: I think it could very well be an artifact.

MASERI: We have evidence that similar ST changes and also changes of much smaller magnitude are consistently associated with transient impairment of left ventricular function. That's one the ways to proof that ECG change was caused by ischemia, regardless of whether the patient did have coronary stenoses and/or a positive stress test.

ROUND TABLE

ROUND TABLE

DONATO: I was the first chairman of the CMSI and I was followed by Professor Shillingford and finally now by Professor Laurent, who is actually running the group. When we speak of perspectives of coronary care units, as a Council for Medical and Public Health Research of the European Community, we must look at it on both sides; the Medical Research side and the Public Health side. Until perhaps the first half of this century, that difference would have been nonsense because progress in health care was strictly linked to progress in medical research. But now in this particular heavily technologically loaded areas of health care, there is some sort of divergency, there is a phylosophical divergency between health care programs and medical research programs. And this unfortunate divergency has essentially an economic reason. When the cost of health care goes up to 10 % of gross national product, then it's obvious that people start to worry and immediately, one of the easiest things is to accuse the scientific community of pollution of technology, of uncontrolled transfer of technology to health care, and of indiscriminate transfer of technology. There is no doubt that the scientific community has to face this reality. The real point is to devise mechanisms that will not stop scientific progress but will not kill the economy of our countries. Now this demands very responsible attitudes, both on the side of health workers and on the side of the scientific community.
This is the real challenge for a group like this, because we have heard here a vast list of technical possibilities, of their implications, and we've heard a lot about their appeal. But this has to be considered on what I would say the cost-benefit analysis. There should not be a global cost-benefit analysis because this is the real problem, and this is the argument on which I would like now first to be very provocative with the chairmen of the various sessions, then ask the audience to come in. We should realize that one thing is the yield and the performance of a given technique in the ideal environment, and quite another thing is the performance of the same technique in the average environment. When we speak of sophisticated technologies and of the good results that they produce in certain centers, we cannot automatically say that the same techniques, transposed to other centers, to the average universe, will yield the same results.
I was impressed by Dr. Holmberg's data showing that also noncardiac cases benefit from his approach. Thus, better care produced better results, whatever the area you are in. If we on the asset side put the reduced mortality, reduced handicaps and also reduced burden on

non specialized departments, then all this may fit into a very nice pattern that justifies the continuous advances in technology, provided we do not imply that any new technology is immediately supplied to the entire community. We should try to make a sort of stratified proposals, define a certain hierarchy of levels in which, corresponding to a different level of medical structure, a different kind of solution should come out. This as far as the distribution of these technological resources. From this point of view, CRM really expects something, some specific suggestion from a meeting like this, and the Committee, CMSI, will have time to evaluate the results, discuss and come up with proposals, since it is difficult to reconduct together Medical Research and Public Health in individual countries, because they are diverging on a national level. This is the costant complaint, of all national Research and Public Health organizations: the attitude of the scientific community is that Health Care problems kill medical research and the attitude of the health community is that Medical Research kills health care. What we are trying to do at the level of the EC is to try to have the two going back together, because no one doubts that the solution to the major health care problems must start at the scientific level. How, in the field of coronary care, should be stratified the approach? Which technical level, which degree of technological sophistication is required at each level? This is something that should come out very clearly to avoid wastage of money. More and more controlled testing will be needed. We must find cooperative ways of doing it. We must devise clinical trials on the technology that we are using and on the procedures that we are using. I hope I've been provocative enough, and I'd like to have your reaction to it.

PANTRIDGE: In a situation like pre-hospital coronary care it was very obvious that you were going to arrive at the results that we have heard, beatifully done but the result is entirely predictable. A different problem is the randomized study that has been going on in England, organized by the Ministry of Health, which purports to show that coronary care in general is irrelevant and the patients do just as well if you leave them at home. I think I am correct in saying it might help our system considerably if this committee made a definitive statement about these randomized studies that are going on at the present time.

JULIAN: In England, certain experiments have been undertaken in circumstances where they could not possibly produce a positive result, because the number of patients studied was not sufficient to demonstrate a result, quite apart from other methodological problems. Now this is, in our view, a malicious device of our Department of Health, so that they can say this study showed no favourable response. Therefore the procedure is no good, which is not a logical deduction, but that is the way that politics works. I think we must be very critical. I think such a committee as this could be very critical, of the sort od control trials which are so designed that they are bound to come up with a negative result.

DONATO: I fully agree with you. You can always design a trial in a sufficient tricky way to get out of it the result that you want. Thus, my plea is costantly the same: the people who know the problem should not leave it to the health care department, but should design the study themselves.

JULIAN: I agree with you in many ways, but there are many situations where the problem does not lend itself to controlled trials. If I fell down here on the floor here now, I would be disappointed if you took out a randomization envelope and opened it up to say whether you were going to defibrillate me or not. So that is one situation where you simply cannot do it. But there are also all the trials that have been done on coronary care, particularly the ones in England, which have only randomized a very small subset, and then extrapolated from that to the whole population.

In a double-blind control trial, you have to select according to quite rigid criteria, a particular subset, which may be only 10, or 15 or 20 % of the whole population. And this is the danger. Actually, Michael Oliver and I wrote an article about the impossibility of doing this 10 years ago, and I think it's still impossible to do it in many circumstances. I don't think that anybody will do this in a hospital now, really.

PANTRIDGE: The problem that we face is this: these trials were designed by the Ministry of Health officials, and they randomized people, patients at the end of the fifth hour to home or hospital care. Now if you make a decision as to whether you send your individual into hospital, say five and a half hours after the onset of his infarct, it will make very little difference. And so they came up with exactly that result, and therefore this is the point that Prof. Julian has been stressing, from these inadequate date, they come to the conclusion that coronary care is of no relevance.

DONATO: There are many procedures that have been examined here during these days, therapeutic procedure, diagnostic procedure. Are they accurate? Provided you obtain the accurate answer, what is the relevance of that answer to the patient? It might not be relevant for a clinical decision but it might be very relevant for better understanding of the disease. Then it is something that should be continued, but in centers of high advanced research, and this is not something - if you are not able to make a clinical decision on that, you should not have it at clinical level. But this kind of question, I mean, should be clearly answered. If this kind of approach, doesn't become an intrinsic, intimate approach in an area so loaded with high costs, we are running for trouble.

HUGENHOLTZ: Do you imagine that by whatever means we gave that clarity to the burocrats, they'd behave any different when they have the evidence? Do you think that somebody in Brussels can tell the

Ministry of Health in England what to do if they give an answer on the European basis, by this committee? Do you think anybody in the Hague would listen to what Brussels would tell? I'd rather propose to this committee to do two things.

First, we should define where our wastage is, where our unnecessary usages are, and I agree with Professor Pantridge that if a balloon pump situation is using too much manpower, then that is something which we seriously should consider. But I think the answers to these questions must be dealt with on a decentralized basis: given answers may be applicable to Glasgow, others are applicable to Rotterdam, others to Pisa. I think we should communicate to each other these answers, and then formulate a number of partial solutions.

Second, we should propose a registration protocol, a common form where we enter every patient that is admitted to our coronary care unit. Until we adopt this common form, we will be talking at different directions because we don't know what the population is that we are having in our hands.

DONATO: I am in full agreement with Professor Hugenholtz, when he speaks about this decentralized approach. It is from a decentralized approach that you should reduce wastage in this area and to exploit to the best what already exists. And I'm not so pessimistic on the burocrats. Because they face a lost battle. If you look at the report of the last WHO assembly, health care costs keep going up. When people start to go back to the problem, well, we need a scientific solution to this problem, the scientific community should get organized to give the proper answer to them. The other point I'd like to stress is that we should not forget that, since we are also interested in medical research, as an instrument for improvement of care: the coronary care units are a fantastic investigational instrument for better understanding of the disease, and they should be used also as such. But let's be very frank, we cannot pretend that this occurs at all levels of coronary care units, or this may become a justification for sophisticated instrumentation. If everyone with two-bed units in district hospitals, having few cases coming in per year, tries to justify the acquisition of costly equipment for research reasons, that is not acceptable. Thus, we must combine scientific appeal with elements of reasoning that have very clear vision of the economical health care problem.

JULIAN: I think as far as the costs are concerned, the costs of just simple coronary care, I can't see any reason for alarm. I think every hospital, every hoospital of a reasonable size, is going to require intensive care for cardiac patients. Whether or not we believe in coronary care for everybody, every hospital needs, and I think it's been recognized in most countries, in every major center of population, such hospitals should have an intensive care area for monitoring of cardiac patients. And it's curious that in England, where there has been this attack on coronary care, all the three centers, Bristol, Nottingham and in Teeside, where they actually produced these reports saying what a bad thing coronary care was, they all have fluorishing coronary care units. Now there is some curious anomaly here. There isn't a single place that has stopped having a coronary care unit. And I think the costs of coronary care are not so very great when one accepts that there's got to be organization of this kind.

MASERI: I believe it is appropriate to conclude that coronary cares are here to stay, they are already very widely distributed and they are necessary.

We should try to provide suggestions on how we could exploit to a greater extent the know-how and the expertise of the staff in the first level routine coronary care for a greater benefit to the community. That's why we brought in the problem of Holter monitoring and of telephone transmission to the coronary care. The new technologies that became available should be evaluated in terms of efficiency and effectiveness in specialized centers on carefully standardized subset of patients selected according to common protocols, before being folded out to community hospitals. Finally, we should identify the research lines that will improve the level of care by increasing our understanding of the pathophysiology of the disease.

APPENDIX A

SURVEY REPORT ON HEMODYNAMIC MONITORING IN CCU

A. Maseri, C. Marchesi, S. Chierchia, M.G. Trivella

A.1. INTRODUCTION

A.1.1. BACKGROUND

This Survey Report is in line with the tasks of the CMSI as a logical offspring of the Survey report in Coronary Care Units (CCU) (1), which has provided an overall information on the diffusion of these Units in the member countries and indicated guidelines on optimal dimensions, staffing and equipment for the various levels of care and for research units.

In 1960 the mortality in patients admitted to hospital for myocardial infarction was 30 to 35%. With the introduction of CCU's, this hospital mortality has been reduced now to about 15%. Such units are well established throughout the world. Although there are a few questions about their value (2-5) there seems to be little doubt that CCU's will continue to be established in many hospitals throughout all countries in the light of international experience (6-15).

The introduction of CCU has contributed to a reduction of mortality directly from the prompt detection and effective treatment of arrhythmias, and indirectly as a fall out of research which has improved understanding of disease processes.

Reduction of infarct size, complications and mortality from pump failure is currently considered as one of the important goals in Monitoring of the Seriously Ill in CCU. In turn, early hemodynamic monitoring, based on invasive and/or non-invasive techniques, with or without computer assistance is considered a possible prerequisite for the choice and the evaluation of therapeutic interventions.

Technological requirements, personnel training and staffing for routine hemodynamic monitoring represent at present a considerable often unrealistic burden for ordinary CCU's. This Survey Report is aimed:

1. to assess the potential benefit to be expected from extensive hemodynamic monitoring in CCU's;
2. to evaluate the possibility of non invasive monitoring;
3. to investigate the forseable impact of advanced technology for future routine improvement of care in CCU's.

For the applications to routine CCU's, the implementation of hemodynamic monitoring will be framed in the general socio-economic problems of medical care in the European countries.

For research coronary cares, the report will indicate guidelines for the most promising lines of research and identify European centers with common interests and available for joint projects.

A.1.2. RATIONALE

Hemodynamic monitoring in CCU's is still mainly confined to relatively few research units without standardization in the selection of
patients to be monitored, of the parameters to be measured nor of
the techniques to be used.
Invasive measurements may be required for critically ill patients,
non invasive measurements may be adequate for uncomplicated patients. While changing situations, intermittent measurements may be
adequate for patients in more stable conditions. The organization
and the skills required for applying invasive measurements without
risk for the patient are less frequently available than those needed
for non invasive measurements and the technology necessary for
continuous, computerized monitoring is so far only accessible to few
highly sophisticated centers.
Therefore we considered appropriate to deal separately with:
1. intermittent hemodynamic measurements, invasive and non invasive;
2. continuous, computerized monitoring.
This survey report is composed of 3 parts:
1. a survey of the literature;
2. a survey of the centers active in the field of CCU monitoring in
   the European countries;
3. the conclusions of a seminar organized in Pisa, December 1978, on
   the perspective of CCU's, aimed to frame the conclusion of our
   report in the present scientific and economic situation of the
   care of coronary patients.

A.2. SURVEY OF THE LITERATURE

A.2.1. INTERMITTENT HEMODYNAMIC MEASUREMENTS

An up to date survey of the literature reveals that a large variety
of invasive and non invasive hemodynamic measurements have been
performed during the acute phase of AMI. They are listed below with
the respective principal bibliographic references:

A.2.1.1. Invasive measurements

1. Right ventricular filling pressure (16-24).
2. Pulmonary artery and wedge pressures (18, 19 and 21-33)
3. Arterial blood pressure (16, 18, 20, 21, 23, 24, 31, 34).
4. Left ventricular pressure (17, 18, 20, 24, 26, 30, 34, 35, 36,
   37).
5. Cardiac output: Fick (38, 39)

- Dyedilution (16, 20, 33, 34, 39)
- Thermodilution (19, 21-24, 32, 33, 39).
- Radioisotopes (39-41).
6. Aortic flow velocity (42, 43)
7. Mixed venous O_2 saturation (19, 29, 31).
8. Arterial blood gases (as an index of pulmonary venous congestion) (38, 44, 45).

A.2.1.2. Non invasive measurements

1. Chest x ray films (as an index of pulmonary vascular congestion) (22, 28 and 46-50);
2. Systolic time intervals (20 and 51-61).
3. Apex cardiogram (54).
4. Echocardiography (24 and 62-71).
5. Radioisotopes (70 and 72-76).
6. Aortovelography (77-79).
7. Impedance cardiography (80).

A.2.1.3. Field of application

The study of the reports in the literature indicates that both invasive and non invasive measurements were performed in specialized research enviroments. These measurements were applied to the complete spectrum of patients with AMI, regardless of the degree of functional impairment, although among non invasive measurements, systolic time intervals, apex cardiogram, echocardiography were scarcely employed in several complicated patients. We were unable to find reports dealing with purely routine applications of hemodynamic measurements with the exception of few centers where the organization developed for research purpose was apparently used for routine (16, 22, 24, 31, 81, 82, 83).

A.2.1.4. Information derived from hemodynamic measurements

The research performed has considerably increased our understanding of the derangements of circulatory function in patients with AMI. However, in our survey we were particularly concerned with the information useful for the practical management of the patient with AMI and with his prognostic evaluation.
A. Value for the management of patients.
There is general consensus that hemodynamic measurements are of considerable help in the management of the patients with AMI because, in addition to the clinical findings, they may provide an

objective, quantitative or semiquantitative basis for the evaluation of the circulatory conditions of the patient and for the choice of the most appropriate treatment. However, the degree of improvement in the management of patients resulting from individual measurements or derived indexes is difficult to assess. We consider of practical importance the following points summarized from our survey:

Invasive measurements.

There is about 80% agreement between the hemodynamic classification of the severity of AMI derived from measurements of systemic and pulmonary pressures and of cardiac output, and the clinical classification (uncomplicate; signs of mild left ventricular impairment; ventricular failure, and cardiogenic shock (or Killips classes 1-4)) (32). The main source of discrepancy are patients with compromised hemodynamics without a corresponding clinical picture or patients in hypovolemic shock (19, 32). Furthermore:

Measurements of central venous pressure (CVP) alone are of little benefit to assess left ventricular function impairment since CVP may be elevated as a consequence of right ventricular involvement by AMI in the presence of a mildly elevated left ventricular filling pressure. Conversely CVP may be nearly normal despite the presence of an elevated left ventricular filling pressure when right ventricular function is good (39).

Pulmonary wedge or diastolic pressure is a good index of left ventricular end-diastolic pressure in the absence of pulmonary arterial hypertension or of mitral stenosis (22, 39).

Measurements of left ventricular pressures and of indexes of ventricular functions derived from the pressure curve do not secur to provide more valuable information that the measurement of arterial and pulmonary pressures (34).

Systemic arterial pressure, left ventricular filling pressure and cardiac output appear so far the most informative parameters (when considered in combination) (34).

Other measurements such as aortic flow velocity, mixed venous O_2 saturation, arterial blood gases, may contribute to an extent yet undefined to the evaluation of the patients when taken in combination with the measurements mentioned in the above point and/or with the clinical findings.

Non invasive measurements.

X ray films represent the most practical non invasive means of assessing objectively the degree of derangement of the cardiac function from cardiac dimensions and contours, and from signs of pulmonary venous congestion and interstitial fluid accumulation (47, 49).

Systolic time intervals, apex cardiogram, echocardiography may be of value for the detection of latent ventricular function impairment in clinically uncomplicated patients, but seem to provide little additional information for complicated cases relative to the clinical assessment.

Among the latest developments: 1) cardiac gated cineangiography with radioisotopes, which can be repeated at frequent intervals for several hours after the injection of the tracer and allows the visualization of dynamic changes of the heart chambers, seems a very promising tool; 2) aortovelography, which provides a non invasive mean of assessing aortic flow velocity, requires more widespread testing and validation.

B. Classification of patients with AMI.

A more precise pathophysiologic classification of patients can be adopted on the basis of the hemodynamic studies particularly for clinically uncomplicated cases and for cases in shock. This classification represents a considerable improvement relative to clinical classifications and thus it can be of help in the therapeutic approach (22, 32, 81).

Apparently uncomplicated patients may fall into 4 categories: 1) hyperdynamic circulation (which can be normalized by betablockers; 2) normal hemodynamics (betablockers may still be of benefit); 3) slightly compromized cardiac function (betablockers, with caution); 4) clearly compromized cardiac function (betablockers controindicates).

Patients in shoch may fall into 2 categories: 1) elevated left ventricular pressure to the level of causing interstitial fluid accumulation and edema in the lung (to be treated with peripheral vasodilators and circulatory assistance); 2) inadequate left ventricular filling pressure, althouth often well above normal (to be treated with fluid infusion).

There is still a considerable non uniformity in the criteria for classification of patients (such as the values of pressures, cardiac or stroke index taken to separate different groups and the definition of shock). This lack of uniformity largely accounts for the variability in the therapeutic results and prognostic expectation among various groups.

C. Prognostic value.

There is consensus that hemodynamic measurements and derived indexes have a considerably greater predictive value in separating survivors from non survivors than any clinical classification (31, 84). Systemic pulse pressure cardiac index, stroke index, end-diastolic pressure and various combination of these parameters appear to have a prognostic accuracy definitely superior to that based on classification of patients in various subsets because of the lack of uniformity in the criteria used for the separation. The prognostic significance of the individual hemodynamic measurements and of the derived indexes may have relevant practical implications for the identification of the most helpful parameters for the definition of the conditions of the patients during continuous monitoring.

A.2.1.5. Practical problems

Invasive measurements.
In spite of the technologic developments such as disposable, special purpose catheters and of gradual improvement in the level of care un CCU, the generalized indiscriminate use of pulmonary artery catheters and of arterial cannulas cannot be considered free of discomfort and of risks of complications for the patient. Both discomfort and risk are inversely related to the level of organization of the CCU and to the skills of the personnel. It can be reasonably assumed that the performance, processing and interpretation of the measurements pose no problems for the teams capable of introducing and maintaining in place the catheters with the minimum risk and discomfort for the patients.
Non invasive measurements.
These measurements have the non negligible advantage of being free from risk although frequently they also cause discomfort to the patient. In general, as opposed to invasive, the organization and skills are not so much required for obtaining measurements as for obtaining measurements of adequate quality.
Nuclear medicine equipment for gated cineangiography which appears the most promising non invasive tool for frequent assessment of cardiocirculatory function in AMI has a considerable cost and is available only to a very limited number of centers.

A.2.1.6. Conclusions on the present routine role of hemodynamic measurements in CCU.

The advance in the understanding of derangement of cardiovascular function in AMI must be considered the most significant achievement of hemodynamic measurements. Furthermore, the introduction of a pathophysiologic classification of patients with AMI, based on the hemodynamic conditions, has indirectly contributed to raise the level of care also in units where hemodynamic measurements are out of reach, by drawing attention to its existance and by suggesting guidelines for treatment.
By contrast, no conclusive effort has been made so far for finding practical ways of facilitating the diffusion of hemodynamic measurements our of R and D CCU's into 2nd level CCU's (1) for the routine management of patients.
The widespread adoption of routine hemodynamic measurements would require:
For invasive measurements.
1. identification of the patients and of the conditions where it may be beneficial for reduction of mortality, complications, infarct size.

2. Improvement of the organization, skills and equipment in CCU up to a level where risks and discomfort for the patients are justified by the improved results of management.

For non invasive measurements.

1. validation of the techniques (with the obvious exception of x-ray films);

2. demonstration that their use is beneficial for the reduction of mortality, complications, infarct size.

The survey of the literature indicates that at present it is extremely difficult to reach convincing evidence that hemodynamic measurements in CCU may affect overall mortality, complications and infarct size because:

1. the more sophysticated units where the best hemodynamic measurements are performed are those with the best skills and organization, a fact which, per se, would be significantly contributory;

2. differences in mortality and complications are hard to assess;

3. reduction in infarct size is still difficult to detect in spite of the tremendous research effort in this direction now produced.

These appear to be also the non official conclusions of the MIRU project in the U.S.A.(*). Thus as a provisional conclusion it appears reasonable to state that although invasive hemodynamic measurements would make therapeutic decisions easier and more precise than the simple clinical observation, the organization and the skills required for its generalized application are out of reach of routine CCU's of the second level (1). Therefore, they should be reserved for special cases where the clinical and the more readily available and reliable non invasive techniques (such as chest x-ray films) result inadequate for a rational therapeutic management.

A.2.2. CONTINUOUS COMPUTERIZED HEMODYNAMIC MONITORING

Continuous computerized invasive hemodynamic monitoring in CCU cannot be considered so far as standardized technique because the systems available were developed in specialized, highly sophisticated centers and taylored to match special research aims and patients care needs. Hemodynamic monitoring is often part of a more "comprehensive" system of computerized patient care in special units, usually post cardiac surgery.

(*) - A complete report of the MIRU study is not published. This is a personal communication of Dr. Rosati-Durham Medical Center, North Carolina (U.S.A.).

A.2.2.1. Characteristics of the principal systems

We have attempted to group in Tables (1-4) the main characteristics of the systems adopted in some well known centers. It is also worth mentioning some commercially available systems. The Hewlett Packard offers an efficient system of storage and retrieval of clinical data, the General Electric offers a flexible structure, comprehensive function analysis, and data presentation, for the Roche system a validation study is now in progress (85).
The Mennen-Greatbach and the Oxford Unibed systems are the most recent. They are based on the concept of distributed processing, achieved by microprocessor technology (86-88). The survey of the literature in the field has suggested us the following provisional consideration.

A.2.2.2. Hardware

For the first systems developed the principal problem was the attempt to proportionate the high costs of the computers to the functions to be implemented, with the consequent tendency to monitor the largest number of patients possible with a relatively small computer power. Thus: 1) special dedicated systems for data collection were preferred to continuous monitoring of the hemodynamic parameters by software confining the computers to a role of data logger; 2) functions normally carried out by medical and paramedical personnel in the intensive care unit were transferred to the computer with the aim of reducing running costs and improving standardization and reliability. Within this optics the trend was towards the choice of medium size computers with multiprogramming operative systems.
More recently the reduced cost of computers has led to a change in the phylosophy of the system design with a transition to multimini-computers with low cost apparatus dedicated to single beds (89, 90), or to multi-micro-computers dedicated to single functions connected to a central computer with control and executive tasks (86).
The present day availability of microprocessor technology is forcing the distribution of processing power at bedside level and to the design of modular, very flexible structures (87, 88, 91).

A.2.2.3. Software

In contrast to the considerable changing trend occurring in hardware no significant changes can be sensed in the general phylosophy of programming, with the exception of the present availability of the sophysticated diagnostic aids represented by the acquisition of large data base with rapid memory access (this aspect will not be dealt in this report).

A number of problems appears adequately solved:

QRS detection. This apparently simple problem has stimulated the development of several solutions among which it is difficult to select the most reliable and most general purpose, also because of the lack of a "gold" standard against which to test the different systems. A similar problem still exist for the classification of the different patterns of the QRS (92) and for the criteria for quality control of the signals.

An updated list of algorithms used for QRS detection and classification is reported in (256).

Analysis of the state of the patient. This is a field scarcely explored. Often the criteria for alarm setting is based on predeterminated thresholds on preselected signals. An improvement is represented by the logical association of alarms from several measurements (93-94). On a more advanced line some studies have attempted to develop multiparametric prognostic indexes computed by statistical techniques based on the monovariate or multivariate analysis (95) or on the discriminant function (45, 96, 97) or on the cluster analysis (98).

All the methods considered above are aimed to detect significant deviation from a given steady state of the patient. Methods capable of following dynamically changing state of a given patient (99) are still in a more preliminary stage of development. A possible advance in this direction may be represented by the development of reliable clinical models which so far appear rather fuzzy with the exception of limited tasks such as the computer controlled infusion (100-103) and of some respiratory function controls (104).

It is important to stress the possible role of this approach in defining an optimal set of features of the patient state, so minimizing redundancy (105).

A.2.2.4 . Data presentation

The most widely adopted method is the time plot with linear cohordinates of the selected measurements over selected periods of time. This solution becomes impractical when the number of parameters becomes large and when the correlation among variations are of interest. Modifications in the cohordinate systems have been used such as logarithmic time scale (106) (in order to compact past events) and adaptation of the ordinate in proportion to the significance of the changes of each variable (107). Another form of data presentation is that based on the use of polar cohordinates (108, 109) which may be practical when the number is large but presents difficulties for the evaluation of transient changes. An ideal model function has also been proposed and the data presented as a deviation from it (45).

A.2.2.5. Conclusions

Also for continuous computerized hemodynamic monitoring it is not yet possible to evaluate the cost-benefit related to their routine use. Specific studies on this aspect are not available. Generally, evaluations of the cost-effectiveness were attempted for "cohomprensive" system and include also the cost of the personnel, thus they not allow an evaluation of the cost of computerized hemodynamic monitoring alone. Anyway the lack of common standards makes very hard the comparison of the performance of different systems and the cost/benefit evaluation of specific functions. Some examples are reported in (44, 85, 110).
The overall presently available information on the results of the computerized hemodynamic monitoring can be derived from tables 3 and 4 .

A.3. REPORT ON THE QUESTIONNAIRE

A.3.1. CRITERIA OF THE SURVEY

This report rather than an exaustive and accurate reflection of all activities in the field of CCU hemodynamic monitoring in the member countries should be considered a basic framework into which additional information can be fed.
The initial problem we were faced with was the more or less general lack of information on the centers active in the field of hemodynamic monitoring. Only for Holland and for Italy a list of CCU's was available, but without specification of the type of activity, equipment and research interest (see enclosed lists). Therefore we contacted the centers which were known to us directly because of their publications, presentations or meetings, personal communications, or indirectly because of indications of other workers in the field in the member countries. In particular we are indepted to the members of CMSI and to Dr. Beneken and Dr. Mester for Holland and to Dr. Fazzini for Italy. Detailed informations for each center which returned us the filled questionnaire are reported in Table 5 (A, B, C).

A.3.2. RESPONSES OF THE QUESTIONNAIRE

A.3.2.1. Basic characteristics of the units

Number of beds	Number of Centers
1 - 5	4
6 - 10	30
11 - 20	8
>20	3

Single rooms	
all	30
partly	8
none	7

Patients are under visual control in 37

Post intensive care unit is available in 39

A blood gas laboratory is available in 31

Fluoroscopy at bedside is available in 35

Cardiac open chest surgery available in 33

A.3.2.2.   Patients material and standard routine procedures upon admission

Patients Total number/p. week	Number of Centers
6 - 10	15
11 - 19	19
20 - 25	7
> 25	4

A.M.I./p. week	
2 - 5	18
6 - 10	24
> 10	3

Unstable angina/p. week	
1	4
1 - 3	33
4 - 6	6
> 6	2

Diagnosis of A.M.I. is established by:

ECG and enzimes: 14 centers

ECG, enzimes and isoenzimes: 23 centers
ECG, enzimes, isoenzimes and isotopic techniques: 6 centers
ECG, enzimes and isotopic techniques: 2 centers.

A.3.2.3. Standard monitoring (hemodynamic measurements)

Non invasive techniques are used only in 5 centers for patients in
Killip class 1, in 4 centers for patients in Killip class 2 and 3,
in 3 centers for patients in Killip class 4.
Routine chest x ray is reported only in 6 centers for all patient
classes. Intensive hemodynamic monitoring is reported for patients
in Killip class 1 only in 1 center, for patients in Killip class 2
in 17 centers, for patients in Killip class 3 in 35 centers, for
Killip class 4 in 40 centers.
Arterial blood gases determination is reported in 2 centers for
patients in Killip class 2, in 3 for patients in Killip class 3 and
4.
Detailed information on the measurements performed is reported below.
Monitoring in Killip class 1

Parameters (*)	Centers
ECG	45
ECT	10
NIH - poligraphy	4
- ECHO	1
XR	6

Monitoring in Killip class 2

Parameters	Centers
ECG	45
ECT	10
NIH - polig.	2
- ECHO	2
PA +	17
$\pm$	4
AP +	6
$\pm$	4
CV	2
CO	8
BG	2
$PaPO_2$	1
XR	6

(*) The list of the abbreviations is reported at the end of the A.3
    paragraph.

Monitoring in Killip class 3

Parameters		Centers
ECG		45
ECT		10
NIH	− polig.	2
	− ECHO	2
PA	+	35
	±	4
PW		1
AP	+	22
	±	3
CV		1
BG		3
XR		6

Monitoring in Killip class 4

Parameters		Centers
ECG		45
ECT		10
NIH	− polig.	1
	− ECHO	1
	− Impedance	1
PA	+	40
	±	2
PW		1
AP	+	32
	±	1
CV		1
BG		3
BT		31
UO		45
XR		6

A.3.2.4. Research activity

A. Arrhythmia detection
Nineteen centers are actively involved on research projects on
computer aided arrhythmia detection, implemented by hardware and by
firmware respectively in 5 centers. Four centers do not specify the
method used. Data bank collection is in the process of being
instituted in 4 centers.
B. Hemodynamic monitoring
Research studies on A.M.I. based on monitoring of different invasive
and non invasive parameters are performed respectively in 25 and 4

centers as reported below:

Invasive	n. of centers
AP	19
PA	25
PW	12
CV	4
LV	1
RV	4
RA	4
CO	22

Non invasive	
Impedance	2
Isotopic techniques	1
Systolic time int.	1

Computer aided hemodynamic research is performed in 12 centers.

Home developed algorithms are used	in 6
Continuous analysis of signals is performed	in 7
Intermittent analysis is performed	in 5
Off line analysis	in 6
On line analysis	in 9
Trend analysis is performed	in 5
Based on multiparametric cryteria	in 2
Prognostic indexes are derived	in 3
Automatic quality control is provided	in 2

C. Reduction of infarct size

Thirty centers evaluate infarct size. Detailed informations on the methods used are reported below.

Methods:	Centers
Enzimes	1
Isoenzimes	2
Enzimes-Isoenzimes	9
Enzimes-ST mapping	2
Enzimes-Isotopic-techniques	1
Enzimes-Isoenzimes-ST mapping	11
Enzimes-Isoenzimes-Isotopic techniques	3
Enzimes-Isoenzimes-ST mapping-Isotopic techniques	1

List of the abbreviations:

ECT	=	Number of ectopics/min
NIH	=	Non invasive hemodynamics
CO	=	Cardiac output
$PaPO_2$	=	Pulmonary artery O_2 partial tension

ST   = ST-mapping
Polig   = Poligraphy
XR   = X-ray
Imp   = Impedance
PA   = Pulmonary artery pressure
PW   = Pulmonary wedge pressure
AP   = Arterial pressure
RA   = Right atrial pressure
LV   = Left ventricular pressure
RV   = Right ventricular pressure
CV   = Central venous pressure
dp/dt   = Pressure first derivative
CBF   = Coronary blood flow
BG   = Blood gases
$AVDO_2$ = Arterial-venous O_2 difference
O_2 MV sat   = Mixed venous O_2 saturation
BT   = Body temperature
UO   = Urine output.
+   = Sistematically
±   = Non sistematically

A.4. CONCLUSIONS OF THE SEMINAR: 'PERSPECTIVES OF CORONARY CARE UNITS'

Sponsored by the Economic European Communities CMSI. Organized in Pisa (Italy) on December 1-2, 1978.

The conclusions of the Seminar are in line with the document XII/201 /74-E-F-N produced by the ad hoc group of the C.M.S.I.

There was unanimous agreement that CCU's have become a well established routine system of care of acute coronary patients fully justified by the experience collected over the years.

It was emphasized that it was essential to separate clearly the problems of Research CCU's from those of Routine CCU's. It was stressed the fact that too often techniques and instrumentation, still in the domain of research and development, are distributed to routine CCU's before their usefulness had been convincingly proved.

SESSION 1 was devoted to: Perspective on arrhythmia monitoring and was developed along two main lines: new understanding of the pathophysiology of arrhythmias and practical implications.

   Pathophysiologic conclusions

1. There appear to be as yet no good predictors of ventricular fibrillation;

2. Computer systems capable of sophisticated recognition of rhythm disturbances are available but at present there is no convincing evidence that they can be of significant advantage for the management of the patient.

   Practical implications. There was a consensus that at present: 1.

Development of equipment for routine use in CCU's should go hand in hand with improvement in training and staffing of medical and paramedical personnel of these units.

2. The use of computer systems in CCU's for arrhythmia detection should be considered as a research project because their cost is still disproportioned to practical benefit to patient management 3. According to the present understanding a simple, reliable system for detection of ventricular fibrillation and asystole would be the most reasonable technological goal for widespread routine use in CCU's.

SESSION 2 was devoted to non invasive haemodynamic measurements and dealt with the application of ultrasounds.

The use of these techniques for the study of coronary patients in particular in the acute phase of their disease, has lagged considerably behind the application to other areas of cardiology, but the studies presented indicated that they may provide considerable information in acute hemodynamic situations.

There was consensus that after continuing appropriate validation in research centers they would be particularly suited for non invasive haemodynamic monitoring in routine CCU's.

SESSION 3 was devoted to invasive hemodynamic monitoring. The discussion was intense and agreement was reached on the following points:

1. Routine CCU's without adequate staffing equipment and expertise should not performe invasive hemodynamic monitoring. Complicated patients should be promptly transferred to specialized units for monitoring;

2. A common form (already available and tested in Rotterdam) should be properly filled in by all centers willing to co-operate in order to get adequate statistics in the current natural history of acute myocardial infarction;

3. An adequate evaluation of the effect of early and extensive hemodynamic monitoring in patients with initial complications should be carried out in specialized research units;

4. A study of the factors conditioning cardiac rupture, now one of the leading causes of death in CCU, and of the possibilities of its prevention is suggested.

Consensus was not reached on whether invasive hemodynamic monitoring should be performed in patients without severe cardiac disfunction outside specialized research units.

SESSION 4 was devoted to clinical aspects and new research lines on preinfarction angina.

Since one of the remarkable fall-outs of CCU's was the improvement in our understanding of the pathophysiology of myocardial infarction which lead by itself to a better therapeutic result, it was suggested that a promising research line could be the study of the caused of angina attacks in patients admitted to CCU's for the severity of their symptoms.

Agreement was not reached ·on this subject, largely because of differences in phylosophy of various centers. The available evidence suggests that, for the centers interested in this problem, this may be a very promising line of research. It makes use of possibilities which are largely available in CCU's and may lead to new pharmacological approach to these patients that are at high risk of developing an acute myocardial infarction.

SESSION 5 was devoted to Pre-Unit care and dealt with two aspects: 1. ambulance system for reducing admission time to CCU; 2. early transfer of shock cases for balloon pumping from peripheral CCU's to central CCU's.

There was consensus that the use of an ambulance system reduces considerably the delay of admission to CCU. However, there was disagreement on whether a specialized or a standard ambulance system with or without a physician should be used. Special emphasis was placed on the political and bureaucratic problems involved in the organization of a mobile unit system. Given the local difficulties it was suggested that the issue should be taken up at the level of the European Community.

There was considerable discussion on: 1. the selection of patients for balloon pumping; 2. on the experties and the facilities required for their application which at present are found only in few centers with good cardiac surgery teams; 3. the possibility of performing randomized studies to test its efficacy and effectiveness.

SESSION 6 was devoted to expanding role of CCU's in the Community and dealt in particular with the possibility of better exploiting the experties of CCU personnel for other activities such as telephone consultations of ECG diagnosis and on analysis of patients with Holter monitoring.

There was consensus that common action should be encouraged for Holter monitoring for S-T segment changes in the following directions:

1. development of tests to be run during the recording for continuous quality control of the recording;

2. evaluation of the significance of ST segment changes;

3. development of programs for automatic data analysis and testing on a data bank of tapes to be collected.

A.5. FORSEABLE CONCERTED ACTIONS

Our survey of the literature, of analysis of the activites and intents of the European centers that answered our questionaire and the conclusions of the Seminar on 'Perspectives of CCU's' that we organized in Pisa indicates that the most promising line of common action at the European level should concern the efficacy and effectiveness of advanced technologies in the management of acute coronary patients.

The dimensions of the socio-economic problem represented by ischemic heart disease require a concentration of effort for its treatment and prevention at least comparable to that in program for neoplastic disease.

It appears a logical conclusion of the work of the CRM an action which obviously cannot be undertaken at a national level for 3 main reasons:

1. the dimension of the problem;
2. the absence of expertises on all the different aspect in individual countries;
3. the difference in patient population and in the phylosophy guiding the approach to coronary patients in different countries.

Review of the recent literature of the survey report on hemodynamic monitoring in coronary care units (document 1979 - PISA) and the results of the recent seminar held in Pisa on "Perspectives of Coronary Care Units" indicate that this field is in the process of rapid transience because of accumulating information which appears to modify substantially traditional concepts concerning patient management and prevention.

Advanced technologies may potentially play a major role not only in diagnostic and therapeutic procedures but also in our understanding of disease processes, thus opening new lines for treatment and prevention.

Our proposition is oriente to:

1. Development and assessment of technologies capable of improving the level of care of acute patients at reduced costs, such as

development and testing of simple monitoring equipment capable of reliable detection of ventricular fibrillation and of asystole;

development and testing of non invasive techniques for the evaluation of the degree of pump function impairment in patients with acute myocardial infarction.

2. Standardized application of new technologies and procedures to prevent and reduce complications in acute coronary patients;

multicenter, systemic investigation of patients with severe angina at rest, aimed to the identification of variables that may permit more specific treatments so as to reduce the incidence of myocardial infarction in this high risk group;

multicenter, systematic investigation of the mechanisms involved in the extension of acute myocardial infarction aimed to identify variables that may permit evaluation of the results of treatments;

multicenter, multinational studies aimed to updated knowledge of the natural history of the acute stages of the disease.

We believe that interventions along these lines will considerably improve the cost effectiveness ratio in Coronary Care Units and will improve our understanding of the disease, which is the key to future rationale therapeutic and preventive interventions.

REFERENCES

1. Survey-Report Coronary Care, second revision for the Commission of the European Communities, Standing Committee "Monitoring of Seriously Ill" of the Ad hoc Group Coronary Care. Doc. XII/380/73 - E 20 November 1973.

2. Mather HG, NG Pearson, KLQ Read et al: Acute myocardial infarction: home and hospital treatment. Br Med J 3: 334, 1971.

3. Colling A, AW Dellipiani, P McGormack et al: Coronary care units. (Annotations) Am Heart J 91: 537, 1976.

4. Lindholm J, N Fabricius-Bjerre, K Astvad et al: Coronary care units. (Annotations). Am Heart J 91: 673, 1976.

5. Hill JD, G Holdstock, JR Hampton: Comparison of mortality of patients with heart attacks admitted to a coronary care unit and an ordinary medical ward. Br Med J 2: 81, 1977.

6. Killip T, JT Kimball: Experience with monitoring myocardial infarction of the New York Hospital-Cornell Medical Center: Comparison of regular hospital care. Proc New Engl Cardiovasc Soc 24: 27, 1965-1966.

7. Hofvendahl S: Influence in a coronary care unit on prognosis in acute myocardial infarction. Acta Med Scand Suppl 519, 1971.

8. Bielsky MT, A Edwards, CK Frieberg et al: Members of study group of coronary heart disease. Resources for the optimal care of patients with acute myocardial infarction. Circulation 43: A-171, 1971.

9. Bloom BS, OL Peterson: End results, cost and productivity of coronary-care units. New Engl J Med 288: 72, 1973.

10. Campus S, A Rappelli, P Russo et al: Considerazioni clinico statistiche su 284 casi di infarto miocardico ricoverati in unità coronarica. Min Cardioang 22: 716, 1974.

11. Stross JK, PW Willis III, EW Reynolds et al: Effectiveness of coronary care units in small community Hospitals. Ann Int Med 85: 709, 1976.

12. Hunt D, G Sloman, D Christie et al: Changing patterns and mortality of acute myocardial infarction in a coronary care unit. Br Med J 1: 795, 1977.

13. Feruglio GA, L Bandera, A Manfroni et al: Sei anni di attività dell'Unità Coronarica. Bilancio e prospettive. Min Med 68: 2193, 1977.

14. Geddes JS: General practitioners and coronary care (letter). Br Med J 6056: 289, 1977.

15. Lie KI, KL Liem, RM Schuilenburg et al: Early identification of patients developing late in Hospital ventricular fibrillation after discharge from the Coronary Care Unit. A 5 year Retrospective and Prospective Study of 1,897 patients. Am J Cardiol 41: 674, 1978.

16. Shubin H, AA Afifi, WM Rand WM et al: Objective index of hemodynamic status for quantitation of severity and prognosis of shock complicating myocardial infarction. Cardiovasc Res 4: 329, 1968.

17. Forrester JS, G Diamond, T McHugh et al: Filling pressures in the right and left sides of the heart in acute myocardial infarction: a reappraisal of central venous pressure monitoring. N Engl J Med 285: 190, 1971.

18. Dowling JT, DV Hunt, RO Russell et al: Intracardiac catheterization in the acute stage of myocardial infarction. Circulation 33 and 44 (Suppl II): 159, 1971.

19. Forrester JS, GA Diamond, HJC Swan: Bedside diagnosis of latent cardiac complications in acutely ill patients. JAMA 222: 59, 1972.

20. Loeb HS, SH Rahimtoola, MR Kenneth et al: Assessment of ventricular function after acute myocardial infarction by plasma volume expansion. Circulation 47: 720, 1973.

21. Mantle JA, EM Strand, SE Wixon et al: Computerized hemodynamic and electrophysiologic clinical studies in a myocardial infarction research unit. Five years experience. Computers in Cardiology p 95, 1975.

22. Forrester JS, G Diamond, K Chatterjee et al: Medical therapy of AMI by application of hemodynamic subsets. Part I. New Engl J Med 295: 1356, 1976.

23. Chatterjee K, HJC Swan, VS Kanshik et al: Effects of vasodilator therapy for severe pump failure in AMI on short-term and late prognosis. Circulation 53: 797, 1976.

24. Rackley CE, RO Russell Jr, RE Moraski et al: Recent advances in hemodynamic studies in patients with acute myocardial infarction. In: Progress in Cardiology. Ed by Yu PN and Goodwin JF. Lea & Febiger, Philadelphia. Chapter 8: 201, 1976.

25. Jenkins BS, RD Bradley, MA Branthwaite: Evaluation of pulmonary arterial and diastolic pressure as an indirect estimate if left atrial mean pressure. Circulation 42: 75, 1970.

26. Hunt D, JF Pombo-Ramos, C Potanin et al: Intravascular monitoring in acute myocardial infarction. Am J Cardiol 25: 104, 1970.

27. Bouchard RJ, JH Gault, J Ross Jr: Evaluation of pulmonary arterial end-diastolic pressure as an estimate of left ventricular end-diastolic pressure in patients with normal and abnormal left ventricular performance. Circulation 44: 1072, 1971.

28. Rutherford BD, WD McCann, TBP O'Donovan: The value of monitoring pulmonary artery pressure for early detection of left ventricular failure following myocardial infarction. Circulation 43: 655, 1971.

29. Hagemeijer F, A De Greve, J Pool et al: Pulmonary capillary wedge pressure (PCW) and venous oxygen saturation (O_2 sat) in acute myocardial infarction. Circulation 45 (Suppl II): II-163, 1972.

30. Rahimtoola SH, HS Loeb, A Ehsani et al: Relationship of pulmonary artery to left ventricular diastolic pressures in acute myocardial infarction. Circulation 46: 283, 1972.

31. Verdouw PO, F Hagemeijer, WG Van Dorf et al: Short-term survival after AMI predicted by hemodynamic parameters. Circulation 52: 413, 1975.

32. Forrester JS, GA Diamond, HJC Swan: Correlative classification of clinical and hemodynamic function after acute myocardial infarction. Am J Cardiol 39: 137, 1977.

33. Weber KT, JS Janicki, RO Russel et al: Identification of high risk of AMI. Derived from the myocardial infarction research units cooperative Study Data Bank. Am J Cardiol 41: 197, 1978.

34. Parmley WW, G Diamond, H Tossoda et al: Clinical evaluation of left ventricular pressures in myocardial infarction. Circulation 45: 358, 1972.

35. Russell RO Jr, CE Rackley, J Pombo et al: Effects of increasing left ventricular filling pressure in patients with acute myocardial infarction. J Clin Invest 49: 1539, 1970.

36. Forrester J, G Diamond, W Ganz et al: Right and left heart pressure in the acutely ill patient. Clin Res 18: 306, 1970.

37. Crexells C, K Chatterjee, JS Forrester et al: Optimal level of filling pressure in the left side of the heart in acute myocardial infarction. N Engl J Med 289: 1263, 1973.

38. Osborn JJ, JO Beaumont, JCA Raison et al: Measurement and monitoring of acutely ill patients by digital computer. Surgery 64: 1057, 1968.

39. Rackley CE, RO Russell Jr: Left ventricular function in acute myocardial infarction and its clinical significance. Circulation 45: 231, 1972.

40. Maseri A, V Pecorini, P Toni et al: Clinical applications of quantitative radiocardiography. II. Results in normal subjects and changes with age. Acta Med Scand 176: 769, 1964.

41. Maseri A, A Pesola, C Contini, et al: Hémodinamique pulmonaire et coronarienne dans la phase aigue de l'infarctus du myocarde Arch Mal Coeur 4: 401, 1973.

42. Mills CJ, JP Shillingford: A catheter tip electromagnetic velocity probe and its evaluation. Cardiovasc Res 1: 263, 1967.

43. Gabe IT, JH Gault, J Ross Jr et al: Measurement of instantaneous blood flow velocity and pressure in conscious man with a cathetertip velocity probe. Circulation 40: 603, 1969.

44. Gardner RM: Computerized intensive care monitoring at LSD hospital. Progress and development. Computers in Cardiology p 97, 1974.

45. Shubin H, MA Weil, P Da Luz et al: Objective assessment of prognosis in shock due to AMI. Computers in Cardiology p 183, 1974.

46. Nixon PGE, MB Durh: Pulmonary oedema with low left ventricular

diastolic pressure in acute myocardial infarction. Lancet July: 146, 1968.

47. McHugh TJ, JS Forrester, L Adler et al: Pulmonary vascular congestion in acute myocardial infarction: Hemodynamic and radio-logic correlations. Ann Intern Med 76: 29, 1972.

48. Turner F, FYK Lau, G Jacobson: A method for the estimation of pulmonary venous and arterial pressures from the routine chest roentgenogram. Am J Roentgenology 116: 97, 1972.

49. Kostuk W, JW Barr, AL Simon et al: Correlations between the chest film and hemodynamics in acute myocardial infarction. Circulation 48: 624, 1973.

50. Meszaros WT: Lung changes in left heart failure. Circulation 47: 857, 1973.

51. Garrard CL, RO Russell Jr, JM Perry et al: Systolic time intervals: a measure of response to alterations in filling pressure in acute myocardial infarction. Circulation 42: (Suppl III): 155, 1970.

52. Dowling JT, G Sloman, C Urquhart: Systolic time interval fluctua-tions produced by acute myocardial infarction. Br Heart J 33: 765, 1971.

53. Heikkila J, K Luomanmaki, K Pyorala: Serial observations on left ventricular dysfunction in acute myocardial infarction. II. Systolic time intervals in power failure. Circulation 44: 343, 1971.

54. Jain SR, J Lindahl: Apex cardiogram and systolic time intervals in acute myocardial infarction. Br Heart J 33: 578, 1971.

55. Hamosh P, J Cohn, K Engelman et al: Systolic time intervals and left ventricular function in acute myocardial infarction. Circu-lation 45: 375, 1972.

56. Hodges M, BL Halpern, GC Friesinger et al: Left ventricular preejection period and ejection time in patients with acute myocardial infarction. Circulation 45: 933, 1972.

57. Perloff J, N Reichneck: value and limitations of systolic time intervals (preejection period and ejection time) in patients with acute myocardial infarction. Circulation 45: 929, 1972.

58. Delahaye JP, JC Chulliat, JP Bons et al: Valeur prognostique de l'étude des intervalles systoliques dans l'infarctus myocardique récent. II. Applications à la métodologie cardiaque. Arch Mal Coeur 67: 421, 1974.

59. Robijns H, D Clement, G Verstreken et al: Left ventricular systolic time intervals during acute myocardial infarction. Eur J Cardiol 2/4: 431, 1975.

60. Luomanmaki K, J Heikkila, M Helin: Assessment of immediate prognosis in acute myocardial infarction by a new noninvasive hemodynamic index. Europ J Cardiol 4/2: 175, 1976.

61. Letac B, JL Cazor, JM Thiron: Etude des temps systoliques par phonomécanocardiographie externe dans l'infarctus du myocarde.

Arch Mal Coeur 69: 367, 1976.

62. Stefan G, RJ Bing: Echocardiographic findings in experimental myocardial infarction of posterior left ventricular wall. Am J Cardiol 30: 629, 1972.

63. Bergeron GA, MV Cohen, LE Teicholz et al: Echocardiographic analysis of mitral valve motion after acute myocardial infarction. Circulation 51: 82, 1975.

64. Corya BC, S Rasmussen, S Knoebel et al: Echocardiography in acute myocardial infarction. Am J Cardiol 36: 1, 1975.

65. Nieminen M, J Heikkila: Echoventriculography in acute myocardial infarction. III. Clinical correlations and implication of the non-infarcted myocardium. Am J Cardiol 38: 1, 1976.

66. Friedewald Jr VE: Coronary artery disease. In: Textbook of echocardiography, Chapter 14. WB Saunders Company Philadelphia-/London/Toronto p 256, 1977.

67. Corya BC: Echocardiography in ischemic heart disease. Am J Med 63: 10, 1977.

68. Fortuin NJ, CGK Pawsey: The evaluation of left ventricular function by echocardiography. Am J Med 63: 1, 1977.

69. Kisslo JA, D Robertson, BW Gilbert et al: A comparison of real time, two dimensional echocardiography and cineangiography in detecting left ventricular asynergy. Circulation 55: 134, 1977.

70. Sharpe DN, EH Botvinick, DM Shames et al: The noninvasive diagnosis of right ventricular infarction. Circulation 5: 483, 1978.

71. Kerber RE, ML Marcus: Evaluation of regional myocardial function in ischemic heart disease by echocardiography. Prog Cardiovasc Dis 20: 441, 1978.

72. Douglas MA, HG Ostrow, MV Freen et al: A computer processing system for ECG-gated radioisotope angiography of the human heart. Computers and Biomedical Research 9: 133, 1976.

73. Bacharach SL, MV Green, JS Borer et al: A real-time system for multi-image gated cardiac studies. J Nucl Biol 18: 79, 1977.

74. Borer JS, SL Bacharach, MV Green et al: Real-time radionuclide cineangiography in the noninvasive evaluation of global and regional left ventricular function at rest and during exercise in patients with coronary-artery disease. New Engl J Med 296: 839, 1977.

75. Pitt B, HW Strauss: Evaluation of ventricular function by radio-isotopic technics. New Engl J Med 296: 1097, 1977.

76. Reduto LA, HJ Berger, LS Cohen et al: Sequential radionuclide assessment of left and right ventricular performance after acute transmural myocardial infarction. Ann Int Med 89: 441, 1978.

77. Sequeira RF, LH Light, G Crosset al: Transcutaneous aortovelography. A quantitative evaluation. Br Heart J 38: 451, 1976.

78. Buchthal A, GC Hanson, AR Peisach: Transcutaneous aortovelography: a possible adjunctive technique in the management of the

critically ill patient. Br Heart J 38: 451, 1976.

79. Light H: Transcutaneous aortovelography. A new window on the circulation? Br Heart J 38: 433, 1976.

80. Stick C, R Buchsel: Impedence cardiography: the reproducibility of stroke volume measurements under conditions of mass examination. Basic Res cardiol 73: 627, 1978.

81. Forrester JS, G Diamond, K Chatterjee K et al: Medical therapy of AMI by application of hemodynamic subsets. Part. II. New Engl J Med 295: 1404, 1976.

82. Tavazzi L, JA Salerno, M Ray et al: Classificazione dell'infarto miocardico acuto. Implicazioni terapeutiche. Atti VII Congresso Nazionale ANMCO Firenze, p 88, 1976.

83. Gorlin R: Practical cardiac hemodynamics. N Engl J Med 296: 203, 1977.

84. Antonini FM et al: Hemodynamic monitoring in AMI: significance of prognostic indexes. To be published in the Proceedings of the EEC Seminar "Perspectives of Coronary Care Units", Pisa December 1-2, 1978.

85. Stevens JM, SH Stone, AE Wechsler: An evaluation of computer-aided patient monitoring of post-cardiac surgery patients. Computers in Cardiology p 119, 1976.

86. Zeelenberg C, WAH Engelse: A hierarchical patient monitoring computer network. Computers in Xardiology. Rotterdam p 439, 1977.

87. Kalinsky D, A Miller: Use of a mobile computer cart for cardiovascular monitoring and clinical investigation. Computers in Cardiology, Rotterdam p 427, 1977.

88. Engelse WAH et al: Lines of development of instrumentation for hemodynamic monitoring in CCU. To be published in the Proceedings of the EEC Seminar "Perspectives of Coronary Care Units", Pisa December 1-2, 1978.

89. Glaeser DH, RF Trost: Distributed system for continuous and discrete monitoring of cardiovascular patients. Computers in Cardiology p 117, 1974.

90. Hugenholtz PG, F Hagemeijer, AC Miller et al: L'ordinateur dans les unités de soins intensifs. Arch Mal Coeur 67: 1095, 1974.

91. Miller A: Summary of the Workshop Distributed Processing in Intensive Care. Computers in Cardiology, Rotterdam p 445, 1977.

92. Feldman CL: Evaluation of arrhythmia detectors. Computers in Cardiology p 21, 1974.

93. Sanders WJ, EL Alderman, DC Harrison: Alarm processing in a computerized patient monitoring system. Computers in Cardiology p 21, 1975.

94. Yanowitz FG, TA Pryor, D Frost: A computerized ECG alarm system for the coronary care unit. Computers in Cardiology p 431, 1976.

95. Lorente P, M Delabre: Use of correspondence analysis in processing hemodynamic data from acute myocardial infarction. Computers and Biomedical Research 10: 213, 1977.

96. Hilberman M, B Kamm, M Lamy et al: Prediction of respiratory adequacy following cardiac surgery. Computers in Cardiology p 171, 1974.

97. Postigal L, PC Chang, MH Weil: Method for the development of prognostic indices for patients in shock. Computers in Cardiology p 389, 1976.

98. Thompson Jr HK, MA Woodbury: Clinical data representation in multidimensional space. Computers and Biomedical Research 3: 58, 1970.

99. Hope CE, CD Lewis, IR Perry et al.: Computed trend analysis in automated patient monitoring systems. Brit. J Anaesth 45: 440, 1973.

100. Sheppard LC, NT Kouchoukos, JW Kirklin: The digital computer in surgical intensive care automation. Computer 6: 29, 1973.

101. Acton JC, LC Sheppard, NT Kouchoukos et al: Automated care systems for critically ill patients following cardiac surgery. Computers in Cardiology p. 111, 1974.

102. Sheppard LC, JW Kirklin: Cardiac surgical intensive care computer system. Computer Conference. Federation Proceedings 33: 2326, 1974.

103. Sheppard LC, NT Kouchoukos: Computers as monitors. Anesthesiology 45: 250, 1976.

104. Kunz J, M Hilberman: Alarm warnings using a respiratory monitoring system. Computers in Cardiology p. 217, 1975.

105. Beneken JEW: Prognostic indexes, trend detection and prediction techniques. To be published in the Proceedings of the EEC Seminar "Perspectives of Coronary Care Units", Pisa December 1-2, 1978.

106. Warner HR: A data-trend log and bar graph display for physiology monitoring. Computers and Biomedical Research 3: 285, 1970.

107. Marchesi C, S Chierchia, A Maseri: Left and right ventricular pressures monitoring in CCU. Methods and significance. Computers in Cardiology, Rotterdam p. 579, 1977.

108. Wolff HS: in Biomedical Engineering. McGraw-Hill, New York p. 16, 1970.

109. Siegel JH, RM Goldwyn, HP Friedman: Pattern and process in the evolution of human septic shock. Surgery 70: 232, 1971.

110. Little AD, Inc: Evaluation of Computer based patient monitoring systems (Summary Volume 1) Contract HSM110-70-406, March 1973.

111. Day HW: An intensive coronary care area. Chest 44: 423, 1963.

112. Brown KWG, RL MacMillan, N Forbath et al: Coronary unit, an intensive care center for AMI. Lancet 2: 348, 1963.

113. Ross J Jr, E Braunwald: The study of left ventricular function in man by increasing resistance to ventricular ejection with angiotensin. Circulation 29: 739, 1964.

114. Lemlich A: Multivariate analysis of clinical and prognostic factors in myocardial infarction. NY State J Med 65: 1209, 1965.

115. Shubin H, MH Weil: Hemodynamic alterations in patients after myocardial infarction, in shock and hypotension: Pathogenesis and treatment. The 12th Hahnemann Symposium. Edited by LC Mills and JH Moyer. Grune & Stratton. p 499, 1965.

116. Kaltman AJ, WH Herbert, RJ Conroy et al: Gradient in pressure across the pulmonary vascular bed during diastole. Circulation 34: 377, 1966.

117. Goble AJ, G Sloman, JS Robinson: Mortality reduction in a coronary care unit. Br Med J 1: 1005, 1966.

118. Weil MH, H Shubin, W Rand: Experience with a digital computer for study and improved management of the critically ill. JAMA 198: 1011, 1966.

119. Shubin H, MH Weil: Efficient monitoring with a digital computer of cardiovascular function in seriously ill patients. Ann Intern Med 65: 453, 1966.

120. Killip T, JT Kimball: Treatment of myocardial infarction in a coronary care unit. A two year experience with 250 patients. Am J Cardiol 20: 457, 1967.

121. Lawrie DM, TW Greenwood, M Goddard et al: A coronary-care unit in the routine management of acute myocardial infarction. Lancet 2: 109, 1967.

122. Lown B, AM Fakhro, WB Hood Jr et al: The coronary care unit. New Perspectives and directions. JAMA 199: 188, 1967.

123. Killip T, JT Kimball: A survey of the coronary care unit: concept and results. Prog Cardiovasc Dis 11: 45, 1968.

124. Weill MH, H Shubin: Shock following acute myocardial infarction. Current understanding of hemodynamic mechanisms. Prog Cardiovasc Dis 11: 1, 1968.

125. Scott PJ: Hospital mortality in acute myocardial infarction. Brit Med J 3: 143, 1968.

126. Sloman G, M Stannard, Aj Goble: Coronary care unit: A review of 300 patients monitored since 1963. Amer Heart J 75: 140, 1968.

127. Kurien VA, MF Oliver: Assessment of the immediate prognosis during acute myocardial infarction. Am Heart J 2: 142, 1968.

128. Warner HR, RM Gardner, AF Toronto: Computer-based monitoring of cardiovascular functions in postoperative patients. Circulation 37, 38 (Suppl II): 68, 1968.

129. Rapaport E, M Scheinman: Rationale and limitations of hemodynamic measurements in patients with acute myocardial infarction. Mod Conc Cardiovasc Dis 38: 55, 1969.

130. L'organisation des unités de soins aux coronariens. Rapport sur une Réunion préparatorie organisée par le Bureau régional de l'Europe de l'Organisation mondiale de la Santé. Copenhague, 3-6 Février, 1969.

131. Swan HJC, JS Forrester, R Danzig et al: Power failure in acute myocardial infarction. Prog Cardiovasc Dis 12: 568, 1970.

132. Scheidt S, R Ascheim, T Killip III: Shock after acute myocar-

dial infarction: a clinical and hemodynamic profile. Am J Cardiol 26: 556, 1970.

133. Hunt D, C Potanin, J Pombo et al: Left ventricular function in clinically uncomplicated myocardial infarction. Clin Res 18: 313, 1970.

134. Russell RO, J Pombo, D Hunt et al: Comparison of left ventricular hemodynamics in patients with anterior and with inferior myocardial infarction. (Abstr) Circulation 42 (Suppl III): III-193, 1970.

135. Feild BJ, RO Russell, D Hunt et al: Clinical usefulness of hemodynamic monitoring in acute myocardial infarction. Am J Cardiol 26: 632, 1970.

136. McHugh TJ, L Adler, D Zion et al: Acute myocardial infarction: Radiologic, clinical and hemodynamic correlations. Circulation 42 (Suppl III): III-31, 1970.

137. Sjogren A: Left heart failure in acute myocardial infarction. Acta Med Scand Suppl 510, 1970.

138. Peterson OL, BJ Duffy: A report on coronary care in the tristate region. Boston, Medical Care and Education Foundation, Inc November 1970.

139. Pantridge JF et al: The effect of early therapy on the hospital mortality from acute myocardial infarction, Q J Med 39: 621, 1970.

140. Harnarayan C, MA Bennet, BL Pentecost et al: Quantitative study of infarcted myocardium in cardiogenic shock. Br Heart J 32: 728, 1970.

141. Shell WE, JK Kjeshus, VE Sobel: Quantitative assessment of the extent of myocardial infarction in the conscious dog by means of analysis of serial changes in serum CPK activity. J Clin Invest 50: 2614, 1970.

142. Raison JCA: Patient monitoring: on-line computing. Postgrad Med J 46: 360, 1970.

143. Diamant B, T Killip: Indirect assessment of left ventricular performance in acute myocardial infarction. Circulation 42: 579, 1970.

144. Leinbach RC, MJ Buckley, WG Austen et al: Effects of intra-aortic balloon pumping on coronary flow and metabolism in man. Circulation 43 and 44 (Suppl I): 77, 1971.

145. Maroko RP, JK Kjekshus, BE Sobel et al: Factors influencing infarct size following experimental coronary artery occlusion. Circulation 43: 67, 1971.

146. Ratshin RA, F Harrell, BJ Field et al: A prognostic index for myocardial infarction from analysis of acute phase hemodynamic data. Circulation 43: (Suppl II): II-214, 1971.

147. Hamosh P, JN Cohn: Left ventricular function in acute myocardial infarction. J Clin Invest 50: 523, 1971.

148. Pombo JF, RO Russell Jr, CE Rackley et al: Comparison of stroke

volume and myocardial infarction. Am J Cardiol 27: 630, 1971.

149. Hughes JL, AF Salel, RA Massumi et al: The electrocardiogram as a predictor of ventricular function and cardiogenic shock in acute myocardial infarction. (Abstr) Circulation 44 (Suppl II): II-179, 1971.

150. Blum R, W Parmley, G Diamond et al: Left ventricular contractile state in acute myocardial infarction. (Abstr) Circulation 44 (Suppl II): 11-97, 1971.

151. Diamond G, H Marcus, T McHugh et al: Catheterization of the left ventricle in the acutely ill patient. Brit Heart J 33: 489, 1971.

152. Dikshit K, J Vyden, R Prakash et al: Extra-renal hemodynamic effetcs of furosemide in acute left ventricular failure. (Abstr) Circulation 44 (Suppl II): II-50, 1971.

153. Hamosh P, JN Cohn: Left ventricular function in acute myocardial infarction. J Clin Invest 50: 523, 1971.

154. Chopra MP, U Thadani, RW Portal et al: Lignocaine therapy for ventricular ectopic activity after acute myocardial infarction: a double-blind trial. Br Med J 3: 668, 1971.

155. Page DL, JB Caulfield, JA Kastor et al: Myocardial changes associated with cardiogenic shock. New Engl Med 285: 133, 1971.

156. Jossot G, L Birman, H Tannebaum et al: Mortalité au stade aigu de l'infarctus du myocarde dans une unité de soins intensifs pour maladies coronaires. J Méd Strasb 10, 775, 1971.

157. Gourgon R, G Motte, J Gueris et al: Etude hémodynamique de 33 cas d'infarctus myocardiques récents. Coeur et Med Int 10: 365, 1971.

158. Lorente P, G Motte, A Fabiato et al: L'exploration hémodynamique au stade aigu de l'infarctus du myocarde. I. Etude critique des paramétres recueillis. Arch Mal Coeur 64: 217, 1971.

159. Motte G, R Gourgon, P Lorente et al: L'exploration hémodynamique au stade aigu de l'infarctus du myocarde. II. Résultats, incidences thérapeutiques et prognostiques. Arch Mal Coeur 64: 217, 1971.

160. Motte G, M Perraolt, P Lorente et al: L'exploration hémodynamique au stade aigu de l'infarctus du myocarde. III. Siége de la nécrose et fonctions ventriculaires. Arch Mal Coeur 64: 1377, 1971.

161. Maseri A, A Pesola, C Contini et al: Congestione venosa polmonare: pressione e volume di sangue nell'infarto miocardico acuto. Boll Soc It Cardiol 17: 275, 1971.

162. Shubin H, MH Weil, N Palley et al: Monitoring the critically ill patient with the aid of a digital computer. Computers and Biomedical Research 4: 460, 1971.

163. Swan HJC, JS Forrester, G Diamond et al: Hemodynamic spectrum of myocardial infarction· and cardiogenic shock: a conceptual model. Circulation 45: 1097, 1972.

164. Sobel BE, GF Bresnahan, WE Shell et al: Estimation of infarct size in man and its relation to prognosis. Circulation 46: 640, 1972.

165. Agress CM, S Wegner, JS Forrester et al: An indirect method for evaluation of left ventricular function in acute myocardial infarction. Circulation 46: 291, 1972.

166. Linhart JW: Atrial pacing in coronary disease, including preinfarction angina and postoperative studies. Am J Cardiol 30: 603, 1972.

167. Russell RO Jr, D Hunt, C Potanin et al: Hemodynamic monitoring in a coronary intensive care unit: Clinical application. Arch Intern Med 130: 370, 1972.

168. Sanghvi VT, F Khaja, AL Mark et al: Effects of blood volume expansion on left ventricular hemodynamics in man. Circulation 46: 780, 1972.

169. Ratshin RA, CE Rackley, RO Russell Jr: Hemodynamic evaluation of left ventricular function in shock complicating myocardial infarction. Circulation 45: 127, 1972.

170. Gunnar RM, HS Loeb: Use of drugs in cardiogenic shock due to acute myocardial infarction. Circulation 45: 1111, 1972.

171. Prakash R, J Forrester, WW Parmley et al: Prognostic implications of left ventricular stroke work index in acute myocardial infarction. Clin Res 20: 391, 1972.

172. Darby MA, MA Sheila, MA Bennet et al: Trial of combined intramuscular and intravenous lignocaine in prophylaxis of ventricular tachyarrhythmias. Lancet 1: 817, 1972.

173. Loeb HS, R Lal, SH Rahimtoola et al: Assessment of ventricular function in acute myocardial infarction. Clin Res 20: 358, 1972.

174. Gourgon R, PH Coumel, CH Masquet et al: Effects hémodynamiques du remplissage vasculaire au stade aigu de l'infarctus du myocarde. Ann Méd Interne 123: 265, 1972.

175. Franciosa JA, NH Wilha, CJ Limas et al: Improved left ventricular function during nitro prusside infusion in acute infarction. Lancet 1: 650, 1972.

176. Maroko PR, P Libby, J Covell et al: Precordial ST segment elevation mapping: an atraumatic method for assessing alterations in the extent of myocardial ischemic injury. The effect of pharmacologic and hemodynamic interventions. Am J Cardiol 29: 223, 1972.

177. Maroko PR, P Libby, BE Sobel et al: Effect of glucose-insulin-potassium infusion on myocardial infarction following experimental coronary artery occlusion. Circulation 45: 1160, 1972.

178. Wolk MJ, S Scheidt, T Killip: Heart failure complicating acute myocardial infarction. Circulation 45: 1125, 1972.

179. Feild BJ, P Russell, JT Dowling et al: Prognostic value of stroke work in acute myocardial infarction. Circulation (Abstr) 46: 4, 2, 1972.

180. Diamond G, JS Forrester, K Chatterjee et al: Mean electromechanical dP/dt. An index of the peak rate of rise of left ventricular pressure. Am J Cardiol 30: 338, 1972.

181. Fabian J, EJ Epstein, N Coulshed et al: Duration of phases of left ventricular systole using indirect methods. II: Acute myocardial infarction. Br Heart J 34: 882, 1972.

182. Lewis RP, H Boundoulas, WF Forrester et al: Shortening of electromechanical systole as a manifestation of excessive adrenergic stimulation in acute myocardial infarction. Circulation 46: 856, 1972.

183. Sobel BE, GF Bresnahan, WE Shell et al: Estimation of infarct size in man and its relation to prognosis. Circulation 46: 640, 1972.

184. Smithen C, C Wharton, E Sowton: Changes in left ventricular wall movement following exercise, atrial pacing and acute myocardial infarction measured by reflected ultrasound. Am J Cardiol 29: 293, 1972.

185. Shubin H, N Palley, MH Weil: Computer surveillance of the seriously ill patient. Journal of the Association for the Advancement of Medical Instrumentation 6: 48, 1972.

186. Epstein SE, DR Redwood, KM Kent: Atrophine and acute myocardial infarction. Circulation 47: 1398, 1973.

187. Heikkila J, PG Hugenholtz, BS Tabakin: Prediction of left heart filling pressure and its sequential change in acute myocardial infarction from the terminal force of the P wave. Br Heart J 35: 142, 1973.

188. Verdouw PD, AVD Vorl, F Hagemeijer et al: Is prognosis of survival following myocardial infarction possible from hemodynamics at the time of admission? Circulation 48 (Suppl IV): IV-227, 1973.

189. Russell RO Jr, D Hunt, CE Rackley: Left ventricular hemodynamics in anterior and inferior myocardial infarction. Am J Cardiol 32: 8, 1973.

190. Chapman BL, CH Gray: Prognostic index for myocardial infarction treated in a coronary care unit. Br Heart J 35: 135, 1973.

191. Bleifeld W, W Merx, KW Heinrich et al: Controlled trial of prophylactic treatment with lidocaine in acute myocardial infarction. Eur J Clin Pharmacol 6: 119, 1972.

192. O'Brien KP, PM Taylor, RS Croxson: Prophylactic lignocaine in hospitalized patients with acute myocardial infarction. Med J Aust (Special Suppl) 2: 36, 1973.

193. Scheidt S, G Wilner, S Fillmore et al: Objective hemodynamic assessment after acute myocardial infarction. Med J Aust (Special Suppl) 2: 36, 1973.

194. Chatterjee K, HJC Swan: Hemodynamic profile in acute myocardial infarction. In myocardial infarction, edited by Corday E, Swan HJC, Baltimore, Williams and Wilkins Publishers, p 51, 1973.

195. Kelly DT, CE Delgado, DR Taylor, et al: Use of phentolamine in acute myocardial infarction associated with hypertension and left ventricualr failure. Circulation 47: 729, 1973.

196. Kiely J, DT Kelly, DR Taylor et al: The role of furosemide in the treatment of left ventricular dysfunction associated with acute myocardial infarction. Circulation 48: 581, 1973.

197. Alonso R, S Scheidt, M Post et al: Pathophysiology of cardiogenic shock; quantification of myocardial necrosis. Clinical, Pathologic and Electrocardiographic correlation. Circulation 48: 588, 1973.

198. Cohn JN: Vasodilator therapy for heart failure. The influence of impedence on left ventricular performance. Circulation 48: 5, 1973.

199. Helmers C: Short and long prognostic indices in acute myocardial infarction. Acta Med Scand (Suppl I): 555, 1973.

200. Kostuk WJ, AA Ehsani, JS Karliner et al: Left ventricular performance after myocardial infarction assessed by radioisotope angiocardiography. Circulation 47: 242, 1973.

201. Pitt B, P Rigo, D Taylor et al: Scintiphotographic evaluation of left ventricular function in patients with acute myocardial infarction. Circulation (Suppl IV) Abstr 7 and 8, 1973.

202. Peterson KL, JB Uther, R Shabetai et al: Istantaneous tension velocity-length. Relations obtained with the aid of an electromagnetic velocity catheter in the ascending aorta. Circulation 47: 924, 1973.

203. Michaud R, E Leclair, A Pohu: Traitement de la phase aigue de l'infarctus du myocarde sous monitorisation constante dans une unité de soins intensifs. Arch Mal Coeur 8: 1009, 1973.

204. Afifi AA, PC Chang, VY Liu et al: Prognostic indexes in acute myocardial infarction complicated by shock. Am J Cardiol 33: 826, 1974.

205. Reid PR, DR Taylor, DT Kelly et al: Myocardial-infarct extension detected by precordial ST segment mapping. N Engl J Med 290: 123, 1974.

206. Astvad K, N Fabricius-Bjerre, J Kjaerulff et al: Mortality from acute myocardial infarction before and after establishment of a coronary care unit. Br Med J 1: 567, 1974.

207. Bloom BS, OL Peterson: Patient needs and medical-care planning. N Engl J Med 290: 1171, 1974.

208. Kolling A: Home or hospital care after myocardial after myocardial infarction: is this the right question? Br J Med 1: 559, 1974.

209. Bleifeld W, D Hanrath, D Mathey et al: Acute myocardial infarction V: left and right ventricular hemodynamics in cardiogenic shock. Br Heart J 36: 822, 1974.

210. Schell WE: Infarct size, the key to mortality. Cardiologie d'aujourd'hui 2: 1, 1974.

211. Hirshfeld JW Jr, JS Borer, RE Goldstein et al: Reduction in

severity and extent of myocardial infarction when nitroglycerin and methoxamine are administered during coronary occlusion. Circulation 49: 291, 1974.

212. Abdelmomen A, AA Afifi, C Potter et al: Prognostic indexes in acute myocardial infarction complicated by shock. Am J Cardiol 33: 825, 1974.

213. Gilgenkrantz JM, F Cherrier, JP Saulnier et al: Etude hémodinamique ventriculaire gauche au stade aigu de l'infarctus du myocarde. II. Corrélations clinico-hémodinamique. Evaluation prognistique. Arch Mal Coeur 67: 757, 1974.

214. Bleifeld W: Un indice de gravité du choc cardiogenique. Communication 7° Congrès Mondial de Cardiologie, Buenos Aires, Septembre 1974.

215. Greene HL, DT Kelly, DR Taylor et al: Hemodynamic effects of plasma volume expansion and prognostic implications in acute myocardial infarction. Circulation 49: 106, 1974.

216. Mathey D, W Bleifeld, P Hanrath et al: Attempt to quantitative relation between cardiac function and infarct size in acute myocardial infarction. Br Heart J 36: 271, 1974.

217. Rackley CE, RO Russell: Right ventricular function in acute myocardial infarction. Am J Cardiol 33: 927, 1974.

218. Rahimtoola SH, RO Russell Jr, CE Rackley: Hemodynamics in myocardial infarction. Am J Cardiol 33: 691, 1974.

219. Sobel BE: Détermination quantitative des lésions du myocarde. Triangle XIV 3, 1974.

220. Daluz PL, MH Weil, VY Liu et al: Plasma volume prior to and following volume loading during shock complicating acute myocardial infarction. Circulation 49: 98, 1974.

221. Strand EM, SE Wixon, RO Russell Jr et al: The computer as an integral part of hemodynamic monitoring. In: Hemodynamic monitoring in a coronary intensive care unit edited by Russel RO Jr and Rackley CE. Futura Publishing Company. Chapter VI: 101, 1974.

222. Rackley CE, RO Russell Jr, JA Mantle: Clinical considerations of hemodynamic measurement and left ventricular function in myocardial infarction. In: Hemodynamic monitoring in a coronary intensive care unit. Edited by Russel RO Jr, and Rackley CE. Futura Publishing Company. Chapter VII: 173, 1974.

223. Rackley CE, RO Russell Jr, JA Mantle: Hemodynamic measurements in patients with clinically uncomplicated myocardial infarction. In: Hemodynamic monitoring in a coronary intensive care unit. Edited by Russell RO Jr and Rackley CE. Futura Publishing Company. Chapter VIII: 191, 1974.

224. Rackley CE, RO Russell Jr, JA Mantle: Hemodynamic measurements of heart failure in patients with myocardial infarction. In: Hemodynamic monitoring in a coronary intensive care unit. Edited by Russell RO Jr and Rackley CE. Futura Publishing

Company. Chapter IX: 203, 1974.

225. Rackley CE, RO Russell Jr, RA Ratshin et al: Cardiogenic shock in patients with myocardial infarction. In: Hemodynamic monitoring in a coronary intensive care unit. Edited by Russel RO Jr and Rackley CE. Futura Publishing Company. Chapter X: 223, 1974.

226. Marchesi C, A Fernandez-Perez De Talens, A Maseri: ECG and pressures waveforms monitoring in CCU by a module-structure sofware. Medinfo 74. North Holland Publishing Company. Intensive Care. Session 3.2. p 741, 1974.

227. Alderman EL, AL Spitz, WJ Sanders et al: A cardiologist's evaluation of a computer cardiac catheterization system. Computers in Cardiology p 81, 1974.

228. Thomas LJ, GJ Blaine, VW Gerth et al: Continuous monitoring of physiologic variables with a dedicated minicomputer. Computers in Cardiology p. 107, 1974.

229. Norris RM, DE Caughey, JC Mercer et al: Prognosis after myocardial infarction. Six years follow-up. Br Heart J 36: 786, 1974.

230. Chatterjee K: Vasodilator therapy for heart failure (editorial) Ann Intern Med 83: 421, 1975.

231. Cairns JA, GA Klassen: Modification of acute myocardial infarction (AMI) By i.v. Propranolol (P). Circulation 51 (Suppl II): 107, 1975.

232. Askenazi J, L Tavazzi, JE Muller et al: Effects of hyaluronidase on electrocardiographic evidence of necrosis in patients with acute myocardial infarction. Circulation 51 (Suppl II): 106, 1975.

233. Henning R, T Lundman: Swedish Co-operative CCU Study. Acta Med Scan Suppl 586, 1975.

234. Robicsek F, PL Reichertz, TN Masters et al: Computerized intensive care of postoperative cardiac surgical patients. Computers in Cardiology p 83, 1975.

235. Hilberman M, B Kamm, M Tarter et al: An evaluation of computer based patient monitoring at Pacific Medical Center. Computers and Biological Medicine 8: 447, 1975.

236. Huntsman LL, E Gams, CC Johnson et al: Transcutaneous determination of aortic blood-flow. Am Heart J 89: 605, 1975.

237. De Luz PL, H Shubin, MH Weil et al: Pulmonary edema related to changes in colloid osmotic and pulmonary artery wedge pressure in patients after acute myocardial infarction. Circulation 51: 350, 1975.

238. Hilberman M, JJ Osborn: An evaluation of computer-based respiratory monitoring in a surgical intensive care unit. Computers in Cardiology p. 89, 1975.

239. Risso WL, KM Kempner, DC Owens et al: A postsurgical intensive care computer system at the National Institute of Health. Computers in Cardiology p.101, 1975.

240. Mantle JA, EM Strand, SE Wixson et al: Computer assisted

intensive care monitoring. Computers in Cardiology p. 237, 1976.

241. Klovekorn WP, F Richter, N Mendler et al: Computer assisted intensive care monitoring. Computers in Cardiology p. 237, 1976.

242. Nygords ME, J Transesjo, JH Atterhog et al: On-line computer processing of pressure data from cardiac catheterizations. Computer Programs in Biomedicine 5: 272, 1976.

243. Arnould JL, A Saasjian, JA Fondarai et al: Approche du prognostic de l'infarctus du myocarde à partir de l'exploration hémodynamique initiale. Arch Mal Coeur 69: 23, 1976.

244. Bourgeois MJ, BK Gilbert, Von Bernuth et al: Continuous determination of beat-to beat stroke volume from aortic pressure pulses in the dog. Circ Res 39: 15, 1976.

245. Rubicsek F, TN Manters: Application of medical logic in computer-based intensive care management of open heart patients. Computers in Cardiology p 139, 1976.

246. Mount Sinai Hospital: Patient Monitoring Unit-Operations Manual. New York 1976.

247. O'Rourke F, B Walsh, M Fletcher et al: Impact of the new generation coronary care unit. Br Med J 2: 837, 1976.

248. Fett JD: Practicality of hemodynamic monitoring (Correspondence). New Engl J Med 296: 757, 1977.

249. White GM, CN Murthy: A computer program for the on-line computation of cardiac output from thermodilution curves. Computer Programs in Biomedicine 7: 37, 1977.

250. Parisi AF, DE Tow, WR Felix Jr et al: Noninvasive cardiac diagnosis (1st of 3 parts) New Engl J Med 296: 316, 1977.

251. Parisi AF, DE Tow, WR Felix Jr et al: Noninvasive cardiac diagnosis (2nd of 3 parts) New Engl J Med 296: 368, 1977.

252. Parisi AF, DE Tow, WR Felix Jr et al: Noninvasive cardiac diagnosis (3rd of 3 parts) New Engl J Med 296: 427, 1977.

253. Chatterjee K, WW Parmley: Vasodilator treatment for acute and chronic heart failure. Br Heart J 39: 706, 1977.

254. Sheppard LC, B McA Sayers: Dynamic analysis of the blood pressure response to hypotensive agents, studied in postoperative cardiac surgical patients. Computers and Biomedical Research 10: 237, 1977.

255. Robicsek F, TN Manters, PL Reichertz et al: Three years' experience with computer-based intensive oare of patients following open heart and major vascular surgery. Surgery 81: 12, 1977.

256. Willems JL, J Peperstraete: Cardiac arrhythmia monitoring. EEC survey report, Doc. 388-77-7 ECI B, October 1978.

APPENDIX B

Table 1. General characteristics

System	Developed at	References	Date	Patients	Beds	Field of appl.			Average stay	Cost/day (US $)
						SICU	RICU	CCU		
1	Los Angeles	119 – 162	1964	–	2	x	x	x	–	–
2	Salt Lake City	128 – 44	1966	6000 (1974)	32	x	x	x	2.4	95 – 329
3	Stanford Pacific Medical Center(duplicated at Mount Sinai Hospital N.Y.C.1973)	38 – 142 235 – 238 246	1966	–	–		x		6.6	–
4	Birmingham	100 – 101 102 – 103	1967	4624 (1974)	8	x			less than 2	100
5	Birmingham (MIRU CCU)	221-21-240	1970	–	7			x	–	–
6	Bethesda	239	1971	–	4	x			–	–
7	Rotterdam	90	1971	–	10	x	x	x	–	–
8	Houston	89	1972	500 (1974)	2	x			2.3	20 – 59
9	St. Louis	228	1973	–	5	x			2.6	10
10	Charlotte (Commercial System)	234-85-245	1974	1200 (1976)	4	x			0.1 – 2.2	75
11	Munchen (Commercial System)	241	1974	–	32	x	x	x	–	–

Table 2. Technical characteristics

System	Computer Size	Continuous Monitoring	Hardware signal preprocessing	Arrhythmia detection	Signal quality control	Includes record Keeping
1	medium size	no	yes	no	yes	yes
2	multi-medium size	no (variable)	–	no	yes	yes
3	medium size	no (every 1-10 minutes)	no	PVC	–	yes
4	medium size	no (every 2 min)	yes	no	–	yes
5	medium size	ECG only other signal every 2-15 min.	no	yes	ECG only	yes
6	medium size	yes	yes	PVC	–	yes
7	multi-mini	no	yes	PVC	no	yes
8	multi-mini	yes	no	PVC	–	yes
9	mini	yes	yes	no	–	yes
10	mini	no	yes	no	–	yes
11	medium size	no	yes	no	no	yes

Table 3. Evaluation

System	Mortality decrease	Stay reduction	Care improvement	Personnel efficiency increase	Personnel reduction is possible	Complications reduction
1	–	–	–	–	–	–
2	no	yes	–	–	–	yes
3	yes	yes (10%)	yes	yes	yes	yes
4	–	yes	yes	yes	yes	yes
5	–	–	–	–	–	–
6	–	–	–	–	–	–
7	–	–	–	–	–	–
8	–	–	no	yes	–	no
9	–	yes (23%)	–	yes	yes	–
10	–	yes	yes	yes	yes	yes (10%)
11	–	–	–	–	–	–

Table 4. Main reasons for positive evaluation

System	Measurements reliability and accuracy	Fast data retrieval	Faster therapeutical intervertion	More informative
1	–	–	–	–
2	yes	yes	–	yes
3	–	–	–	–
4	yes	yes	yes	yes
5	–	–	–	–
6	–	–	–	–
7	–	–	–	–
8	–	–	–	–
9	–	–	–	–
10	yes	–	yes	yes
11	–	–	–	–

T A B L E 5A.

	DENMARK						FRANCE										
	1	2	3	4	5	6	7	8	9	10	11	12	13	14	15	16	17
	Amtssygehuset Gentofte Hellerup	Odense Sygehus Odense	Bispebjerg Hospital Copenhagen	Kommunehospitalet Copenhagen	Copenhagen County Hospital-Glostrup	Hvidovre Hospital Hvidovre	Hôpital Cardiologique, B.P.Lyon-Monchat-Lyon	Hôpital Charles Nicolle Rouen	Hôpital Lariboisière Paris	Hôpital Beaujon Clichy	Hôpital Saint Eloi Montpellier	Hôpital Necker Paris	Cardiologie Clinique et Expérimentale-Toulouse	Centre Cantini Marseille	Hôpital du Tondu Bordeaux	Hôpital Central Nancy	Hôpital A. Paré Boulogne
CCU FACILITIES																	
Beds N.	10	22	20	7	21	20	16	10	14	10	8	17	8	6	12	10	8
Single rooms	2	5	20	7	2	20	12	10	7	10	8	17	8	6		10	8
Visual control					+	+	+		+	+	+	+	+		+	+	+
Postintensive CU		+	+	+		+			+	+	+	+	+	+		+	+
Blood gas laboratory	+	+	+		+	+	+			+		+	+	+		+	+
Fluoroscopy at bed side	+	+	+				+	+	+	+	+		+	+		+	+
Cardiac open chest surgery	+	+	+	+	+	+	+	+		+	+		+		+	+	+
PERSONNEL																	
Physicians - A	2	2	1	1	1	1	2	1	1	2	5	2	1	3	2	3	2
" - B	5	2		2	8	1	4	3	3	1	4	2	1	3	2	3	7
Pts per week - average n. — Total	13.7	20	30	13	25	10	30	20	20	15	35	15	10	8	13	10	13
- A.M.I.	7	10	10	7	10	7	12	10	10	9	15	6	7	4	4	5	10
- Unstable Angina	1	0.5	2	1		1	6	3	3	4	8	3	2	1	2	2	2
- Others	5.7	10	18	5	15	2	12	7	7	2	12	6	1	3	7	3	1
Median admission time for A.M.I.		3h	3h	5	15	4	13	6	24	8			6		30	6-8	10

TABLE 5A.

	UNITED KINGDOM						BELGIUM				GERMANY	
	Hammersmith Hospital London (18)	The Royal Infirmary Edinburgh (19)	National Heart Institute London (20)	Kings College Hospital London (21)	Royal Sussex County Hospital – Brighton (22)	Royal Victoria Hospital Belfast (23)	Belgium Hôpital S.Pierre Bruxelles (24)	St.Pieters Hospital Leuven (25)	Universitett Hospital Leuven (26)	Hôpital de Bavière Liège (27)	Hannover Medical School Hannover (28)	German Heart Center Munich (29)
CCU FACILITIES												
Beds N.	3	8	8	6	4	10	6	7	8	8	9	8
Single rooms		8	8		4	10	4	7	8	4	9	8
Visual control	+	+	+	+	+	+	+	+	+	+	+	+
Postintensive CU	+					+	+	+		+		+
Blood gas laboratory		+	+	+	+	+	+	+	+		+	+
Fluoroscopy at bed side	+	+		+	+	+	+	+		+	+	+
Cardiac open chest surgery	+	+	+			+	+	+	+	+	+	+
PERSONNEL												
Physicians – A	2	2	1	1	1	1		1	2		1	2
" – 3		2	2	1.5		1		1	2		1	2
Pts per week – average n. – Total	5	20	20	14	12	21	10	8	14	12	13	11
– A.M.I.	2	8	5	10	6	11	5	2.5	7	6		2
– Unstable Angina	1	3	5	2	3	4	1.5	3	5	1-2		2
– Others	2	9	10	2	3	6	3.5	3.5	2	5	10	6
Median admission time for A.M.I.				3		1.40	6	8	2-3			4

TABLE 5A.

	ITALY										NETHERLANDS					
	Ospedali Riuniti di Trieste - Trieste	Divisione Cardiologica "De Gasperis"-Milano-Niguarda	Ospedale Regionale Udine	Policlinico S. Matteo Pavia	Ospedale Cardiologico Regionale "G.M.Lancisi"-Ancona	Istituti Ospedalieri Verona	Arcispedale di S.Maria Nuova Careggi - Firenze	Ospedale Maggiore della Carità - Novara	Ospedale di S.Maria Nuova Firenze	Fisiologia Clinica Pisa	Academisch Ziekenhuis Groningen - Groningen	Wilhelmina Gasthuis Amsterdam	Academic Hospital Amsterdam	Gemeente Ziekenhuis Arnhem	Torax Centrum Rotterdam	Sint Anthonius Hospital Utrecht
	30	31	32	33	34	35	36	37	38	39	40	41	42	43	44	45
CCU FACILITIES																
Beds M.	6	8	7	6	5	8	6	8	8	3	6	12	22	8	8	8
Single rooms	6	8		6	5	2	6	8	8	3		12	22		8	
Visual control	+	+	+	+	+	+		+		+	+	+		+	+	+
Postintensive CU	+	+	+	+		+	+	+		+	+	+			+	
Blood gas laboratory		+	+	+		+	+	+		+		+	+		+	
Fluoroscopy at bed side	+	+	+	+	+	+	+	+	+	+		+	+	+	+	
Cardiac open chest surgery	+	+	+	+	+	+	+	+	+	+	+	+	+	+	+	+
PERSONNEL																
Physicians - A	1	2	1	2		1		1		1	1	2	2		1	
" - B	1	2	1	1	1	1		2		1	2	3	2		4	
Pts per week - average n.																
- Total	14	11	10	7	10	8.5	14	10	9		12	50	15	6	25	15
- A.M.I.	8	4	4	4.6	4	5.3	7	6	5		6	6.7	5	2	8	7
- Unstable Angina	4	2	1	1.4	2	0.5	3	0.5	1		2	6.7	3	2	1	3
- Others	2	5	5	1	4	2.7	4	3.5	3		4	38	7	2	16	5
Median admission time for A.M.I.	9		7	9		9						3.5	30'	20'	6	

T A B L E 58.

STANDARD ROUTINE PROCEDURES

	1	2	3	4	5	6	7	8	9	10	11	12	13	14	15
1. Diagnosis of A.M.I.															
E.C.G.															
Enzimes	+	+	+	+	+	+	+	+	+	+	+	+	+	+	+
Isoenzimes	+	+	+	+	+	+	+	+	+	+	+	+	+	+	+
99mTe PYP													+	+	+
201Tl												+	+		
Others													VCG		
2. Monitoring for pts Killip cl.1															
E.C.G. (scope)	+	+	+	+	+	+	+	+	+	+	+	+	+	+	+
Ectopics N.	+	+	+	+					+						
Non invasive haemodynamic						Polig.									
3. Monitoring for pts Killip cl.2															
E.C.G. (scope)	+	+	+	+	+	+	+	+	+	+	+	+	+	+	+
Ectopics N.	+								+						
Non invasive haemodynamic						Polig.									ECHO
Pulmonary artery											+	+	+	+	+
Arterial pressure								+			+		+	+	+
Others													∞		∞
4. Monitoring for pts Killip cl.3															
E.C.G. (scope)	+	+	+	+	+	+	+	+	+	+	+	+	+	+	ECHO
Ectopics N.	+	+							+						
Non invasive haemodynamic	+	+				Polig.			+			+	+	+	+
Pulmonary artery pressure	+				+	+	+	+	+	+	+	+	+	+	+
Arterial pressure					+					∞			∞		∞
Others															
5. Monitoring for pts Killip cl.4															
E.C.G. (scope)	+	+	+	+	Imp.	Polig.	+	+	+	+	+	+	+	+	ECHO
Ectopics N.	+								+						
Non invasive haemodynamic	+	+	+	+	+	+	+	+	+	+	+	+	+	+	+
Pulmonary artery pressure	+	+	+	+	+	+	+	+	+	+	+	+	+	+	+
Arterial pressure	+	+	+	+	+			+			+	,		+	+
Body temperature	+	+	+	+	+	+	+	+	+	+	+	+	+	+	+
Urine output	+	+	+	+									+	+	+
Others										∞			∞	†	∞

TABLE 58.

STANDARD ROUTINE PROCEDURES

	16	17	18	19	20	21	22	23	24	25	26	27	28	29	30
1. Diagnosis of A.M.I.															
E.C.G.	+	+	+	+	+	+	+	+	+	+	+	+	+	+	+
Enzimes	+	+	+	+	+	+	+	+	+	+	+	+	+	+	+
Isoenzimes	+	+	+	+	+	+	+1	+	+	+	+	+	+	+	+
99mTe PYP	+		+	+		+		+	+		+	+	+	+	+
201Tl	+						+		+			+		+	
Others			ST												
2. Monitoring for pts Killip cl.1															
E.C.G. (scope)	+			+	+		+	+	+	+	+		+		+
Ectopics N.			+	+	+			+	+	+	+				
Non invasive haemodynamic								XR							
3. Monitoring for pts Killip cl.2															
E.C.G. (scope)	+		+	+	+	+	+	+	+	+	+	+	+	+	+
Ectopics N.				+				+	+	+	+				
Non invasive haemodynamic		+						XR	+	+	+	+		+	
Pulmonary artery								+1		+	+1	+			
Arterial pressure												+			
Others		BG							∞	∞	∞	∞PA-PO2	CVP	∞	
4. Monitoring for pts Killip cl.3															
E.C.G. (scope)	+	+	+	+	+	+	+	+	+	+	+	+	+	+	+
Ectopics N.				+	+			+	+	+	+				
Non invasive haemodynamic								XR							
Pulmonary artery pressure	+	+		+	+	+	+	+1	+	+	+	+	+	+	+1
Arterial pressure	+	+								+		+PA-PO2			+1
Others		BG							∞	∞	∞		∞	∞	
5. Monitoring for pts Killip cl.4															
E.C.G. (scope)	+	+	+	+	+	+	+	+	+	+	+	+	+	+	+1
Ectopics N.				+	+			+	+	+	+				+1
Non invasive haemodynamic								XR							
Pulmonary artery pressure	+	+	+	+	+	+	+	+1	+	+	+	+	+	+	+
Arterial pressure	+	+	+	+	+	+	+	+	+	+	+	+	+	+	+
Body temperature															
Urine output	+	+	+	+	+				+						
Others		BG							∞	∞	∞	∞PA-PO2	CO.PN	∞	

T A B L E   5B.

STANDARD ROUTINE PROCEDURES

	31	32	33	34	35	36	37	38	39	40	41	42	43	44	45
1. Diagnosis of A.M.I.															
E C.G.	+														
Enzimes	+	+	+	+	+	+	+	+	+	+	+	+	+	+	+
Isoenzimes	+|	+	+	+	+	+	+	+	+|	+	+	+	+	+	+
99mTc PYP								+	+|	+	+	+			+
20' Tl										+|	+				
Others									ST VCG	VCG					
2. Monitoring for pts Killip cl.1															
E.C.G. (scope)	+	+	+	+	+	+	+	+	+	+	+	+	+	+	+
Ectopics N.	+	+	+	+		+		+	+					+	+
Non invasive haemodynamic	ECHO	ECHO			Polig.	Polig.	XR		XR.BG		XR				XR
3. Monitoring for pts Killip cl.2															
E.C.G. (scope)	+	+	+	+	+	+	+	+	+	+	+	+	+	+	+
Ectopics N.	ECHO	ECHO	+	+	+		XR	+	XR	+|	XR	+	+		XR
Non invasive haemodynamic	+|	+	+	+	+|		+|	+	+|	+	+	+			+
Pulmonary artery	+|	+	+	+	+|		+|	+			+				
Arterial pressure															
Others	CO	CVP	CO				CO		BG						
4. Monitoring for pts Killip cl.3															
E.C.G (scope)	+	+	+	+	+	+	+	+	+	+	+	+	+	+	+
Ectopics N.	ECHO	ECHO	+	+		+		+	+					+	+
Non invasive haemodynamic	ECHO	ECHO					XR		XR		XR				XR
Pulmonary artery pressure	+|	+	+	+	+		+	+	+|	+	+	+		+	+
Arterial pressure	+|	+	+	(+)	+|		+	+	(+)	+		+		+	-
Others	CO	CVP	CO				CO		BG						CO
5. Monitoring for pts Killip cl.4															
E.C.G. (scope)	+	+	+	+	+	+	+	+	+	+	+	+	+	+	+
Ectopics N.	ECHO	ECHO	+	+		+		+	+					+	+
Non invasive haemodynamic	ECHO	ECHO					XR		XR		XR				XR
Pulmonary artery pressure	+	+	+	+	+	+	+	+	+	+	+	+	+	+	+
Arterial pressure	+	+	+	+	+		+		+	+	+	+	+	+	+
Body temperature	+	+	+	+	+	+	+	+			+	+	+	+	+
Urine output	+	+	+	+	+	+	+	+			+	+	+	+	+
Others	CO	CVP.BG RA.CO					CO		BG.CO o2 mvCat	o2 mvCat					CO

TABLE 5C.

RESEARCH ACTIVITY	1	2	3	4	5	6	7	8	9	10	11	12	13	14	15	16	17
A. RESEARCH PROJECTS ON A.M.I.																	
1. Arrhythmia detection																	
Beds N.			2		2	8	8		4			4			4		8
Computer analysis	+		+	+	+	+	+		+			+		+	+		
Hardware			+				+		+								
Firmware			+		Imp.		+		+						+		
Databank collection	+		+		+	+	+		+								
2. Haemodynamic monitoring																	
Beds N.			2		2	6	8		2			4			4	3	8
Invasive			AP.CVP		CVP.PA CO	CVP.PA CO	PA.AP CO		PA.PW AP			PW.PB			PB.AP CO	PB.AP CO	PB.PB
Non invasive			BT		Imp.							Isot. Imp.			ECHO		
Computerized	+		+	+	+	+	+	+	+			+		+	+	+	+
Home developed									+								
a. Continuous analysis			+	+	+	+			+								
Intermittent analysis			+		+	+	+	+	+								
b. Off line analysis				+	+	+		+	+								
On line analysis			+	+	+				+								
Pattern recognition																	
- software																	
- hardware																	
- mixed approach			+			+	+		+								
d. Automatic data quality control?																	
e. Cycles associated to arrhythmias rejected							+		+								
f. Trend analysis																	
On multiparametric basis?																	
g. Prognostic indexes	+		+	+	+	+	+	+	+			+		+	+	+	+
3. Reduction of infarct size																	
Method to evaluate I.S.:																	
Enzimes		+	+	+	+	+	+	+	+			+	+	+	+	+	+
Isoenzimes		+	+	+	+	+	+	+	+				+	+	+	+	+
ST mapping		+	+	+					+								
Isotopes												+			+	+	
Others																	
B. Study of "PREINFARCTION SYNDROME"		+	+	+	+	+	+	+	+			+	+	+	+	+	+
Haemodynamic monitoring			+		+	+	+	+	+			+		+	+	+	+

TABLE 5C.

	18	19	20	21	22	23	24	25	26	27	28	29	30	31
RESEARCH ACTIVITY														
A. RESEARCH PROJECTS ON A.M.I.														
1. Arrhythmia detection														
Beds N.		8	8	6			4	4						
Computer analysis		+	+	+		+	+	+						
Hardware		+				+	+	+						
Firmware		+	+											
Databank collection			+	+		+	+	+						
2. Haemodynamic monitoring														
Beds N.	3	8	4	6		1	6		3	4	3	4		4
Invasive	PA.PW	PW	PA.CO	AP,PW,CO		PA.PW	PA.AP	PA.AP		PW,PA,RV PA.CO	CO,PA,PW AP	PA,PA Ap,CO,PvO2		PA,AP CO
Non invasive														
Computerized			+⁻					+	+		+	+		
Home developed								+	+			+		
a. Continuous analysis														
Intermittent analysis			+						+			+		
b. Off line analysis														
On line analysis								+	⁻			⁻		
Pattern recognition														
- software								+				+		
- hardware														
- mixed approach				+					+	+		+		
d. Automatic data quality control?								+	+					
e. Cycles associated to arrhythmias rejected								+	+		+	+		
f. Trend analysis								+	+		+	+		
On multiparametric basis?								+	+					
g. Prognostic indexes								+						
3. Reduction of infarct size														
Method to evaluate I.S.:														
Enzimes	+	+	+	+		+		+	+	+	+	+		+
Isoenzimes	+	+	+	+				+	+	+	+	+		+
ST mapping	+	+										+		+
Isotopes										+		+		
Others														
B. Study of "PREINFARCTION SYNDROME"														
Haemodynamic monitoring		+	+	+		+		+				+		+

TABLE 5C.

	32	33	34	35	36	37	38	39	40	41	42	43	44	45
RESEARCH ACTIVITY														
A. RESEARCH PROJECTS ON A.M.I.														
1. Arrhythmia detection														
Beds N.	7					6					12		8	1
Computer analysis	+					+					+		+	+
Hardware													+	+
Firmware														+
Databank collection														
2. Haemodynamic monitoring														
Beds N.	2	2	1			4	2	1	2		2		8	
Invasive	PA CVP AP	PA AP	PA AP			PA PW	PA PW CO	PA PW	PA PW PA				PA AP PW CO	
Non invasive	ECHO POLIG.	ECHO POLIG	ECHO POLIG					Others						
Computerized							+	+			+		+	
Home developed								+						
a. Continuous analysis				+		+	+	+					+	+
Intermittent analysis								+						
b. Off line analysis														
On line analysis							+	+					+	
Pattern recognition														
- software														
- hardware								+						
- mixed approach							+							
d. Automatic data quality control?														
e. Cycles associated to arrhythmias rejected										+				
f. Trend analysis						+		+	+				+	+
On multiparametric basis?										+				
g. Prognostic indexes						+		+	+				+	
3. Reduction of infarct size														
Method to evaluate I.S.:														
Enzymes	+	+	+	+		+		+	+			+		+
Isoenzymes	+	+	+	+		+		+		+				+
ST mapping	+	+	+	+		+		+				+		
Isotopes										+				
Others														+
B. Study of "PREINFARCTION SYNDROME"	+	+	+	+				+					+	+
Haemodynamic monitoring	+	+	+	+				+					+	